Pathology and Laboratory Medicine

nova
Medicine & Health
New York

Pathology and Laboratory Medicine

Pathogenesis of Neurotrauma and Stroke: New Directions for Neuroprotective and Neuroregenerative Treatments
Jacek M. Kwiecien, DVM, MSc, PhD (Editor)
2022. ISBN: 979-8-88697-365-5 (Softcover)
2022. ISBN: 979-8-88697-429-4 (eBook)

Advances in Neuropathology
John O. McCarthy (Editor)
2022. ISBN: 978-1-68507-620-7 (Softcover)
2022. ISBN: 978-1-68507-701-3 (eBook)

An Outline of Office-Based Bladder and Prostate Biopsy Pathology
David Y. Zhang, MD, PhD (Editor)
2019. ISBN: 978-1-53615-248-7 (Hardcover)
2019. ISBN: 978-1-53615-249-4 (eBook)

Clinical Flow Cytometry: Approaches, Principles, and Applications
Jason Howard Kurzer, M.D., Ph.D.
and Olga Kagan Weinberg, M.D. (Editors)
2019. ISBN: 978-1-53614-643-1 (Hardcover)
2019. ISBN: 978-1-53614-644-8 (eBook)

Rattus norvegicus – A Review and Directions for Research
Ana Isabel Rocha Faustino
and Antonieta Maria Alvarado Muñoz (Editors)
2019. ISBN: 978-1-53614-685-1 (Softcover)
2019. ISBN: 978-1-53614-686-8 (eBook)

More information about this series can be found at
https://novapublishers.com/product-category/series/pathology-and-laboratory-medicine/

Richard A. Prayson
Editor

Central Nervous System Pathologies in Hereditary Tumor Syndromes

nova
Medicine & Health
New York

DOI: https://doi.org/10.52305/HDHV6059.

NOTICE TO THE READER

Library of Congress Cataloging-in-Publication Data

ISBN: 979-8-88697-620-5

Published by Nova Science Publishers, Inc. † New York

Contents

Preface

The central nervous system can be affected in many hereditary tumor syndromes, also sometimes referred to as familiar tumor syndromes, genetic tumor syndromes or cancer predisposition syndromes. Although a few of these have been recognized for a long period of time and have been well delineated with regard to clinical presentations and genetic abnormalities, some have been only recently defined. These disorders are highly complex and patients are best cared for in specialized centers which have broad interdisciplinary expertise to handle the wide array of phenotypic manifestations of these disorders. This book contains a collection of chapters which focus on a subset of these syndromes. The focal of the chapters in this text is on the neuropathologic features associated with the various syndromes that are highlighted.

Chapter 1 - Neurofibromatosis type 2 (NF2) is an autosomal dominant hereditary tumor predisposition disorder caused by germline mutations in the NF2 gene located on chromosome 22. NF2 is classically associated with the development of bilateral vestibular schwannomas. Additionally, patients commonly develop meningiomas, ependymomas, as well as peripheral, spinal, and cranial nerve schwannomas. Other characteristics manifestations include meningioangiomatosis, glial microhamartomas, ocular lesions, and neuropathies. Histologically, tumors resemble their sporadic counterparts with some minor differences. NF2-associated schwannomas are typically multicentric, display higher proliferative indices, and are more invasive. In NF2-associated meningiomas, all major histological variants can be observed, with the most common subtype being the fibroblastic variant. NF2-associated meningioangiomatosis is typically multifocal and may be associated with glial microhamartomas, a pathognomonic finding. NF2-associated ependymomas are identical to their sporadic counterparts. This chapter will review the clinicopathologic features of this disorder, with a primary focus on the central nervous system associated pathology.

Chapter 2 - Tuberous sclerosis is an autosomal dominant genetic disease, marked by hamartomas and benign neoplasms that affect multiple body systems with a wide degree of variability. Patients with tuberous sclerosis typically present with skin lesions, seizures, and hamartomas in the heart, brain, and kidneys. Tuberous sclerosis is characterized by three types of neuropathological lesions: cortical tubers, subependymal nodules and subependymal giant cell astrocytomas. Histologically, tubers are marked by a disorganized cortical architecture with balloon cells that have mixed glioneuronal characteristics. Tuberous sclerosis is due to loss of function mutations in TSC1 or TSC2 tumor suppressor genes that lead to a failure to regulate mTOR pathway-mediated cellular growth and differentiation. This chapter will review the key clinical and pathologic features of tuberous sclerosis and highlight the neuropathological findings associated with this disorder.

Chapter 3 - Von Hippel-Lindau syndrome is an autosomal dominant disorder due to germline variants of the VHL tumor suppressor gene situated on chromosome 3p25.3. Manifestation of the disease outside the central nervous system includes pancreatic cysts and islet cell tumors, renal cysts and renal cell carcinomas, papillary cystadenomas of the epididymis and uterine broad ligament, pheochromocytomas, endolymphatic sac tumors and retinal hemangioblastomas. Within the central nervous system, patients present with hemangioblastomas, either solitary or multiple. The majority of hemangioblastomas of the central nervous system arise in the cerebellum and present with symptoms of increased intracranial pressure, hemorrhage, dysmetria, ataxia and secondary polycythemia vera due to erythropoietin production. The tumor presents as a circumscribed lesion (cystic mass with enhancing mural nodule configuration on imaging) and is marked by a proliferation of epithelioid clear to foamy stromal cells with intermixed capillary vessels. The tumors are considered low grade, World Health Organization grade 1 neoplasms. Immunostaining with inhibin antibody allows for distinction from a metastatic renal cell carcinoma, which is the main differential diagnostic consideration in the setting of von Hippel-Lindau syndrome. Tumors have been treated with surgery, vascular embolization and stereotactic radiosurgery. This chapter will review the features of von Hippel-Lindau syndrome with a focus on hemangioblastoma, the main neuropathologic finding of the syndrome.

Chapter 4 - Sturge-Weber syndrome or encephalofacial angiomatosis is a disorder marked by coexistence of cutaneous and central nervous system lesions. Classically, patients have a nevus flammeus or port-wine stain, typically in the trigeminal nerve distribution, combined with leptomeningeal angiomatosis. The brain parenchyma underlying the leptomeningeal angiomatosis is marked by cortical atrophy due to loss of neurons and microcalcifications, accounting for a characteristic radiographic appearance. Occasionally, other malformative lesions of the central nervous system including angiomatous and meningothelial proliferation of the choroid plexus, polymicrogyria and heterotopias may be seen. The disorder is due to somatic activating mutations in the GNAQ gene located on chromosome 9q21.2. This chapter will review the clinicopathologic features of this disorder, with a primary focus on the central nervous system associated pathology.

Chapter 5 - Cowden disease is a hereditary tumor syndrome marked by an autosomal dominant pattern of inheritance and associated with mutations of the PTEN tumor-suppressor gene located on chromosome 10q23.3. The disorder is marked by the development of hamartomatous lesions derived from any of the three germ cell layers and mucocutaneous lesions. Patients are also at risk of developing cancers in the thyroid, breast, uterus, kidney and colon. In the central nervous system, the classic pathologic manifestation is the dysplastic cerebellar gangliocytoma (Lhermitte-Duclos disease). Patients with this cerebellar tumor most commonly present with dysmetria, cerebellar signs, and symptoms related to obstructive hydrocephalus. Histologically, the lesion is marked by an increased number of large ganglion cells with a relative preservation of the cerebellar architecture. Calcifications and dilated vessels are not uncommon concomitant findings. The lesion is generally cured by surgical resection, although recurrent lesions have been reported. This chapter will review the features of Cowden's syndrome with a focus on the dysplastic cerebellar gangliocytoma.

Chapter 6 - Schwannomatosis is a hereditary tumor predisposition syndrome characterized by the development of multiple schwannomas in the absence of bilateral vestibular nerve involvement typical of neurofibromatosis type 2. With an estimated incidence of 1/40,000 to 1/70,000 births, its molecular pathogenesis is driven by a four-hit process that results in biallelic loss of function of either SMARCB1 or LZTR1 and NF2 on chromosome 22q. The disease generally presents in the second to third decade of life with pain as the dominant symptom and may be diagnosed by a combination of clinical and molecular criteria. Magnetic resonance (MR) imaging with and without contrast is the preferred modality to identify schwannomas and exclude bilateral vestibular nerve involvement. Histologic morphology of schwannomas typically reveals Antoni A pattern with spindle-shaped cells and Verocay bodies and molecular characterization shows loss of SMARCB1 on immunohistochemistry for schwannomatosis-associated tumors. Treatment is symptomatic and involves multimodal pharmacologic pain medication and surgical resection of tumors causing significant pain or neurologic deficits. Schwannomatosis is associated with significant diminished quality of life but has not been shown to reduce life expectancy.

Chapter 7 - Li-Fraumeni syndrome (LFS) is an inherited disorder caused by various alterations in the TP53 gene located on chromosome 17p13.1. It has an autosomal dominant pattern of inheritance with variable penetrance and expressivity. The protein product of the TP53 gene (p53) serves as an important cell cycle regulator and its pathologic alteration leads to cell cycle dysregulation and eventually – neoplastic transformation. LFS manifests with a variety of neoplasms in all age groups, most commonly breast carcinoma, sarcomas, central nervous system (CNS) neoplasms and adrenocortical carcinomas. In the CNS, medulloblastomas (SHH-activated, TP53 mutated), astrocytic neoplasms and choroid plexus carcinomas are most commonly encountered. Several criteria for the clinical recognition of patients with possible LFS have been developed, with genetic testing for pathogenic variants of the TP53 gene being the gold standard for making the diagnosis. This chapter will review the etiopathogenesis, the clinical and the pathologic features of LFS with emphasis on its CNS manifestations.

Chapter 8 - Carney complex is a very rare multiple neoplasia and lentiginosis syndrome characterized primarily by cutaneous, endocrine, and cardiac manifestations. Although there is a high degree of phenotypic variability amongst patients, the most common features include spotty pigmentation, cutaneous myxomas, thyroid lesions, primary pigmented nodular adrenocortical disease, large cell-calcifying Sertoli cell tumors, and cardiac myxomas. The main neuroclinical features of Carney complex are growth hormone (GH)-secreting pituitary neuroendocrine tumors (adenomas) and melanotic schwannomas. In the majority of cases, disease is caused by inactivating, heterozygous mutations of the PRKAR1A gene located on 17q24.2-24.3. This chapter will review the genetics, clinical presentation, imaging findings, histopathologic features, treatment, and prognosis of Carney complex, with a primary focus on the nervous system-associated clinical and histopathologic findings.

Chapter 9 - Lynch syndrome, previously referred to as hereditary nonpolyposis colorectal cancer, is characterized primarily by colorectal and endometrial cancers. Germline mutations in mismatch repair proteins MLH1, MSH2, MSH6, and PMS2 result in microsatellite instability and increased risk for malignancies, including several extra-colonic malignancies. Lynch syndrome confers a four-fold increase in the lifetime risk for neurologic cancers, especially high-grade astrocytoma (glioblastoma). Similar to sporadic neurologic cancers, the prognosis for Lynch syndrome associated neurologic malignancies is poor. However, the true biologic behavior of Lynch syndrome associated glioblastoma is challenging to characterize and distinguish from sporadic cases given their overall low prevalence and high mortality. This chapter will review the clinicopathologic features of Lynch syndrome, highlighting central nervous system associated pathology.

Chapter 10 - Retinoblastoma is a malignancy that arises from the retina and is the most common childhood eye cancer. Patients generally present in infancy with leukocoria. Some hereditary cases may be characterized as trilateral retinoblastoma, in which retinoblastoma is accompanied by a primary neuroectodermal tumor that is most commonly a pineoblastoma. The study of retinoblastoma led to the first discovered tumor suppressor gene, RB1, and thus paved the way for development of Knudson's two-hit hypothesis. Germline mutations of RB1 result in familial retinoblastoma which is inherited in an autosomal dominant fashion. Imaging and histopathology will characteristically demonstrate an intraocular tumor with calcifications. While it is generally a curable malignancy in the setting of early screening and detection, trilateral disease is often fatal. This chapter will review the presentation and diagnosis of familial retinoblastoma and trilateral retinoblastoma with an emphasis on neuropathologic findings common in these conditions.

Chapter 11 - Fanconi anemia is a clinically heterogeneous disorder which results in clinical manifestations in all organ systems due to genetic instability. Patients with Fanconi anemia have deficits in homologous recombination and repair of DNA crosslinking due to germline mutations in the FANC genes. Clinical features include growth retardation, abnormal thumbs, absent radii, café-au-lait spots, progressive bone marrow failure, increased cancer risk, triangular facies, microcephaly, abnormal kidneys, and decreased fertility. Fanconi anemia can occur in patients without these diagnostic clues, resulting in remarkable phenotypic variability, partially explained by genetic heterogeneity. Genetic instability in Fanconi anemia contributes to tumorigenesis, including medulloblastoma. Biallelic variants of BRCA2 or PALB2 most significantly predispose to medulloblastoma. Anaplastic/large cell subtypes of medulloblastoma are frequently found in Fanconi anemia. This chapter presents a review of Fanconi anemia's clinical presentation, genetics, neural manifestations, and histopathology.

Chapter 12 - Paragangliomas are neuroendocrine tumors of the autonomic nervous system. Familial paraganglioma syndromes are a group of genetic conditions in which the development of paragangliomas is one of the possible tumor manifestations. There have been over 20 identified susceptibility genes associated with the development of these tumors. The most common of these syndromes are Neurofibromatosis Type 1, von Hippel-Lindau and Multiple Endocrine Neoplasia Type II. Pheochromocytomas arise from the adrenal medulla, and are the most common subtype of paragangliomas, accounting for 80-85% of all paragangliomas. The remaining 15-20% of paragangliomas occur outside of the adrenal medulla in the spine, head, neck, chest, heart, abdomen, pelvis, or bladder. The classic presentation of a paraganglioma involves signs and symptoms of catecholamine excess including hypertension, tachycardia, palpitations, sweating and anxiety. Not all paragangliomas actively secrete catecholamines, and in this case the tumors are usually discovered incidentally or secondary to symptoms of mass effect. Though all familial paraganglioma syndromes share the possibility of paraganglioma development, features of the tumors differ depending on the molecular consequences of the mutations causing them. The goal of this chapter is to review the spectrum of familial paraganglioma syndromes, focusing on the clinical picture, genetics and histopathology of the paraganglioma tumors that arise in these syndromes.

Chapter 13 - Melanoma-astrocytoma syndrome is a rare tumor predisposition syndrome caused by a germline mutation of the CDKN2A gene. People who carry the mutation are more likely to develop cutaneous melanoma, nervous system tumors, pancreatic cancer, nerve sheath tumors, and oropharyngeal squamous cell carcinoma. Astrocytoma is the most frequent nervous system tumor arising in this syndrome. The neoplastic risk of this syndrome has not been determined due to the small number of families reported. Early detection of melanoma improves outcomes. Nervous system tumors arising in this setting typically have a dismal prognosis depending on type, location, and stage. This chapter will review the clinicopathologic features of this rare syndrome, with a focus on the central nervous system pathology.

Chapter 14 - Familial adenomatous polyposis (FAP1) is an autosomal dominant genetic syndrome caused by a pathogenic, inactivating sequence variant in the tumor suppressor gene APC. While FAP1 is predominantly characterized phenotypically by the development of gastrointestinal neoplasia, formation of primary brain tumors also occurs in a small subset of these patients, a phenomenon termed brain tumor polyposis syndrome 2 (BTP2).

Medulloblastomas are the only tumor type definitively associated with BTP2. Development of these tumors is mediated by activation of the WNT signaling pathway, as a result of APC loss. Although syndromic medulloblastoma due to germline APC mutation makes up a small fraction (roughly 5%) of WNT activated medulloblastomas, both somatic and germline variants are associated with early onset (peak incidence within the first decade of life) and excellent prognosis (5-year survival > 95%). The goal of this chapter is to describe the clinical features of FAP1, histopathologic characteristics of BTP2, and unique molecular findings associated with medulloblastomas arising in this context, as well as diagnostic and prognostic information pertaining to this rare neurologic manifestation.

Chapter 15 - *BAP1* tumor predisposition syndrome (*BAP1*-TPDS) is a syndrome caused by autosomal dominant germline variants of *BAP1*, which lead to *BAP1* protein loss of tumor suppressing function. The syndrome is associated with a predisposition for the development of a variety of tumors including uveal and cutaneous melanomas, mesotheliomas, and meningiomas, among others. Meningiomas are the primary central nervous system tumors associated with *BAP1*-TPDS and are typically high grade and have rhabdoid morphology. This chapter will review *BAP1*-TPDS and its associated tumors, with a focus on the neuropathological features of its associated meningiomas.

Chapter 16 - ELP1-medulloblastoma syndrome is an autosomal dominant disorder caused by mutations in the ELP1 gene. ELP1 is the most common medulloblastoma predisposition gene with a prevalence of 30% among pediatric patients with the sonic hedgehog-activating subtype. The inactivation of ELP1 characterizes the pathogenesis of this syndrome due to somatic loss of chromosome 9q. Additionally, most of these medulloblastomas also exhibit alteration in PTCH1, leading to biallelic inactivation along with amplification of PPM1D and MDM4 which are components that regulate p53 signaling. The median age of diagnosis of ELP1-associated medulloblastomas is 6.3 years with favorable clinical outcomes seen in preliminary data. This chapter will review the clinicopathologic features of this disorder, with a primary focus on central nervous system-associated pathology.

Chapter 17 - Nevoid basal cell carcinoma syndrome, also known as Gorlin syndrome, is a rare neurocutaneous disorder that is marked by developmental anomalies such as dyskeratotic palmar and plantar pitting, rib anomalies, basal cell carcinomas and odontogenic keratocysts of the jaw. Classically, Gorlin syndrome is inherited in an autosomal dominant fashion and characterized by increased tumorigenesis from an early age, prone to developing basal cell carcinomas and medulloblastoma. The syndrome occurs usually because of a frameshift, missense, or nonsense mutation in PTCH1, a human homologue of Drosophila. As a member of the highly conserved hedgehog signaling pathway that modulates cell growth and development, PTCH1 dysfunction gives rise to not only developmental anomalies but also the diverse tumors observed in nevoid basal cell carcinoma syndrome. This chapter will review the clinicopathologic features of this disorder, with a primary focus on the central nervous system associated pathology.

Chapter 18 - Constitutional mismatch repair deficiency syndrome (CMMRD) is a rare genetic cancer syndrome characterized by early-onset central nervous system (CNS), gastrointestinal, and hematologic malignancies. CMMRD is caused by autosomal recessive mutations in DNA mismatch repair genes. Loss of mismatch repair function results in microsatellite instability and accumulation of mutations, predisposing patients to the development of multiple ultramutated cancers in childhood and young adulthood. Children with CMMRD typically present with café-au-lait cutaneous macules, pilomatrixomas, and skin pigmentation changes. CNS and gastrointestinal cancers typically develop within the first decade of life, and one third of patients are diagnosed with a hematologic malignancy. The most common CNS pathology is high-grade glioma, typically manifesting as glioblastoma. Other rare CNS tumors have also been described in CMMRD patients. Prognosis is poor; the most common cause of death is CNS malignancy. Management consists of surveillance for cancers and treatment of malignancy with surgery, radiation, and chemotherapy.

Chapter 19 - Rhabdoid Tumor Predisposition Syndrome (RTPS) is characterized by the development of malignant rhabdoid tumors (MRTs). The most common tumor type found in RTPS is the atypical teratoid and rhabdoid tumor (AT/RT) that occur in the brain, which can co-occur with rhabdoid tumors in other parts of the body, especially the kidney. Patients with RTPS present with an array of neurologic symptoms such as headaches, seizures and cranial nerve palsies. Heterogeneity on imaging studies is characteristic of these large, cystic tumors, which show preference for growth in the cerebellopontine angle region. Constitutional mutations in either the SMARCB1 or SMARCA4 gene on chromosome 22q11.2 and 19p13.2 respectively cause RTPS. Focusing on central nervous system pathology, this chapter will discuss the salient clinicopathologic features of this disorder.

Chapter 20 - DICER1 syndrome occurs when the functionality of the endoribonuclease, DICER, is affected either via direct genetic mutations or secondary site mutations, predisposing the individual to developing multiple types of cancers. Of these cancers, the major brain tumor that presents from DICER1 mutations are pineoblastomas. These are highly aggressive, WHO Grade 4 neuroectodermal tumors, which most commonly affect children and adolescents. The Dicer protein, which regulates miRNA biogenesis, plays an essential role in the development of these tumors. These tumors present with varying mass effect symptoms in the pineal gland region, including vomiting, headache, altered mental status and obstructive hydrocephalus. On imaging, pineoblastomas present as large, poorly defined masses in the pineal gland region with hemorrhagic, necrotic or cystic foci and high rates of seeding to the rest of the neural axis. On histology, these tumors are comprised of poorly differentiated cells with high nuclear to cytoplasmic ratios, frequent mitotic figures, nuclear molding, rosette formation, and sheet-like cells with positive synaptophysin and chromogranin marker staining. Prognosis for the tumor is poor; the tumor is commonly managed with open surgical resection and adjuvant radiotherapy and chemotherapy.

Chapter 21 - Multiple endocrine neoplasia Type I (MEN1) is a rare autosomal dominant inherited disorder that results from germline mutations of the tumor suppressor gene, MEN1. The MEN1 gene encodes menin, a scaffolding protein implicated in a variety of cell processes, including cell division and transcription. An abnormal MEN1 gene leads to the formation of functioning/non-functioning endocrine tumors involving the pancreas, the parathyroid, anterior pituitary, duodenum, and thymus. Tumors of the entero-pancreatic axis, anterior pituitary, and parathyroid are more commonly noted in MEN1. Clinically, MEN1 is defined by findings of two or more MEN1-associated neoplasms or by the presence of a single tumor and a first-degree relative diagnosed with MEN1. The histopathological and radiological indications of MEN1-associated tumors are identical to non-MEN1-related counterparts. Similar to sporadic cases, commonly used stains include Ki-67, Chromogranin A (CgA), and synaptophysin (SYN). Behind parathyroid-associated MEN1 adenomas, pituitary neuroendocrine tumors (adenomas) make up about 40% of all MEN1 cases, with the majority being functioning pituitary neuroendocrine tumors. They are more commonly found in females compared to males and can cause hyperprolactinemia, acromegaly, and Cushing's disease. Pharmacological approaches have been proven effective in managing the symptoms of certain MEN1 disorders. However, the first line of treatment is surgical intervention due to the drug-resistant and aggressive nature of MEN1 pituitary neuroendocrine tumors. The life expectancy of individuals with MEN1 is substantially less than the general population, averaging 55 years. This chapter provides an overview of the clinical characteristics of MEN1 with a focus on its pathology, including the impact on the pituitary gland.

Chapter 22 - Noonan syndrome is a multisystem disorder that was first fully described by Dr. Jacqueline Noonan. It is a genetic disorder that displays variable expressivity, and it is generally marked by an autosomal dominant pattern of inheritance, except for the LZTR1 variant which is inherited in an autosomal recessive fashion. The molecular pathway most implicated in Noonan syndrome is the RAS/MAPK pathway which plays a role in cell proliferation, differentiation, survival, and metabolism. Clinical features described in the condition include short stature, congenital heart defects, hematologic abnormalities, musculoskeletal deformities, and neurological problems. A huge fraction of neuropathologic findings in Noonan are low-grade gliomas/glioneuronal tumors; these include pilocytic astrocytomas, pilomyxoid astrocytomas dysembryoplastic neuroepithelial tumors and rosette forming glioneuronal tumors. High grade gliomas are rare but reported cases have included anaplastic astrocytoma and a case of a spinal cord glioblastoma. The prognosis of these neurological tumors in Noonan syndrome are fairly similar to those arising outside the syndrome. Treatment often involves a multidisciplinary team approach. This chapter will review the clinical features of Noonan syndrome, with an emphasis on the central nervous system-associated pathology.

Chapter 23 - L-2-hydroxyglutaric aciduria is a rare autosomal recessive inborn error of metabolism caused by a homozygous or compound heterozygous mutation in the L-2-hydroxyglutarate dehydrogenase (L2HDGH) gene located on chromosome 14q22.1. This disease is associated with elevated L-2-hydroxyglutaric acid levels in the urine, cerebrospinal fluid, and plasma. Patients with this disorder often present early in life with neurologic signs and symptoms including hypotonia, tremors, intellectual disability, macrocephaly, choreodystonia, and seizures. Disease course is slowly progressive, and patients rarely present with acute metabolic disturbances. Neuroimaging studies demonstrate a distinctive pattern on magnetic resonance imaging T2/FLAIR; abnormalities present as bilateral and symmetric subcortical leukoencephalopathy, atrophy of the cerebellum and signal changes in the putaminal and dentate nuclei. A number of patients have been reported to develop a variety of central nervous tumors in this setting including astrocytomas (low and high grade), anaplastic ependymomas, and medulloblastomas. This chapter will review the neuropathologic findings described in the setting of this rare metabolic disorder.

Chapter 1

Neurofibromatosis Type 2: Central Nervous System Pathology

Darren Liu[1], BS, BA
and Richard A. Prayson[*,2], MD, MEd
[1] Cleveland Clinic Lerner College of Medicine, Cleveland, OH, USA
[2] Department of Anatomic Pathology, Cleveland Clinic, Cleveland, OH, USA

Abstract

Neurofibromatosis type 2 (NF2) is an autosomal dominant hereditary tumor predisposition disorder caused by germline mutations in the *NF2* gene located on chromosome 22. NF2 is classically associated with the development of bilateral vestibular schwannomas. Additionally, patients commonly develop meningiomas, ependymomas, as well as peripheral, spinal, and cranial nerve schwannomas. Other characteristics manifestations include meningioangiomatosis, glial microhamartomas, ocular lesions, and neuropathies.

Histologically, tumors resemble their sporadic counterparts with some minor differences. NF2-associated schwannomas are typically multicentric, display higher proliferative indices, and are more invasive. In NF2-associated meningiomas, all major histological variants can be observed, with the most common subtype being the fibroblastic variant. NF2-associated meningio-angiomatosis is typically multifocal and may be associated with glial microhamartomas, a pathognomonic finding. NF2-associated ependy-momas are identical to their sporadic counterparts.

---

[*] Corresponding Author's Email: praysor@ccf.org.

In: Central Nervous System Pathologies in Hereditary Tumor Syndromes
Editor: Richard A. Prayson
ISBN: 979-8-88697-620-5

This chapter will review the clinicopathologic features of this disorder, with a primary focus on the central nervous system associated pathology.

Introduction

In June of 1819, a 21-year-old male with a history of macrocephaly, amblyopia, and a tendency to fall easily was seen by surgeon John H. Wishart with complaints of gradual hearing loss affecting both ears [1]. Over the last four years, the patient complained of frequent episodes of headaches and vomiting. On examination, a protruding occipital tumor was excruciatingly painful to the touch. Over the course of months, the tumor would progressively increase in size. He had become deaf, blind, and began experiencing paroxysms of pain and rigidity preceded by a disagreeable smell followed by periods of profound sleepiness—symptoms consistent with seizures. An attempt to resect the tumor was unsuccessful with his post-operative course complicated by septicemia that would prove to be fatal.

On autopsy, Dr. Wishart described multiple tumors of different sizes adherent to the dura mater. He noted tumors arising from the 5th, 7th, and 11th cranial nerve as well as the medulla spinalis. This would be the first known detailed clinical description of neurofibromatosis type 2 (NF2). Due to overlapping central nervous system, peripheral nervous system, and cutaneous manifestations, it would not be until 1987 before NF1 and NF2 were recognized as separate entities [2, 3].

This chapter will review the clinical and pathologic features of NF2, focusing on the neuropathological findings that have been described in this syndrome.

Genetics of NF2

NF2 is an autosomal dominant tumor predisposition disorder due to inactivation of the NF2 gene. In 1993, two different labs simultaneously identified a novel type of tumor suppressor NF2 that encodes for the protein Merlin, also known as Schwannomin [4, 5]. NF2 is located on chromosome 22q12. Merlin belongs to the ezrin-radixin-moesin family of band 4.1 proteins which link membrane-associated proteins and to the cytoskeleton—playing an essential role in regulating signal transduction from the extracellular milieu [6].

Merlin is a tumor suppressor that has functions at the plasma membrane, cytoplasm, and nucleus. In response to intercellular adhesion or attachment to the extracellular matrix, Merlin becomes dephosphorylated and localizes to adherens junctions leading to contact-dependent inhibition of cellular proliferation [7-9]. There is also evidence that Merlin interacts with protein found within various intracellular signaling pathways such as MAPK, Rac/PAK, PI3k/Akt, FAK/Src signaling, and negatively regulates EGFR-Ras-ERK pathway [10-13]. In addition, Merlin translocates to the nucleus where it inhibits the E3 ubiquitin ligase CRL4DCAF1 that regulates oncogenic gene expression via activation of the Hippo signaling pathway.

General Clinical Features

Cutaneous manifestations are common in patients with NF2. Café-au-lait spots are well defined flat, hyperpigmented areas of skin and are a nonspecific finding observed in up to half of patients with NF2 [14-18]. The café-au-lait spots in NF2 are typically fewer in numbers compared to NF1 and are not associated with freckling. Additionally, patient may present with plaque-like lesions that may display hyperpigmentation and increased hair. Skin tumors, generally due to schwannomas, are observed in approximately 70% of patients that may present as subcutaneous nodules.

Ophthalmological manifestations are also highly characteristics of NF2. Loss of visual acuity is common in patients with NF2 due to various etiologies such as cataracts, optic nerve meningiomas, and retinal hamartomas [14, 15, 18]. Retinal tufts, dysplasia, and epiretinal membranes are also seen.

Neurologic Clinical Features

Patients with NF2 typically present with symptoms in their early 20s [17, 19]. Presenting symptoms vary depending on age. The most common presenting clinical feature in adults is hearing loss related to vestibular schwannomas (VS) [17-21]. Hearing loss is typically unilateral and often accompanied by tinnitus and imbalance. In contrast, the most common presenting symptoms in pediatric patients are ophthalmological abnormalities, followed by cutaneous features, and non-VS related neurological symptoms [17, 22]. Nearly all patients with NF2 develop bilateral VS by their fourth decade of life. However, nonvestibular schwannomas are also a common feature, often affecting other cranial, spinal, and peripheral nerves. Peripheral and spinal schwannomas nerves are often asymptomatic but can lead to motor and sensory dysfunction [15, 17, 18, 23]. Non-tumor-related neuropathies are also common. Adults may present with a progressive generalized polyneuropathy that may progress to muscle wasting. In contrast, children have a tendency to develop a mononeuropathy, with a predilection for the facial nerve causing a Bell's-like palsy [21].

Meningiomas are the second most common tumor related to NF2, with the incidence increasing with age [18, 24]. Nearly 50% of patient with NF2 will develop intracranial meningiomas and approximately 20% of patients develop intradural extramedullary spinal meningiomas [18]. Intracranial meningiomas can present with headaches or seizures, while spinal tumors present with pain, weakness, and paresthesia [21].

While schwannomas and meningiomas are the most common types of spinal tumors, gliomas are less common tumors seen in NF2 [25, 26]. The majority of histologically diagnosed gliomas are determined to be ependymomas [28]. These tumors are characterized by multiple intramedullary, indolent, asymptomatic masses that typically occur in the cervicomedullary junction or cervical spine [25-28].

Additionally, NF2 is associated with meningioangiomatosis, a plaque-like or nodular lesion due to proliferation of perivascular meningothelial and fibroblast-like cells that typically develops within the cerebral cortex [29, 30]. Meningioangiomatosis can occur sporadically as well. Sporadic cases are typically characterized by a single lesion that presents with seizures or persistent headaches in young adults or children. In comparison, NF-2 associated meningioangiomatosis is typically asymptomatic, may be multifocal, and typically discovered on autopsy.

The clinical diagnostic criteria for NF2 has undergone many revisions since being established at the National Institute of Health (NIH) consensus meeting in 1987 [31]. Due to overlapping clinical features, it can be challenging to differentiate between NF2 and schwannomatosis as the phenotype of these conditions span a phenotypic continuum that is difficult to delineate. Thus, a new consensus was reached in 2022 that proposes the umbrella term—schwannomatosis—in the updated criteria [32]. The subtypes of schwannomatosis are then further classified by molecular genetic testing, with NF2 now termed as "NF2-related schwannomatosis."

The diagnosis of NF2-related schwannomatosis can be made when an individual has one of the following: 1) bilateral vestibular schwannomas, 2) an identical NF2 pathogenic variant in at least 2 anatomically distinct NF2-related tumors, or 3) either 2 major or 1 major and 2 minor criteria as described in the following.

Major Criteria

- Unilateral VS
- First-degree relative other than sibling with *NF2*-related schwannomatosis
- Two or more meningiomas
- *NF2* pathogenic variant in an unaffected tissue such as blood

Minor Criteria

It can count >1 of a type (e.g., 2 distinct schwannomas would count as 2 minor criteria).

- Ependymoma, meningioma (Note: multiple meningiomas qualify as a major criteria), schwannoma (Note: if the major criterion is unilateral VS, at least 1 schwannoma must be dermal in location)

It can count only once (e.g., bilateral cortical cataracts count as single minor criteria).

- Juvenile subcapsular or cortical cataract, retinal hamartoma, epiretinal membrane in a person age < 40 years, meningioma

Imaging Findings

Bilateral VS on radiographic imaging is highly suggestive of NF2 [33]. NF2-associated VS typically demonstrate as multiple discrete tumor nodules that arise from both the superior and inferior branch of the vestibular nerve equally. In contrast, sporadic VS is typically a single tumor arising from the vestibular nerve at the porus acousticus. Tumors are often difficult to characterize on computed tomographic (CT) studies due to the adjacent petrous temporal bone, but may show widening of the internal acoustic canal [33, 34]. Thus, magnetic resonance imaging (MRI) is the preferred imaging modality. On MRI, small tumors appear solid and homogenous while large tumors tend to be more heterogeneous with a cystic component [35]. VS are typically hypo- or isointense to the adjacent brain parenchyma with avid post-contrast enhancement on T1-weighted scans [33, 35]. Intralesional hemorrhage may demonstrate T1 hyperintense signaling. In addition, cystic lesions lead to T2 hyperintense signal and variable T1 signal.

MRI is the image modality of choice for the diagnosis of meningiomas. Meningiomas are typically well-circumscribed extra-axial masses that homogenously enhance [18]. They are best visualized with contrast-enhanced T1-weighted scans. A characteristic imaging finding is the dural tail sign, a region of enhancement that extends from the tumor along the dura. Peritumoral edema and cysts can be visualized on T2-weighted scans or FLAIR sequences.

On CT imaging, meningioangiomatosis is typically characterized as hypodense lesions with heterogeneous contrast enhancement [36]. Calcifications are a common finding that may aid in diagnosis. On T1-weighted MRI images, lesions are hypo- to isointense and hyperintense on FLAIR and T2-weighted images [36].

NF2-associated spinal ependymomas are most commonly located in the cervical spine or cervicomedullary junction, followed by the thoracic spine and lumbar spine [25-27]. Radiographs of patients with spinal ependymomas may demonstrated scoliosis or canal widening [18, 37]. On CT imaging, spinal ependymomas are iso- or hyper-attenuated compared to normal spinal cord. Additionally, nonspecific cord enlargement may be observed. On MRI, majority of these tumors are iso- or hypointense relative to the spinal cord on T1-weighted images, and hyperintense on T2-weighted images. Additionally, cysts are a common feature observed on MRI.

Neuropathologic Findings

Schwannomas

Histologically, schwannomas display a characteristic biphasic pattern known as Antoni A and Antoni B regions. Antoni A areas are compact hypercellular regions with elongated cells with interlacing fascicles (Figure 1) [38]. These areas often also have nuclear palisading around fibrillary processes known as

Verocay bodies (Figure 2). Antoni B areas are hypocellular regions that are much less compact than Antoni A areas. They are characterized by disorderly arranged spindle cells arranged in a myxoid or hyalinized stroma (Figure 3).

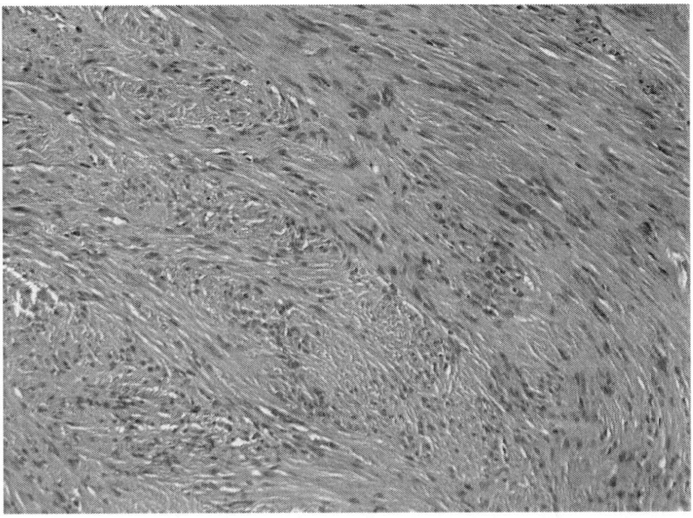

Figure 1. This cerebellopontine angle schwannoma, WHO grade 1, is marked by spindled cells with tapered nuclei. The compact arrangement of cells is typical of the Antoni pattern of tumor (hematoxylin and eosin, original magnification 200X).

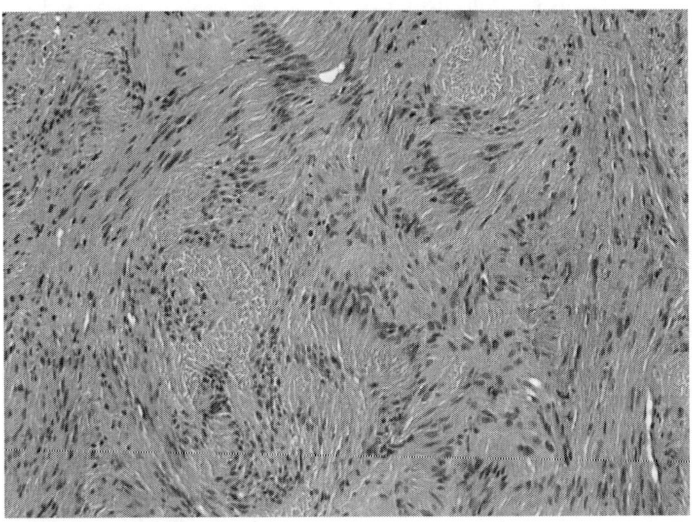

Figure 2. The palisaded pattern of a Verocay body in a schwannoma (hematoxylin and eosin, original magnification 200X).

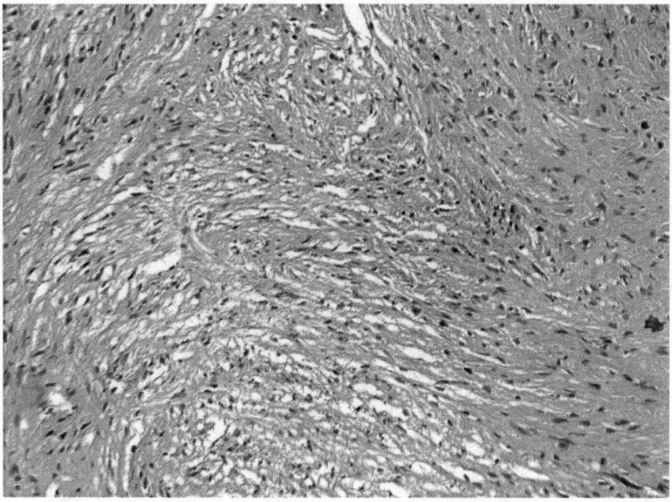

Figure 3. An Antoni B pattern region of a schwannoma marked by a looser arrangement of tumor cells (hematoxylin and eosin, original magnification 200X).

In addition, nuclear atypia may be present with cystic degeneration and hemosiderin deposition. Hyalinized vessels, thromboses, and collagenous scarring are often observed. Pseudoglandular spaces are cystic spaces lined by Schwann cells that may represent degenerated Verocay bodies that represent a very rare morphological variant of schwannomas [39]. NF2-associated schwannomas generally appear microscopically similar to their sporadic counterparts with a few exceptions. NF2-associated schwannomas are typically multicentric, demonstrate a grape-like nodularity, display higher proliferative indices, and are more invasive [40].

Differential consideration of NF-2 associated schwannomas include neurofibroma and the fibroblastic variant of meningioma. Antoni B regions of schwannomas may appear histologically similar to neurofibromas. On close inspection, schwannomas typically have larger cells, foci of Antoni A areas, and Verocay bodies. Fibroblastic meningiomas display significant morphological overlap with schwannomas. For example, classic meningioma features such as the whorl pattern can be encountered in schwannomas. While rare, the presence of psammoma bodies can help favor the diagnosis of meningioma. However, immunohistochemistry may be required to delineate between fibroblastic meningioma and schwannomas.

On immunohistochemistry (IHC), schwannomas demonstrate strong and diffuse staining of S-100 protein and abundant pericellular type IV collagen in almost all cases [41]. Schwannomas frequently stain positive for podoplanin, calretinin, and SOX10. A subset of schwannomas also demonstrate immunoreactivity to glial fibrillary acid protein (GFAP) [42]. These cells are typically in the perivascular region of hyalinized blood vessels. Furthermore, schwannomas typically stain negatively for epithelial membrane antigen (EMA). In contrast, while most fibroblastic meningiomas are S-100 positive, they display a patchy rather than diffuse pattern. Additionally, fibroblastic meningiomas stain negatively for GFAP and SOX10, display patchy EMA positivity, and stain positively for progesterone receptor and somatostatin receptor 2a (SSTR2a), the latter being a highly specific meningioma marker [43]. SOX10 and SSTR2a are highly sensitivity and specific markers for differentiating schwannomas from meningiomas that are recommended in the initial IHC assessment.

Meningiomas

The most common histological variant of sporadic meningiomas is the meningothelial variant, characterized by cells arranged in a lobulated architecture, often forming characteristic meningothelial whorls (Figure 4).

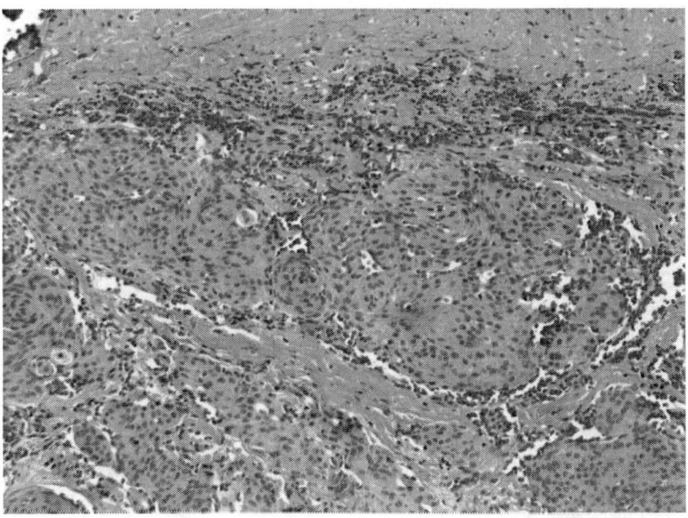

Figure 4. A meningothelial meningioma, WHO grade 1, arising from the frontal dura (top) in a patient with neurofibromatosis type 2 (hematoxylin and eosin, original magnification 200X).

The cells are typically round to polygonal shaped with uniform nuclei and eosinophilic cytoplasm. While all major histological subtypes of meningiomas can be observed in the setting of NF2, the most common histological subtypes of meningioma include the fibroblastic and transitional variants [36, 44]. NF2-associated meningiomas are commonly located within the falx cerebri, tentorium cerebelli, and cerebral and cerebellar convexities [44]. Fibroblastic meningiomas histologically resemble schwannomas; the cells appear spindle-like with elongated nuclei and are intertwined with thick bundles of collagen. Transitional meningiomas display a mixture of histological feature of both meningothelial and fibroblastic variants. In contrast to their sporadic counterparts, NF2-associated meningiomas may be associated with increased frequency of high-grade subtypes [45].

The primary differential for meningiomas is schwannomas (see previous section for differences in staining patterns). Commonly used immune-histochemistry markers for meningiomas include SSTR2a (Figure 5), progesterone receptor (PR), and EMA [43]. Almost all meningiomas demonstrate diffuse staining for SSTR2a and PR, and patchy staining for EMA. A subset of meningiomas, particularly fibrous meningiomas, display patchy S-100 protein staining. Negative stains include GFAP, SOX10, STAT6, and inhibin.

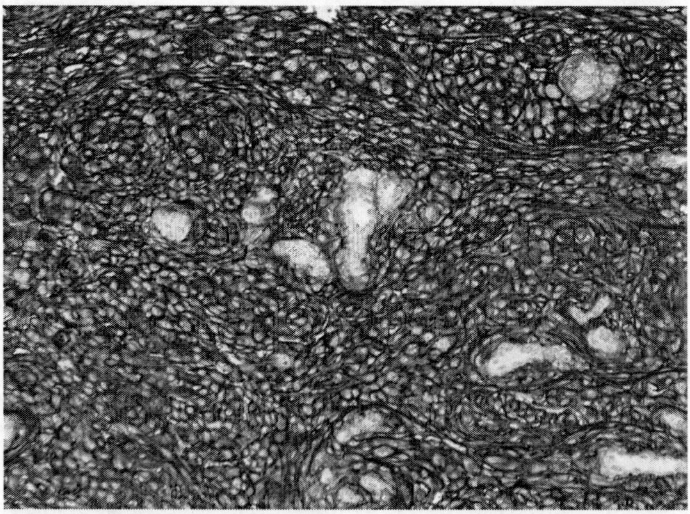

Figure 5. Diffuse SSTR2a immunostaining in a meningothelial meningioma (original magnification 200X).

Meningioangiomatosis

Both sporadic and NF2-associated meningioangiomatosis share overlapping histological features that include a proliferation of blood vessels timed by collars of meningothelial-like, and fibroblastic cells with variable cellularity, hyalinization, and calcification (Figure 6) [30, 36]. Reactive gliosis and neurodegenerative changes, such as neurofibrillary tangles, may be present. Psammoma bodies and meningothelial whorls may be present as well. Mitotic activity is rare. Neoplastic cells are typically well differentiated with the absence of necrosis and pleomorphism. Compared to their sporadic counterpart, NF2-associated meningioangiomatosis is associated with the presence of glial microhamartomas in the cortex or subcortical gray matter—a pathognomonic finding for NF2 [30]. Glial microhamartomas are limited to the gray matter and are mitotically active. They also lack characteristic features of balloon cells—glassy eccentrically placed eosinophilic cytoplasm—seen in cortical tubers and focal cortical dysplasia seen in tuberous sclerosis.

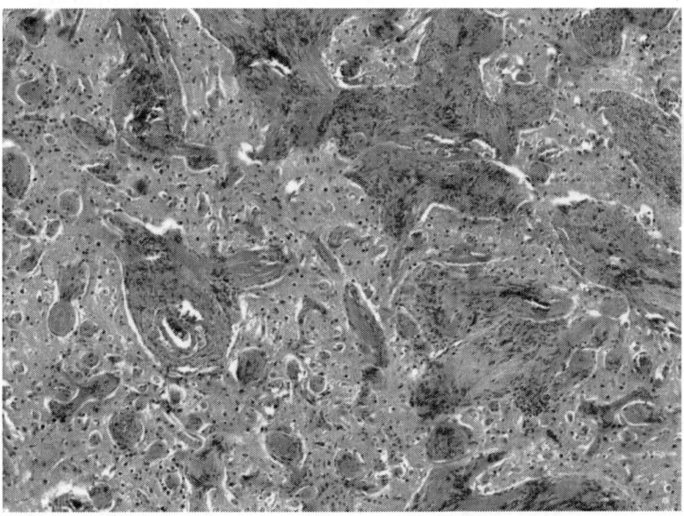

Figure 6. Meningioangiomatosis is marked by a proliferation of blood vessel within the brain parenchyma surrounded by collars of meningothelial cells (hematoxylin and eosin, original magnification 100X).

Immunohistochemistry for meningioangiomatosis is typically unhelpful for diagnosis. Proliferating blood vessels and perivascular fibroblast-like cells stain positively for vimentin uniformly [46]. Other markers such as EMA, S-100, and GFAP have demonstrated inconsistent immunoreactivity among cases. Differential consideration includes vascular malformation, atypical meningioma, or perivascular fibrosis. Vascular malformations can be differentiated by the lack of perivascular meningothelial elements. Meningiomas may demonstrate increased mitotic activity, increased cellularity, high nuclear-to-cytoplasm ratio, or sheet-like growth or necrosis [47].

Gliomas

The majority of NF2-associated spinal gliomas represent ependymomas [28]. Histologically, NF2-associated spinal ependymomas demonstrate classical growth patterns similar to their sporadic counterparts. Ependymomas are well-circumscribed tumors that consist of monomorphic cells with round to oval shaped nuclei. Mitotic figures are usually absent. A classic finding of ependymomas are pseudovascular rosettes that consist of tumors cells radially arranged around a central vessel (Figure 7). A much rarer finding are true ependymal rosettes in which tumor cells arrange themselves around an empty central lumen. On electron microscopy, tumor cells resemble normal ependymal cells that consist of numerous elongated intercellular adherens-type junctions, blepharoplasts, microvilli, and cilia—often arranged in a 9 + 2 pattern [48, 49].

Ependymomas stain positively for GFAP, S-100 protein, and vimentin on immunohistochemistry [49-51]. Additionally, tumors stain positively with EMA, appearing as a perinuclear dot-like pattern of staining. In the setting of NF2, the primary differential considerations is astrocytoma [26, 28]. Histological variants such as tanycytic ependymomas can be challenging to differentiate from astrocytoma. Tanycytic ependymomas lack classic histological features such as pseudorosettes and ependymal rosettes [28]. EMA immunostaining is typically useful in the distinction between ependymomas and astrocytomas. There are, however, cases where astrocytomas express EMA in a dot-like pattern and ependymomas that are EMA-negative. Thus, ultrastructural analysis with electron microscopy to identify ependymal features may be required for definitive diagnosis.

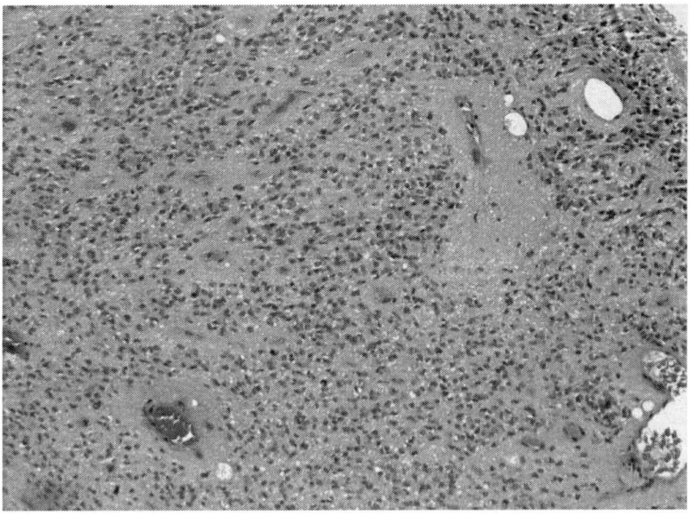

Figure 7. This cervical spinal low grade ependymoma, WHO grade 2, is marked by perivascular pseudorosette formations (hematoxylin and eosin, original magnification 200X).

Treatment and Prognosis

Treatment of patients with NF2 is focused on maintaining function and quality of life while managing tumor load. Due to complexity of clinical care, patients are best managed at specialized multidisciplinary centers [52]. Monitoring for the development and progression of neurological symptoms plays a central role in clinical management. Depending on symptom severity, tumor size, and tumor growth rate, as well as patient preference, management includes conservative management, surgical excision, radiotherapy, typically stereotactic radiosurgery, and more recently, medical therapy. Due to improvements in management, life expectancy of patients with NF2 has improved over the years. The median life expectancy of patients with NF2 is 69 years; patients diagnosed after 1990 lived approximately 15 years longer compared to those diagnosed before 1985 [53]. Despite relatively good life expectancy, this statistic disguises the peaks of deaths that occur in the 2nd and 3rd decade of life due to the widely variable clinical phenotype of NF2.

Historically, patients with NF2 were classified into two phenotypic groups termed "Wishart" (severe) and "Gardner" (mild) type. The Wishart variant typically presents in childhood and is marked by a with high tumor burden;

the Gardner variant typically presents in adulthood with bilateral vestibular schwannomas [52]. Genotype-phenotype correlations regarding NF2 disease severity are well documented. In general, missense mutations, splice-site mutations, large deletions, and somatic mosaicism are associated with milder disease severity compared to those with nonsense or frameshift mutations (54-58). Additionally, mutations that in more upstream exons were associated with more severe phenotypes such as increased intracranial meningiomas [55, 57, 58].

Conclusion

Neurofibromatosis type 2 is a rare autosomal dominant condition marked by germline mutations in the NF2 gene. It is associated with a spectrum of neuropathologic findings including schwannomas, meningiomas, ependymomas, meningioangiomatosis and glial microhamartomas. The pathology of these lesions is similar to their pathology when they arise outside the setting of Neurofibromatosis type 2.

References

[1] Wishart J H. Case of tumours in the skull, dura mater, and brain. *Edinb. Med. Surg. J.* 1822; 18(72): 393-397.

[2] Seizinger B R, Rouleau G A, Ozelius L J, et al. Genetic linkage of von Recklinghausen neurofibromatosis to the nerve growth factor receptor gene. *Cell.* 1987; 49(5): 589-594.

[3] Rouleau G A, Wertelecki W, Haines J L, et al. Genetic linkage of bilateral acoustic neurofibromatosis to a DNA marker on chromosome 22. *Nature.* 1987; 329(6136): 246-248.

[4] Rouleau G A, Merel P, Lutchman M, et al. Alteration in a new gene encoding a putative membrane-organizing protein causes neuro-fibromatosis type 2. *Nature.* 1993; 363(6429): 515-521.

[5] Trofatter J A, MacCollin M M, Rutter J L, et al. A novel moesin-, ezrin-, radixin-like gene is a candidate for the neurofibromatosis 2 tumor suppressor. *Cell.* 1993; 72(5): 791-800.

[6] McClatchey A I, Giovannini M. Membrane organization and tumorigenesis--the NF2 tumor suppressor, Merlin. *Genes Dev.* 2005; 19(19): 2265-2277.

[7] Lallemand D, Curto M, Saotome I, et al. NF2 deficiency promotes tumorigenesis and metastasis by destabilizing adherens junctions. *Genes Dev.* 2003; 17(9): 1090-1100.

[8] Morrison H, Sherman L S, Legg J, et al. The NF2 tumor suppressor gene product, merlin, mediates contact inhibition of growth through interactions with CD44. *Genes Dev*. 2001; 15(8): 968-980.

[9] Okada T, Lopez-Lago M, Giancotti F G. Merlin/NF-2 mediates contact inhibition of growth by suppressing recruitment of Rac to the plasma membrane. *J. Cell Biol*. 2005; 171(2): 361-371.

[10] Cooper J, Giancotti F G. Molecular insights into NF2/Merlin tumor suppressor function. *FEBS Lett*. 2014; 588(16): 2743-2752.

[11] Li W, You L, Cooper J, et al. Merlin/NF2 suppresses tumorigenesis by inhibiting the E3 ubiquitin ligase CRL4(DCAF1) in the nucleus. *Cell*. 2010; 140(4): 477-490.

[12] Hamaratoglu, F., Willecke, M., Kango-Singh, M. et al. The tumour-suppressor genes NF2/Merlin and Expanded act through Hippo signalling to regulate cell proliferation and apoptosis. *Nat. Cell Biol*. 2006. 8: 27–36.

[13] McClatchey A I, Giovannini M. Membrane organization and tumorigenesis--the NF2 tumor suppressor, Merlin. *Genes Dev*. 2005; 19(19): 2265-2277.

[14] Ruggieri M, Iannetti P, Polizzi A, et al. Earliest clinical manifestations and natural history of neurofibromatosis type 2 (NF2) in childhood: a study of 24 patients. *Neuropediatrics*. 2005; 36(1): 21-34.

[15] MacCollin M, Mautner V F. The diagnosis and management of neurofibromatosis 2 in childhood. *Semin. Pediatr. Neurol*. 1998; 5(4): 243-252.

[16] Evans D G, Birch J M, Ramsden R T. Paediatric presentation of type 2 neurofibromatosis. *Arch. Dis. Child*. 1999; 81(6): 496-499.

[17] Evans, D G, Huson S M, Donnai D, et al. "A clinical study of type 2 neurofibromatosis." *Quart. J. Med*. 1992; 84(304): 603-18.

[18] Asthagiri A R, Parry D M, Butman J A, et al. Neurofibromatosis type 2. *Lancet*. 2009; 373(9679): 1974-1986.

[19] Forde C, King AT, Rutherford S A, et al. Disease course of neurofibromatosis type 2: a 30-year follow-up study of 353 patients seen at a single institution. *Neuro Oncol*. 2021; 23(7): 1113-1124.

[20] Martuza R L, Eldridge R. Neurofibromatosis 2 (bilateral acoustic neurofibromatosis). *N. Engl. J. Med*. 1988;318(11):684-688.

[21] Evans DG. Neurofibromatosis type 2 (NF2): a clinical and molecular review. *Orphanet. J. Rare Dis*. 2009; 4:16.

[22] Gugel I, Grimm F, Teuber C, et al. Presenting symptoms in children with neurofibromatosis type 2. *Childs Nerv. Syst*. 2020; 36(10): 2463-2470.

[23] Stemmer-Rachamimov A O, Ino Y, Lim Z Y, et al. Loss of the NF2 gene and merlin occur by the tumorlet stage of schwannoma development in neurofibromatosis 2. *J. Neuropathol. Exp. Neurol*. 1998; 57(12): 1164-1167.

[24] Louis D N, Ramesh V, Gusella J F. Neuropathology and molecular genetics of neurofibromatosis 2 and related tumors. *Brain Pathol*. 1995; 5(2): 163-172.

[25] Patronas N J, Courcoutsakis N, Bromley CM, et al. Intramedullary and spinal canal tumors in patients with neurofibromatosis 2: MR imaging findings and correlation with genotype. *Radiology*. 2001; 218(2): 434-442.

[26] Mautner V F, Tatagiba M, Lindenau M, et al. Spinal tumors in patients with neurofibromatosis type 2: MR imaging study of frequency, multiplicity, and variety

[published correction appears in *AJR Am. J. Roentgenol.* 1996 May;166(5):1231]. *AJR Am. J. Roentgenol.* 1995; 165(4): 951-955.

[27] Plotkin SR, O'Donnell CC, Curry WT, et al. Spinal ependymomas in neurofibromatosis Type 2: a retrospective analysis of 55 patients. *J. Neurosurg. Spine.* 2011; 14(4): 543-547.

[28] Hagel C, Stemmer-Rachamimov A O, Bornemann A, et al. Clinical presentation, immunohistochemistry and electron microscopy indicate neurofibromatosis type 2-associated gliomas to be spinal ependymomas. *Neuropathology.* 2012; 32(6): 611-616.

[29] Stemmer-Rachamimov A O, Horgan M A, Taratuto A L, et al. Meningioangiomatosis is associated with neurofibromatosis 2 but not with somatic alterations of the NF2 gene. *J. Neuropathol. Exp. Neurol.* 1997; 56(5): 485-489.

[30] Perry A, Kurtkaya-Yapicier O, Scheithauer B W, et al. Insights into meningioangiomatosis with and without meningioma: a clinicopathologic and genetic series of 24 cases with review of the literature. *Brain Pathol.* 2005; 15(1): 55-65.

[31] Seizinger B R, Martuza R L, Gusella J F. Loss of genes on chromosome 22 in tumorigenesis of human acoustic neuroma. *Nature.* 1986; 322(6080): 644-647.

[32] Plotkin S R, Messiaen L, Legius E, et al. Updated diagnostic criteria and nomenclature for neurofibromatosis type 2 and schwannomatosis: An international consensus recommendation [published online ahead of print, 2022 Jun 8]. *Genet Med.* 2022; S1098-3600(22): 00773-0.

[33] Stivaros S M, Stemmer-Rachamimov A O, Alston R, et al. Multiple synchronous sites of origin of vestibular schwannomas in neurofibromatosis Type 2. *J. Med. Genet.* 2015; 52(8): 557-562.

[34] Gentry LR, Jacoby CG, Turski PA, et al. Cerebellopontine angle-petromastoid mass lesions: comparative study of diagnosis with MR imaging and CT. *Radiology.* 1987; 162(2): 513-520.

[35] Mulkens T H, Parizel P M, Martin J J, et al. Acoustic schwannoma: MR findings in 84 tumors. *AJR Am. J. Roentgenol.* 1993; 160(2): 395-398.

[36] Coy, S., Rashid, R., Stemmer-Rachamimov, A. et al. An update on the CNS manifestations of neurofibromatosis type 2. *Acta Neuropathol.* 2020; 139: 643–665.

[37] Koeller KK, Rosenblum RS, Morrison AL. Neoplasms of the spinal cord and filum terminale: radiologic-pathologic correlation. *Radiographics.* 2000; 20(6): 1721-1749.

[38] Sobel R A. Vestibular (acoustic) schwannomas: histologic features in neurofibromatosis 2 and in unilateral cases. *J. Neuropathol. Exp. Neurol.* 1993; 52(2): 106-113.

[39] Ud Din N, Ahmad Z, Ahmed A. Schwannomas with pseudoglandular elements: clinicopathologic study of 61 cases. *Ann. Diagn. Pathol.* 2016; 20: 24-28.

[40] Dewan R, Pemov A, Kim H J, et al. Evidence of polyclonality in neurofibromatosis type 2-associated multilobulated vestibular schwannomas. *Neuro. Oncol.* 2015; 17(4): 566-573.

[41] Rodriguez F J, Folpe A L, Giannini C, et al. Pathology of peripheral nerve sheath tumors: diagnostic overview and update on selected diagnostic problems. *Acta Neuropathol*. 2012; 123(3): 295-319.

[42] Kawahara E, Oda Y, Ooi A, et al. Expression of glial fibrillary acidic protein (GFAP) in peripheral nerve sheath tumors. A comparative study of immunoreactivity of GFAP, vimentin, S-100 protein, and neurofilament in 38 schwannomas and 18 neurofibromas. *Am. J. Surg. Pathol*. 1988; 12(2): 115-120.

[43] Boulagnon-Rombi C, Fleury C, Fichel C, et al. Immunohistochemical approach to the differential diagnosis of meningiomas and their mimics. *J. Neuropathol. Exp. Neurol*. 2017; 76(4): 289-298.

[44] Fountain D M, Smith M J, O'Leary C, et al. The spatial phenotype of genotypically distinct meningiomas demonstrate potential implications of the embryology of the meninges [published correction appears in *Oncogene*. 2021 Oct; 40(42): 6139]. *Oncogene*. 2021; 40(5): 875-884.

[45] Perry A, Giannini C, Raghavan R, et al. Aggressive phenotypic and genotypic features in pediatric and NF2-associated meningiomas: a clinicopathologic study of 53 cases. *J. Neuropathol. Exp. Neurol*. 2001; 60(10): 994-1003.

[46] Wiebe S, Munoz D G, Smith S, et al. Meningioangiomatosis. A comprehensive analysis of clinical and laboratory features. *Brain*. 1999; 122(4): 709-726.

[47] Perry A, Stafford S L, Scheithauer B W, et al. Meningioma grading: an analysis of histologic parameters. *Am. J. Surg. Pathol*. 1997; 21(12): 1455-1465.

[48] Baloyannis SJ, Baloyannis IS. The fine structure of ependymomas. *CNS Oncol*. 2014; 3(1): 49-59.

[49] Miettinen M, Clark R, Virtanen I. Intermediate filament proteins in choroid plexus and ependymal and their tumors. *Am. J. Pathol*. 1986; 123(2): 231-240.

[50] Kunishio K, Shiraishi T, Mishima N, et al. Immunohistochemical study for choroid plexus papillomas and ependymomas. *Neuro Med Chir*. 1991; 31(13): 859-866.

[51] Yung W K, Luna M, Borit A. Vimentin and glial fibrillary acidic protein in human brain tumors. *J. Neurooncol*. 1985; 3(1): 35-38.

[52] Lloyd S K, Evans D G. Neurofibromatosis type 2 (NF2): diagnosis and management. *Handb. Clin. Neurol*. 2013; 115: 957-967.

[53] Wilding A, Ingham S L, Lalloo F, et al. Life expectancy in hereditary cancer predisposing diseases: an observational study. *J. Med. Genet*. 2012; 49(4): 264-269.

[54] Baser ME, Kuramoto L, Joe H, et al. Genotype-phenotype correlations for nervous system tumors in neurofibromatosis 2: a population-based study. *Am. J. Hum. Genet*. 2004; 75(2): 231-239.

[55] Mérel P, Hoang-Xuan K, Sanson M, et al. Screening for germ-line mutations in the NF2 gene. *Genes Chromosomes Cancer*. 1995; 12(2): 117-127.

[56] Kluwe L, Bayer S, Baser M E, et al. Identification of NF2 germ-line mutations and comparison with neurofibromatosis 2 phenotypes [published correction appears in *Hum Genet* 1997 Feb; 99(2): 292]. *Hum. Genet*. 1996; 98(5): 534-538.

[57] Kluwe L, MacCollin M, Tatagiba M, et al. Phenotypic variability associated with 14 splice-site mutations in the NF2 gene. *Am. J. Med. Genet*. 1998; 77(3): 228-233.

[58] Kluwe L, Mautner VF. A missense mutation in the NF2 gene results in moderate and mild clinical phenotypes of neurofibromatosis type 2. *Hum. Genet*. 1996; 97(2): 224-227.

[59] Smith M J, Higgs J E, Bowers N L, et al. Cranial meningiomas in 411 neurofibromatosis type 2 (NF2) patients with proven gene mutations: clear positional effect of mutations, but absence of female severity effect on age at onset. *J. Med. Genet*. 2011; 48(4): 261-265.

Chapter 2

Tuberous Sclerosis: Central Nervous System Pathology

Alissa Becerril[1], BA
and Richard A. Prayson[2,*], MD, MEd
[1] Cleveland Clinic Lerner College of Medicine, Cleveland, OH, USA
[2] Department of Anatomic Pathology, Cleveland Clinic, OH, USA

Abstract

Tuberous sclerosis is an autosomal dominant genetic disease, marked by hamartomas and benign neoplasms that affect multiple body systems with a wide degree of variability. Patients with tuberous sclerosis typically present with skin lesions, seizures, and hamartomas in the heart, brain, and kidneys.

Tuberous sclerosis is characterized by three types of neuropathological lesions: cortical tubers, subependymal nodules and subependymal giant cell astrocytomas. Histologically, tubers are marked by a disorganized cortical architecture with balloon cells that have mixed glioneuronal characteristics. Tuberous sclerosis is due to loss of function mutations in TSC1 or TSC2 tumor suppressor genes that lead to a failure to regulate mTOR pathway-mediated cellular growth and differentiation.

This chapter will review the key clinical and pathologic features of tuberous sclerosis and highlight the neuropathological findings associated with this disorder.

[*] Corresponding Author's Email: praysor@ccf.org.

In: Central Nervous System Pathologies in Hereditary Tumor Syndromes
Editor: Richard A. Prayson
ISBN: 979-8-88697-620-5

Introduction

The broad spectrum of pathology seen in tuberous sclerosis mirrors its expansive history of discovery [1]. The characterization of tuberous sclerosis began in 1835 when Pierre François Olive Rayer published illustrations of facial "végétations vasculaires," renamed adenoma sebaceum by Pringle in 1890. In 1862, Friedrich von Recklinghausen's published a case report of a newborn with cardiac myomas and cerebral sclerosis who died within minutes after birth. However, the first clear description of tuberous sclerosis is credited to Parisian neurologist Désiré-Magloire Bourneville, thus leading to the eponym Bourneville's disease. In 1879, he cared for a 15-year-old girl with seizures, psychomotor retardation and a "vesiculo-papular eruption on her nose, cheeks and forehead." When post-mortem gross examination revealed opaque, firm and nodular tumors in the cerebral gyri, Bourneville coined the term *tuberous sclerosis* based on resemblance of the lesions (i.e., "tubers") to potatoes. Although Bourneville also found kidney masses in the patient, it was not until 1905 that renal tumors were associated with tuberous sclerosis along with cerebral, cardiac, and dermal lesions [1].

Three years later, Heinrich Vogt established the clinical "triad" that served to make a clinical diagnosis which had previously only been made by postmortem exam. The clinical features that consisted of epilepsy, mental retardation, and adenoma sebaceum defined the condition for the next 60 years, until radiographic images greatly improved the diagnostic process. In 1979, Spanish-American neurologist Manuel Gómez described the full clinical spectrum of tuberous sclerosis and established a new set of diagnostic criteria to replace the Vogt triad [2]. The late 20th century also saw the discovery of the two genes linked with tuberous sclerosis, which led to further efforts to understand the molecular basis of the disease [1].

This chapter will outline the clinical and pathological features of TSC, highlighting the neuropathological findings that have been described in this syndrome.

Genetics of Tuberous Sclerosis

Tuberous Sclerosis is an autosomal dominant disorder caused by mutations in either the TSC1 or TSC2 tumor-suppressor genes [3]. TSC1 is located on chromosome 9q34 and encodes for the *hamartin* protein; TSC2 is located on chromosome 16p13.3 and encodes the *tuberin* protein [4]. Both hamartin and tuberin are widely expressed and form heterodimers that function to inhibit mTOR. Disruption of the protein complex causes upregulation of the mTOR pathway and increases cellular growth and proliferation and disrupts cell migration [5]. Approximately two-thirds of tuberous sclerosis cases are sporadic. Of the one third of cases that are inherited, high penetrance but considerable phenotypic variability is observed [6].

General Clinical Features

Tuberous sclerosis is characterized by the development of benign tumors in a wide range of organs, and thus clinical presentations are highly variable. The classic Vogt triad of facial angiofibromas, epilepsy and mental retardation is only observed in 30-40% of cases [3].

Table 1. Diagnostic criteria for tuberous sclerosis

Definite Tuberous Sclerosis
Two major features[a] or one major and two or more minor features
Possible Tuberous Sclerosis
Either one major feature or ≥2 minor features
Major Features
Angiofibromas (≥3) or fibrous cephalic plaque
Ungual fibroma ≥2)
Hypomelanotic macules (i.e., ash-leaf spots [≥3], at least 5 mm diameter)
Shagreen patch (connective tissue nevus)
Multiple retinal hamartomas
Cortical dysplasias (includes tubers and cerebral white matter radial migration lines)
Subependymal nodule
Subependymal giant cell astrocytoma (SEGA)
Cardiac rhabdomyoma, single or multiple
Lymphangiomyomatosis
Angiomyolipoma (≥2)*
Minor Features
Multiple randomly distributed pits in dental enamel (≥3)
Intraoral fibromas (≥2)
Nonrenal hamartomas
Retinal achromatic patch
"Confetti" skin lesions
Multiple renal cysts
Sclerotic bone lesions

Modified from Northrup H, Aronow ME, Bebin EM, et al. Updated International Tuberous Sclerosis Complex Diagnostic Criteria and Surveillance and Management Recommendations. Pediatr Neurol. 2021;123:50-66.

*A combination of the two major clinical features lymphangioleiomyomatosis and angiomyolipomas without other features does not meet the criteria for a definite diagnosis.

Skin lesions are detected in all ages of more than 90% of patients with tuberous sclerosis, the most common cutaneous lesion of tuberous sclerosis is hypomelanotic macules with irregular borders ("ash leaf spots") [7]. Another common cutaneous manifestation is facial angiofibromas (previously called "adenoma sebaceum"), which is seen as erythematous papules distributed over the nose and malar region of the face. Although less specific to tuberous sclerosis, other cutaneous manifestations include ungual fibromas and shagreen patches [8]. Renal angiomyolipomas develop by age 10 years in as many as 80% of patients with tuberous sclerosis [9]. Approximately two-thirds of individuals have rhabdomyomas; they are usually present at birth and regress with time [10]. Pulmonary lymphan-gioleiomyomatosis presents after puberty in as many as 40% of women; this can present with progressive shortness of breath, recurrent pneumothoraxes, and deterioration in lung function [11, 12].

Retinal hamartomas are observed in 30-50% of tuberous sclerosis patients. Less common findings are hamartomatous rectal polyps, bone cysts, and gingival fibromas. Diagnosis of Tuberous Sclerosis is based on meeting the 2018 updated diagnostic criteria, shown in Table 1 [13].

Neurologic Clinical Features

Epilepsy is the most common neurological symptom of tuberous sclerosis [14]. It is present in 80-90% of cases and can begin as early as infancy with focal seizures or infantile spasm [15]. Seizure control is difficult and the epilepsy is intractable in 50% of cases despite pharmacological and surgical treatment. Like early-onset epilepsy in general, intellectual disability in tuberous sclerosis often is associated with early onset and refractory epilepsy. About 50% of patients with tuberous sclerosis have cognitive impairment, ranging from mild to severe [16].

In addition to intellectual disability, over 60% of patients with tuberous sclerosis have a combination of behavior and psychiatric dysfunction known as tuberous sclerosis-associated neuro-psychiatric disorders (TAND), which include autism spectrum disorders, mood disorders, aggressive behaviors, and learning differences [17]. Cortical subependymal giant cell astrocytomas (SEGA) can affect 10-20% of patients with tuberous sclerosis and clinically manifests with symptoms of obstructive hydrocephalus (lethargy, emesis, headache, limited upward gaze, increased seizure frequency) [7]. These slow-growing tumors are typically located in the lateral and/or third ventricles near the foramen of Monro. SEGAs are most frequently identified clinically in the early teen years, with a mean age presentation of 13 years [13, 18].

Imaging Findings

Medical imaging plays an important role in the diagnosis and monitoring of central nervous system lesions in tuberous sclerosis [19, 20]. These lesions include cerebral cortical tubers, white matter glioneuronal heterotopia, subependymal nodules, and SEGAs. Both computed tomography (CT) and magnetic resonance imaging (MRI) both detect cortical tubers, although MRI is considered the standard for defining CNS involvement in tuberous sclerosis. On MRI, lesions in adults have low T1 signal and high T2 or FLAIR signal [13, 21]. In young infants, the pattern is reversed because of the high water content in the surrounding unmyelinated brain. Diffusion tensor imaging (DTI) and metabolic studies using positron emission tomography (PET) are useful in localizing epileptic lesions. Higher apparent diffusion coefficients and lower fractional anisotropy on DTI, and hypometabolism on PET have increased epileptogenic potential compared to other lesions [20]. Radial glioneuronal heterotopias are best seen on MRI and have similar signal characteristics to cortical tubers, with low signal on T1-weighted images and high signal on T2-weighted images. Although the lesions are classically linear, they can also be wedge-shaped; both represent cellular elements that arrested during cortical migration [20, 22].

The intrinsic imaging properties of subependymal nodules and SEGAs based on MRI sequences are very similar. Following the administration of contrast agents, both show intense enhancement [23, 24]. The most distinguishing feature between these two lesions is their size and growth patterns. SEGAs are diagnosed by size greater than 10 mm, demonstrable growth, or the production of symptoms of hydrocephalus [25].

Neuropathologic Findings

Cortical tubers, subependymal nodules and SEGAs represent the main neuropathological lesions of tuberous sclerosis. On gross pathology, cortical tubers are tan-white expansions within the cortex and/or subcortical white matter and have a firm or rubbery, potato-like quality due to prominent gliosis

(Figure 1). Substantial calcifications render tubers chalky on the surface (Figure 2).

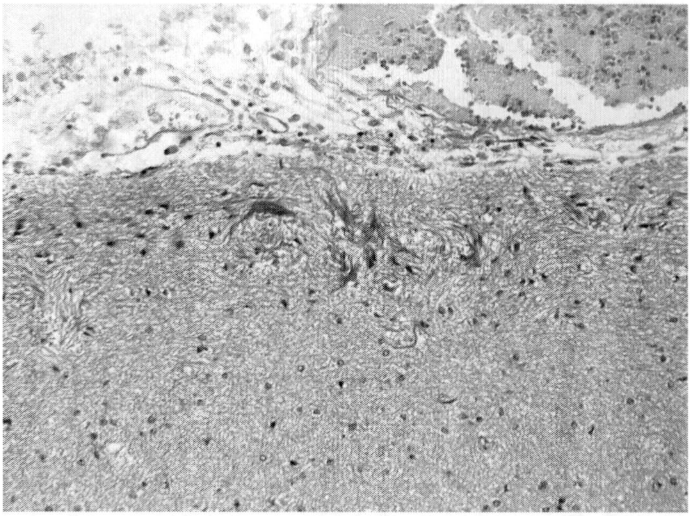

Figure 1. Cortical tuber with prominent subpial gliosis (hematoxylin and eosin, original magnification 200x).

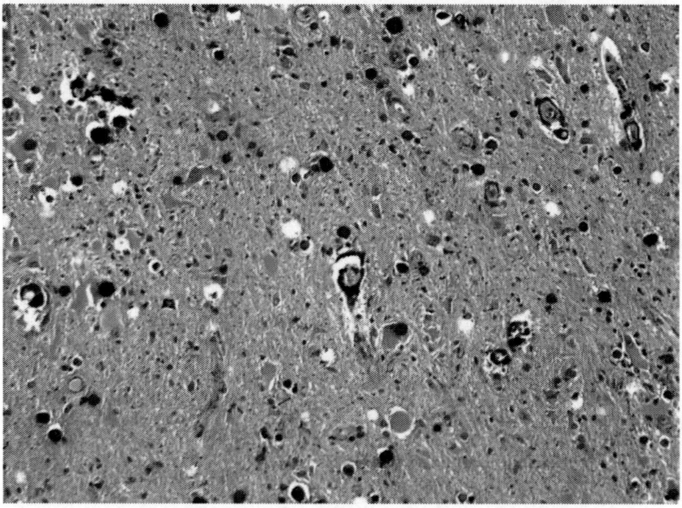

Figure 2. Prominent microcalcifications maybe seen in cortical tubers (hematoxylin and eosin, original magnification 200X).

Histologically, cortical tubers consist of areas of cortical dyslamination and contain different cell types: dysmorphic neurons, reactive astrocytes, and most distinctively, balloon cells (Figure 3) [26]. Dysmorphic neurons demonstrate migrational and maturational abnormalities [27]. These cells exhibit aberrantly directed dendrites and accumulation of argyrophilic fibrils within their perikarya and may be seen in all cortical layers and in underlying white matter [28]. This pattern of distribution leads to radial glioneuronal heterotopias, which extend through the white matter in a linear or wedge-shape manner [29].

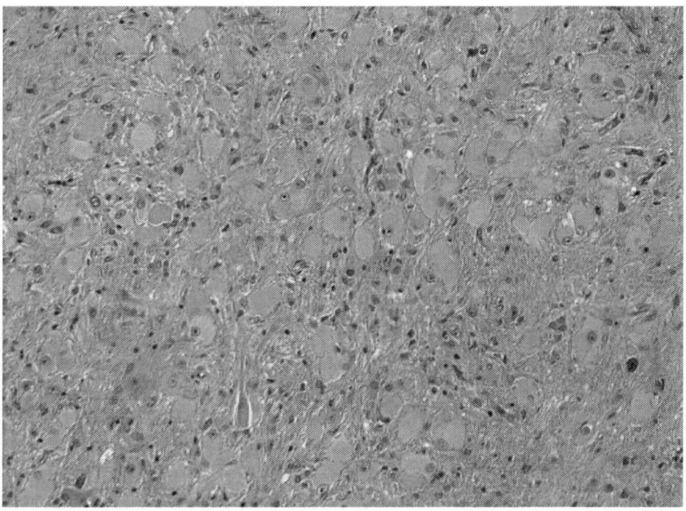

Figure 3. Cortical tuber marked by large balloon cells in the cortex of the tuber (hematoxylin and eosin, original magnification 200X).

Balloon cells are characterized by their large size, abundant pink cytoplasm and eccentric nuclei; sometimes the cells are multinucleated. Some balloon cells may resemble neurons and others may resemble gemistocytic astrocytes. Notably, immunohistochemically markers characteristic of glial and neuronal phenotypes suggest a mixed glioneuronal origin of these cells [26, 30].

Subependymal nodules grossly resemble wax drippings ("candle-guttering"); they diffusely line the ventricular walls and are precursor legions of SEGAs. Both subependymal nodules and SEGAs are histologically indistinguishable and are composed of spindled, epithelioid or gemistocyte-like cells that form sweeping fascicles and ependymoma-like perivascular pseudorosettes. Similar to the cortical tubers, they often contain dystrophic calcification and have mixed glio-neuronal features with neuron-like nuclei and astrocyte-like cytoplasm. SEGAs have a well-demarcated border with the adjacent brain parenchyma; they grow directly under the ependymal surface of the lateral ventricle without infiltration. They are marked by a proliferation of large, generally rounded, sometimes elongated cells with abundant eosinophilic cytoplasm (Figures 4-6). Occasionally, mitotic figures and necrosis are observed, but these features do not suggest more aggressive behavior. Inflammatory cells are also seen, including intratumoral mast cells and lymphocytes [29, 31]. These tumors are considered low grade, World Health Organization (WHO) grade 1 neoplasms.

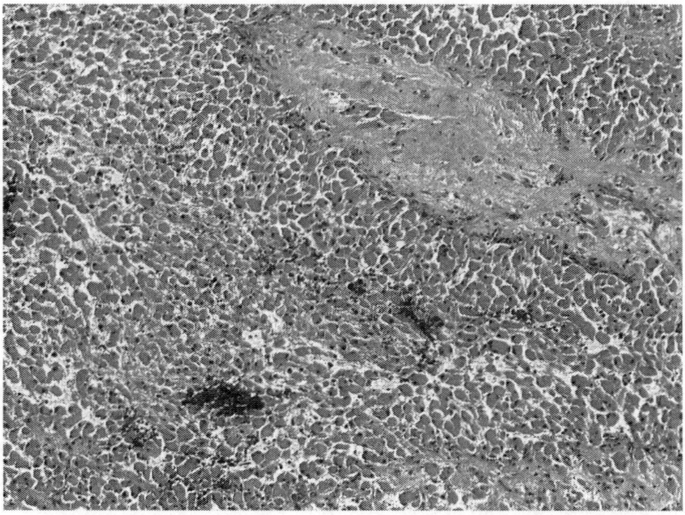

Figure 4. Subependymal giant cell astrocytoma marked by a proliferation of large rounded astrocytic cells (hematoxylin and eosin, original magnification 100X).

Immunohistochemically, the dysplastic cells of tubers express neuronal and glial antigens in a variable fashion [32, 33]. They may show positivity for glial fibrillary acidic protein (GFAP) along with positivity for neuronal markers such as synaptophysin, neurofilament protein and NeuN. Other cell types stain for neither glial or neuronal makers, likely representing a more primitive progenitor phenotype. Large dysplastic neurons typically show neurofilament positive cell bodies. Tumor nuclei in SEGAs may be positive for thyroid transcription factor 1 (TTF-1) and mast cells can be stained with c-kit/CD117 [34, 35].

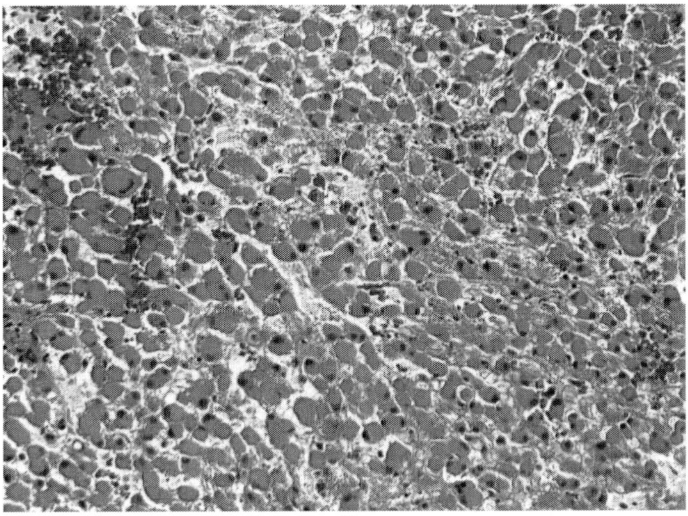

Figure 5. Subependymal giant cell astrocytoma tumor cells generally appear rather monomorphic (hematoxylin and eosin, original magnification 200X).

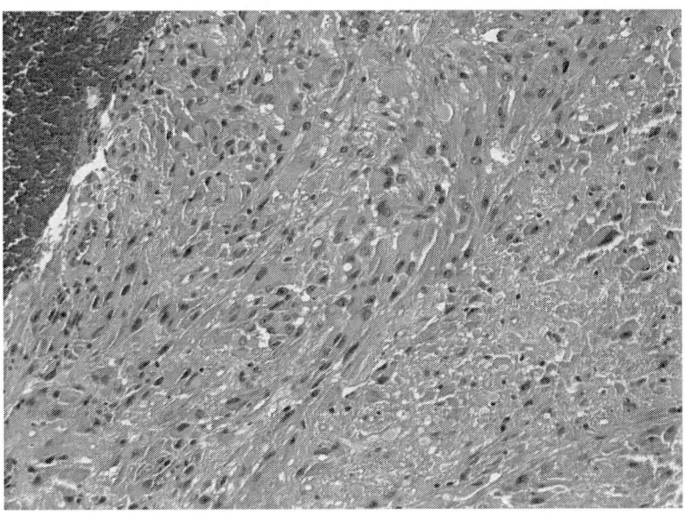

Figure 6. In areas of a subependymal giant cell astrocytoma, tumor cells may have a more spindled appearance (hematoxylin and eosin, original magnification 200X).

Differential Diagnosis

Importantly, cortical tubers seen in tuberous sclerosis are histologically identical to International League Against Epilepsy (ILAE) focal cortical dysplasia type IIb lesions; the latter are isolated or sporadic and do not have other signs of tuberous sclerosis [36].

With regard to the differential diagnosis of SEGAs, this can be approached by location and histology. Other tumors that occur in the ventricular system near the foramen of Monro include ependymoma/ subependymoma, meningioma, chordoid glioma, central neurocytoma and germ cell tumors; each of these lesions have histologic features that distinguish them from SEGAs. Although SEGAs can mimic ependymoma with perivascular pseudorosettes, the strong uniform GFAP expression and lack of gemistocyte-like and ganglionic cells distinguish ependymoma from SEGAs. In comparison to SEGAs, chordoid gliomas have regions with a more prominent chordoid appearance with myxoid stroma and strong GFAP expression. Central neurocytoma are often distinguished by its uniform expression of neuronal markers like synaptophysin and by its delicate neuropil [37].

Treatment and Prognosis

Treatment of patients with tuberous sclerosis includes a focus on symptom management. The γ-aminobutyric acid inhibitor, vigabatrin, is recommended as the first line treatment in early onset seizures because it stops tuberous sclerosis-related infantile spasms in the majority of cases [38, 39]. Early treatment of epilepsy can improve long-term outcomes of patients with tuberous sclerosis, including reduced symptoms of autism and cognitive impairment [40]. Surgical resection of epileptogenic foci is indicated when seizures remain inadequately controlled with a trial of two anti-seizure medications. Additionally, treatment with mTOR inhibitor, sirolimus, has been shown to cause tumor regression of SEGA and renal angiomyolipomas and was FDA approved in 2012 for the treatment of both the neurological and non-neurological manifestations of tuberous sclerosis. Since then, mTOR inhibitors have largely replaced surgery as the primary therapeutic option for the management of SEGA, with the exception of acute hydrocephalus that is still managed with surgery [41].

The prognosis of patients with tuberous sclerosis varies with the type and degree of organ involvement [42]. Renal disease and status epilepticus are the major causes of death, although pulmonary and cardiac lesions are also potential sources [43]. In a recent study of 284 patients with tuberous sclerosis, the median age of death was 33 years old (interquartile range 26-46 years); this study demonstrated that mortality was more common in patients with learning disabilities [44].

Conclusion

Tuberous sclerosis is an autosomal dominant condition due to loss of function mutations on the TSC1 or TSC2 tumor suppressor genes that lead to failure to regulate mTOR pathway mediated cell grow and differentiation. Neuropathologic conditions associated with tuberous sclerosis included cortical tubers, which represent a form of focal cortical dysplasia, subependymal giant cell astrocytomas (WHO grade 1 tumors), and subependymoma nodules.

References

[1] Gómez MR. History of the tuberous sclerosis complex. *Brain Dev.* 1995;17 Suppl:55-57. doi:10.1016/0387-7604(94)00130-8.

[2] Gomez MR. *Tuberous Sclerosis*. 1st ed. New York; 1979.

[3] Maria BL, Deidrick KM, Roach ES, et al. Tuberous sclerosis complex: pathogenesis, diagnosis, strategies, therapies, and future research directions. *J Child Neurol.* 2004;19(9):632-642. doi:10.1177/08830738040190090201.

[4] Kandt RS, Haines JL, Smith M, et al. Linkage of an important gene locus for tuberous sclerosis to a chromosome 16 marker for polycystic kidney disease. *Nat Genet.* 1992;2(1):37-41. doi:10.1038/ng0992-37.

[5] Tee AR, Fingar DC, Manning BD, et al. Tuberous sclerosis complex-1 and -2 gene products function together to inhibit mammalian target of rapamycin (mTOR)-mediated downstream signaling. *Proc Natl Acad Sci U S A.* 2002; 99(21): 13571-13576. doi:10.1073/pnas.202476899.

[6] Short MP, Richardson EPJ, Haines JL, et al. Clinical, neuropathological and genetic aspects of the tuberous sclerosis complex. *Brain Pathol.* 1995;5(2):173-179. doi:10.1111/j.1750-3639.1995.tb00591.x.

[7] Crino PB, Nathanson KL, Henske EP. The tuberous sclerosis complex. *N Engl J Med.* 2006;355(13):1345-1356. doi:10.1056/NEJMra055323.

[8] Datta AN, Hahn CD, Sahin M. Clinical presentation and diagnosis of tuberous sclerosis complex in infancy. *J Child Neurol.* 2008;23(3):268-273. doi:10.1177/0883073807309250.

[9] Ewalt DH, Sheffield E, Sparagana SP, et al. Renal lesion growth in children with tuberous sclerosis complex. *J Urol.* 1998;160(1):141-145.

[10] Bader RS, Chitayat D, Kelly E, et al. Fetal rhabdomyoma: prenatal diagnosis, clinical outcome, and incidence of associated tuberous sclerosis complex. *J Pediatr.* 2003;143(5):620-624. doi:10.1067/S0022-3476(03)00494-3.

[11] Costello LC, Hartman TE, Ryu JH. High frequency of pulmonary lymphangioleiomyomatosis in women with tuberous sclerosis complex. *Mayo Clin Proc.* 2000;75(6):591-594. doi:10.4065/75.6.591.

[12] Hancock E, Tomkins S, Sampson J, et al. Lymphangioleiomyomatosis and tuberous sclerosis. *Respir Med.* 2002;96(1):7-13. doi:10.1053/rmed.2001.1206.

[13] Northrup H, Aronow ME, Bebin EM, et al. Updated International Tuberous Sclerosis Complex Diagnostic Criteria and surveillance and management recommendations. *Pediatr Neurol.* 2021;123:50-66. doi:10.1016/j.pediatrneurol.2021.07.011.

[14] Thiele EA. Managing epilepsy in tuberous sclerosis complex. *J Child Neurol.* 2004;19(9):680-686. doi:10.1177/08830738040190090801.

[15] Cotter JA. An update on the central nervous system manifestations of tuberous sclerosis complex. *Acta Neuropathol.* 2020;139(4):613-624. doi:10.1007/s00401-019-02003-1.

[16] Prather P, de Vries PJ. Behavioral and cognitive aspects of tuberous sclerosis complex. *J Child Neurol.* 2004;19(9):666-674. doi:10.1177/08830738040190090601.

[17] de Vries PJ, Whittemore VH, Leclezio L, et al. Tuberous sclerosis associated neuropsychiatric disorders (TAND) and the TAND Checklist. *Pediatr Neurol.* 2015;52(1):25-35. doi:10.1016/j.pediatrneurol.2014.10.004.

[18] Adriaensen MEAPM, Schaefer-Prokop CM, Stijnen T, et al. Prevalence of subependymal giant cell tumors in patients with tuberous sclerosis and a review of the literature. *Eur J Neurol.* 2009;16(6):691-696. doi:10.1111/j.1468-1331.2009.02567.x.

[19] Baskin HJJ. The pathogenesis and imaging of the tuberous sclerosis complex. *Pediatr Radiol.* 2008;38(9):936-952. doi:10.1007/s00247-008-0832-y.

[20] Russo C, Nastro A, Cicala D, et al. Neuroimaging in tuberous sclerosis complex. *Child's Nerv Syst.* 2020;36(10):2497-2509. doi:10.1007/s00381-020-04705-4.

[21] Rovira À, Ruiz-Falcó ML, García-Esparza E, et al. Recommendations for the radiological diagnosis and follow-up of neuropathological abnormalities associated with tuberous sclerosis complex. *J Neurooncol.* 2014;118(2):205-223. doi:10.1007/s11060-014-1429-y.

[22] Baumer FM, Peters JM, Clancy S, et al. Corpus callosum white matter diffusivity reflects cumulative neurological comorbidity in tuberous sclerosis complex. *Cereb Cortex.* 2018;28(10):3665-3672. doi:10.1093/cercor/bhx247.

[23] Arca G, Pacheco E, Alfonso I, et al. Characteristic brain magnetic resonance imaging (MRI) findings in neonates with tuberous sclerosis complex. *J Child Neurol*. 2006;21(4):280-285. doi:10.1177/08830738060210042301.

[24] Ridler K, Suckling J, Higgins N, et al. Standardized whole brain mapping of tubers and subependymal nodules in tuberous sclerosis complex. *J Child Neurol*. 2004;19(9):658-665. doi:10.1177/08830738040190090501.

[25] Kaplan J, De Domenico I, Ward DM. Chediak-Higashi syndrome. *Curr Opin Hematol*. 2008;15(1):22-29. doi:10.1097/MOH.0b013e3282f2bcce.

[26] Mizuguchi M, Takashima S. Neuropathology of tuberous sclerosis. *Brain Dev*. 2001;23(7):508-515. doi:10.1016/s0387-7604(01)00304-7.

[27] Huttenlocher PR, Heydemann PT. Fine structure of cortical tubers in tuberous sclerosis: a Golgi study. *Ann Neurol*. 1984;16(5):595-602. doi:10.1002/ana.41016 0511.

[28] Marcotte L, Aronica E, Baybis M, et al. Cytoarchitectural alterations are widespread in cerebral cortex in tuberous sclerosis complex. *Acta Neuropathol*. 2012;123(5): 685-693. doi:10.1007/s00401-012-0950-3.

[29] Hirose T, Scheithauer BW, Lopes MB, et al. Tuber and subependymal giant cell astrocytoma associated with tuberous sclerosis: an immunohistochemical, ultrastructural, and immunoelectron and microscopic study. *Acta Neuropathol*. 1995;90(4):387-399. doi:10.1007/BF00315012.

[30] Mizuguchi M. Abnormal giant cells in the cerebral lesions of tuberous sclerosis complex. *Congenit Anom (Kyoto)*. 2007;47(1):2-8. doi:10.1111/j.1741-4520.2006. 00134.x.

[31] Shepherd CW, Scheithauer BW, Gomez MR, et al. Subependymal giant cell astrocytoma: a clinical, pathological, and flow cytometric study. *Neurosurgery*. 1991;28(6):864-868.

[32] Crino PB, Trojanowski JQ, Dichter MA, et al. Embryonic neuronal markers in tuberous sclerosis: single-cell molecular pathology. *Proc Natl Acad Sci U S A*. 1996;93(24):14152-14157. doi:10.1073/pnas.93.24.14152.

[33] Jozwiak J, Jozwiak S, Skopinski P. Immunohistochemical and microscopic studies on giant cells in tuberous sclerosis. *Histol Histopathol*. 2005;20(4):1321-1326. doi:10.14670/HH-20.1321.

[34] Hewer E, Vajtai I. Consistent nuclear expression of thyroid transcription factor 1 in subependymal giant cell astrocytomas suggests lineage-restricted histogenesis. *Clin Neuropathol*. 2015;34(3):128-131. doi:10.5414/NP300818.

[35] Bielle F, Villa C, Giry M, et al. Chordoid gliomas of the third ventricle share TTF-1 expression with organum vasculosum of the lamina terminalis. *Am J Surg Pathol*. 2015;39(7):948-956. doi:10.1097/PAS.0000000000000421.

[36] Solomon DA, Perry A. Familial tumor syndromes. In: *Practical Surgical Neuropathology: A Diagnostic Approach*. 2nd ed. Philadelphia: Elsevier; 2018: 505-545.

[37] Brat DJ, Perry A. Nondiffuse astrocytoma variants. In: *Practical Surgical Neuropathology: A Diagnostic Approach*. 2nd ed. Philadelphia; 2018:125-143.

[38] Curatolo P, Specchio N, Aronica E. Advances in the genetics and neuropathology of tuberous sclerosis complex: edging closer to targeted therapy. *Lancet Neurol.* 2022;21(9):843-856. doi:10.1016/S1474-4422(22)00213-7.

[39] Curatolo P, Nabbout R, Lagae L, et al. Management of epilepsy associated with tuberous sclerosis complex: Updated clinical recommendations. *Eur J Paediatr Neurol EJPN Off J Eur Paediatr Neurol Soc.* 2018;22(5):738-748. doi:10.1016/j.ejpn.2018.05.006.

[40] Kilincaslan A, Kok BE, Tekturk P, et al. Beneficial effects of everolimus on autism and attention-deficit/hyperactivity disorder symptoms in a group of patients with tuberous sclerosis complex. *J Child Adolesc Psychopharmacol.* 2017;27(4):383-388. doi:10.1089/cap.2016.0100.

[41] Ebrahimi-Fakhari D, Franz DN. Pharmacological treatment strategies for subependymal giant cell astrocytoma (SEGA). *Expert Opin Pharmacother.* 2020; 21(11): 1329-1336. doi:10.1080/14656566.2020.1751124.

[42] Shepherd CW, Gomez MR, Lie JT, et al. Causes of death in patients with tuberous sclerosis. *Mayo Clin Proc.* 1991;66(8):792-796. doi:10.1016/s0025-6196(12)61196-3.

[43] Parthasarathy S, Mahalingam R, Melchiorre J, et al. Mortality in tuberous sclerosis complex. *Epilepsy Behav.* 2021;121(Pt A):108032. doi:10.1016/j.yebeh.2021.108032.

[44] Amin S, Lux A, Calder N, Laugharne M, et al. Causes of mortality in individuals with tuberous sclerosis complex. *Dev Med Child Neurol.* 2017;59(6):612-617. doi:10.1111/dmcn.13352.

Chapter 3

Neuropathologic Features of von Hippel-Lindau Syndrome

Richard A. Prayson*[,1], MD, MEd and Elizabeth E. O'Toole[2], MD

[1] Department of Anatomic Pathology, Cleveland Clinic, OH, USA
[2] MetroHealth Medical Center, Cleveland, OH, USA

Abstract

von Hippel-Lindau syndrome is an autosomal dominant disorder due to germline variants of the VHL tumor suppressor gene situated on chromosome 3p25.3. Manifestation of the disease outside the central nervous system includes pancreatic cysts and islet cell tumors, renal cysts and renal cell carcinomas, papillary cystadenomas of the epididymis and uterine broad ligament, pheochromocytomas, endolymphatic sac tumors and retinal hemangioblastomas.

Within the central nervous system, patients present with hemangioblastomas, either solitary or multiple. The majority of hemangioblastomas of the central nervous system arise in the cerebellum and present with symptoms of increased intracranial pressure, hemorrhage, dysmetria, ataxia and secondary polycythemia vera due to erythropoietin production.

The tumor presents as a circumscribed lesion (cystic mass with enhancing mural nodule configuration on imaging) and is marked by a proliferation of epithelioid clear to foamy stromal cells with intermixed capillary vessels. The tumors are considered low grade, World Health Organization grade 1 neoplasms.

---

* Corresponding Author's Email: praysor@ccf.org.

In: Central Nervous System Pathologies in Hereditary Tumor Syndromes
Editor: Richard A. Prayson
ISBN: 979-8-88697-620-5

Immunostaining with inhibin antibody allows for distinction from a metastatic renal cell carcinoma, which is the main differential diagnostic consideration in the setting of von Hippel-Lindau syndrome. Tumors have been treated with surgery, vascular embolization and stereotactic radiosurgery.

This chapter will review the features of von Hippel-Lindau syndrome with a focus on hemangioblastoma, the main neuropathologic finding of the syndrome.

Introduction

von Hippel-Lindau syndrome was named after Eugene von Hippel and Arvid Lindau. In 1904, von Hippel, a German ophthalmologist, first described the retinal lesion associated with the syndrome, which he termed retinal angiomatosis [1]. In 1926, the Swedish pathologist, Lindau, described a morphologically identical tumor in the cerebellum [2]. Lindau recognized the association of the cerebellar and retinal lesions and their hereditary predilection. By the mid-1930s, the two names were associated with the name of the syndrome.

This chapter will review the clinical and genetic features of von Hippel-Lindau syndrome and discuss in detail the major neuropathologic finding in the syndrome, the hemangioblastoma.

Genetics of von Hippel-Lindau Syndrome

von Hippel-Lindau syndrome is an autosomal dominant condition with a penetrance estimated at 90% and with about 20% of patients presenting as sporadic cases with no known family history [3, 4]. The VHL gene is a tumor suppressor gene which is situated on the short arm of chromosome 3 (3p25) and includes 3 highly conserved exons [4]. The gene codes for a protein involved in cellular signalling pathways. There are two isoforms of the VHL protein, a 30-kDa protein and a 19-kDa isoform which results from internal translational initiation [5, 6]. Both isoforms appear to be important for the tumor suppressor effects of the VHL gene. Frameshifts, missense mutations and inactivating gene deletions of the VHL gene have been seen in the syndrome.

Similar to the Knudson's two-hit hypothesis, affected individuals have germline mutations of the gene present in all cell types of the body and cell types with a somatic inactivation of the normal allele are prone to develop tumors [6, 7]. The pVHL multiprotein complex regulates a variety of hypoxia-inducible factor transcripts. High levels of this complex can stimulate angiogenic growth factors, such as vascular endothelial growth factor (VEGF) and platelet-derived growth factor B (PDGF-B), which may explain the hypervascularity seen in some von Hippel-Lindau associated lesions such as hemangioblastoma [8, 9].

There have been over 300 germline mutations of the VHL gene that have been described in families with von Hippel-Lindau syndrome [4]. A classification schema has been constructed based on specific genotype-phenotype correlations in affected families [6, 10, 11]. The schema consists of four subtypes:

1) *Type 1 (decreased risk for pheochromocytoma)* – associated with retinal and central nervous system hemangioblastomas, renal cell carcinoma, pancreatic cysts and neuroendocrine tumors and associated with truncating or missense mutations;
2) *Type 2A (increased risk for pheochromocytoma and low risk of renal cell carcinoma)* – associated with pheochromocytoma, retinal hemangioblastoma and central nervous system hemangioblastoma and associated with missense mutations;
3) *Type 2B (increased risk for pheochromocytoma and high risk for renal cell carcinoma)* – associated with pheochromocytoma, renal cell carcinoma, retinal hemangioblastoma, central nervous system hemangioblastoma, pancreatic cysts and neuroendocrine tumors;
4) *Type 2C* –associated with pheochromocytomas only.

The picture is complicated by reports of homozygous missense VHL gene mutations being associated with congenital polycythemia syndromes without evidence of von Hippel-Lindau disease [12, 13].

For example, patients with so-called Chuvash polycythemia homozygous for VHL 598 C > T mutation present with polycythemia, pulmonary hypertension, varicose veins, vertebral hemangiomas and elevated vascular endothelial growth factor (VEGF) levels; they do not appear to be at increased risk of developing hemangioblastomas or renal cell carcinomas [13].

General Clinical Features

There are a variety of extra-central nervous system findings that can occur in patients with von Hippel Lindau syndrome. Retinal angiomatosis (hemangioblastomas) occur in about half of all von Hippel-Lindau patients and are frequently bilateral [3, 14]. Larger size tumors are associated with exudation, retinal traction or hemorrhage, which can compromise vision. Clinical management is focused on the early detection of asymptomatic lesions in order to prevent complications. Laser photocoagulation or cryotherapy can be used to treat retinal tumors; antiangiogenic agents have also been employed as a treatment option in some patients [10, 15, 16].

Renal cysts and renal cell carcinomas are often multifocal and bilateral in patients with von Hippel Lindau syndrome. The lifetime risk of developing renal cell carcinoma in some of the subtypes (Types 1 and 2A) is about 70% [17, 18]. The mean age at the time of diagnosis for renal cell carcinomas is about 40 years, although asymptomatic tumors may be detected much earlier in patients under surveillance. Clinical findings include a renal mass with hematuria or flank pain [6, 10, 19]. Histologic examination of kidneys from von Hippel-Lindau individuals typically show multiple microscopic tumor foci in the kidneys [20]. Patients with renal cysts often likewise have multiple cysts, which in most cases do not interfere with renal function. Some of these cysts may demonstrate a dysplastic epithelial lining or carcinoma in situ microscopically. Regular surveillance and a nephron-sparing approach is the usual strategy in managing these patients with a subset of cases requiring more extensive surgery [20]. About 25% of von Hippel-Lindau patients with larger renal cell carcinomas (>3cm) are more likely to develop metastatic disease [21].

About 20% of von Hippel-Lindau patients develop pheochromocytomas [6]. The mean age of diagnosis of pheochromocytoma in this clinical setting is about 30 years [10]. Only rare cases are malignant in this setting. The tumors present often with symptoms related to excessive norepinephrine production including tachycardia, hypertension, headaches, palpitation, sweating nausea and pallor [7, 22]. Surgical resection of pheochromocytomas with pharmacologic alpha-adrenergic and beta-adrenergic blockade is typically employed in treatment.

Pancreatic abnormalities are seen in 35-70% of von Hippel-Lindau patients [6]. Pancreatic tumors, which typically are solid non-secretory islet cell tumors, occur in about 5-10% of cases [10]. The neuroendocrine tumors can become malignant in 8% of patients [19]. Benign pancreatic cysts usually do not require surgical resection unless there are obstructive symptoms due to the cysts. Tumors, especially those presumed to be malignant, require surgical resection.

Epididymal and broad ligament cystadenomas have also been noted with increased frequency in von Hippel-Lindau patients. Epididymal lesions may be seen in anywhere from 25-60% of male patients [6]. These lesions are benign and are often asymptomatic.

Endolymphatic sac tumors develop in about 2-11% of von Hippel-Lindau patients within the vestibular aqueduct [4, 23]. Patients present with ear fullness, hearing loss or disequilibrium [6]. Larger lesions can involve the facial nerve and cause facial paresis [19, 23]. They are benign tumors which may be locally aggressive but do not typically metastasize; surgical excision is the typical approach to treatment.

Neurologic Clinical Features

Hemangioblastoma represents the primary central nervous system pathology encountered in von Hippel-Lindau syndrome. About three quarters of hemangioblastomas arising in this setting do so in the infratentorial region, mostly involving the cerebellum; the remaining quarter of cases may arise in the spinal cord, brainstem and lumbosacral nerve roots. Multifocal hemangioblastomas are more common in this clinical setting. Tumors arising in this setting also tend to present at a younger age than spontaneous hemangioblastomas.

Patients may present with signs and symptoms related to compression of adjacent structures or related to hydrocephalus [10]. Dysmetria and ataxia may also be encountered. About 75% of tumors are partially cystic and cyst fluid may be amber in color [3]. Tumors with an associated cyst tend to become symptomatic sooner than those that do not [24]. Due to erythropoietin production, a subset of hemangioblastomas are associated with secondary polycythemia [25]. Hemangioblastoma are hypervascular tumors on angiography and contrast enhancing, as such, on other imaging modalities [4, 7, 10, 19]. Their common solid and cystic appearance is also often evident on imaging.

Neuropathologic Findings

Hemangioblastomas are usually well-circumscribed, pseudoencapsulated tumors that may be entirely solid or more commonly have a cystic component grossly [24]. Tumors may appear yellow to red in coloration.

Histologically, the tumor is marked by a stromal cell component comprised of epithelioid cells with abundant clear to foamy cytoplasm intermixed with a prominent capillary vasculature (Figure 1). Nuclear pleomorphism may be evident in some tumors but has no known clinical significance (Figure 2).

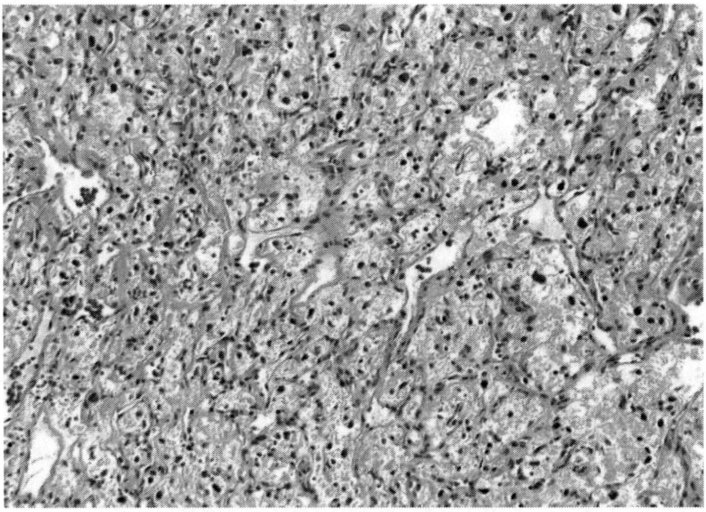

Figure 1. Hemangioblastoma is marked by a proliferation of stromal cells with clear cytoplasm and a prominent intermixed vasculature (hematoxylin and eosin, original magnification 200X).

In some tumors or areas of tumor, the stromal cell component may predominate and in others, the vascular component may appear prevalent (Figure 3). In many tumors, cysts, ranging in size from small microscopic ones to large, grossly evident ones, are present (Figure 4). Mitotic figures are relatively infrequent. The adjacent tissue is commonly marked by piloid gliosis with reactive astrocytes and Rosenthal fibers. Areas of hemorrhage and hemosiderin deposition may be seen.

The tumors generally show low rates of cell proliferation, as evidenced on Ki-67 or MIB-1 immunostaining. The stromal cells do not stain with endothelial-associated immunomarkers, such as CD34, CD31, ERG and von Willebrand factor [26]. The stromal cells may stain with antibodies to inhibin, D2-40 and brachyury (Figure 5) [27, 28].

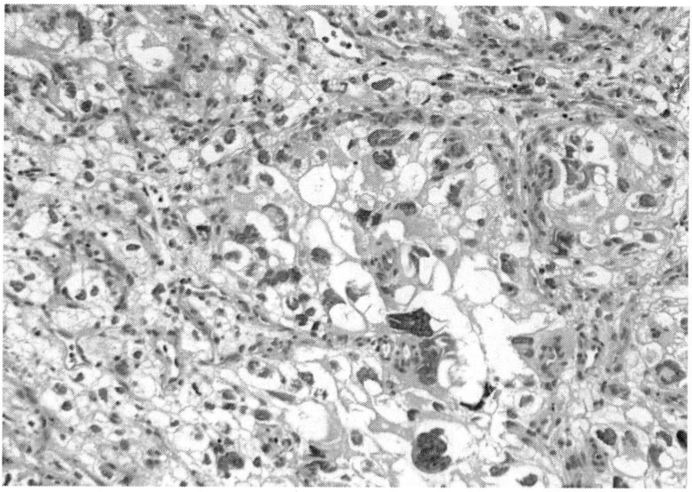

Figure 2. Nuclear pleomorphism of stromal cells may be seen in some hemangioblastomas (hematoxylin and eosin, original magnification 200X).

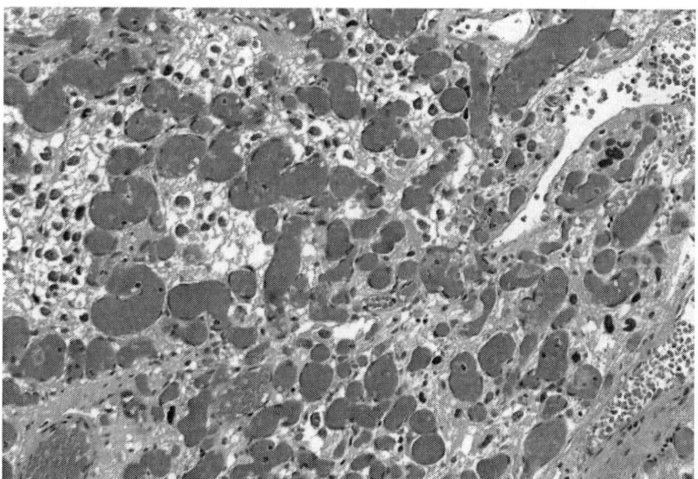

Figure 3. In some hemangioblastomas, the vasculature may be quite prominent (hematoxylin and eosin, original magnification 200X).

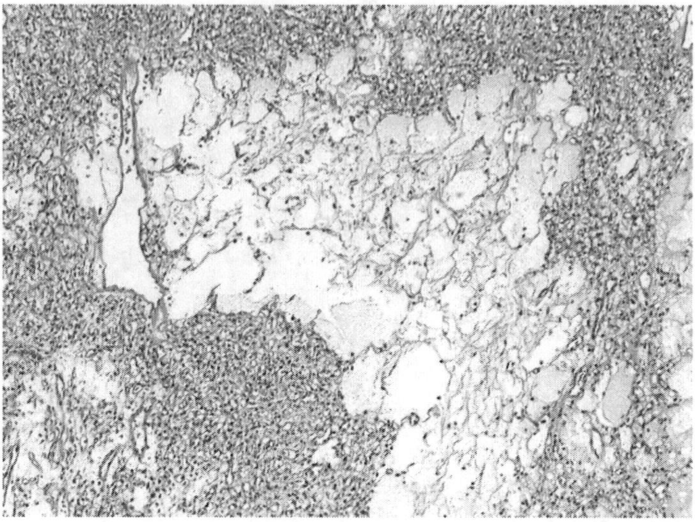

Figure 4. Microcystic areas or sometimes grossly evident cysts may be present in hemangioblastoma (hematoxylin and eosin, original magnification 100X).

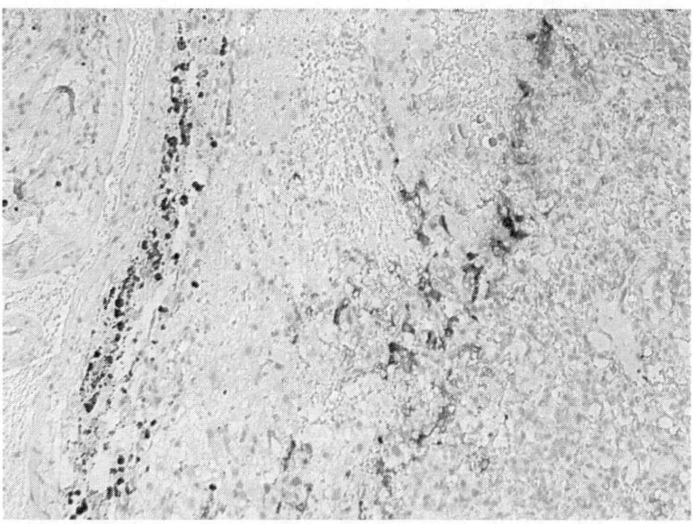

Figure 5. Focal positive staining with antibody to inhibin is seen in this hemangioblastoma. Hemosiderin pigment is also seen in this tumor on the left (original magnification 200).

Probably the most significant differential diagnostic consideration with hemangioblastoma in the setting of von Hippel-Lindau disease is a metastatic clear cell renal cell carcinoma. The metastasis similarly consists of epithelioid cells with clear cytoplasm (Figure 6). The metastases often have a prominent vascularity as well. Immunostains can be useful in making the distinction. In addition to the immunomarkers mentioned previously that characteristically stain hemangioblastomas, immunomarkers that characteristically stain renal cell carcinoma, such as epithelial membrane antigen (EMA), RCC, CD10 and PAX 8 can be useful in making the distinction. Occasionally, hemangioblastoma may resemble an angiomatous meningioma. Meningiomas do not stain with inhibin antibody and often stain with EMA, somatostatin receptor 2a (SSTR2a) and progesterone receptor antibody.

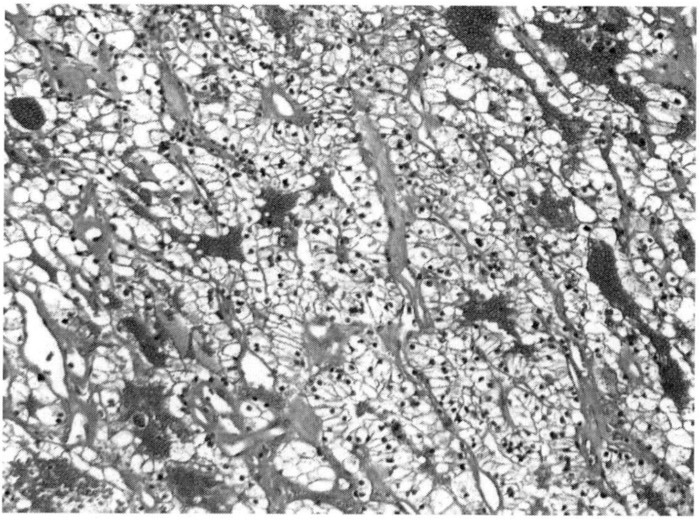

Figure 6. Patients with non von Hippel Lindau syndrome may also develop renal cell carcinomas which can metastasize to the cerebellum (seen in this image) and resemble hemangioblastoma (hematoxylin and eosin, original magnification 200X).

Treatment and Prognosis

Hemangioblastomas are low grade, World Health Organization (WHO) grade 1 tumors, and generally have an excellent prognosis following gross total surgical excision. Tumors that are incompletely excised, may persist [29]. There is no routine role for radiotherapy or chemotherapy.

Conclusion

von Hippel-Lindau syndrome is an autosomal dominant disorder associated with germline alterations of the VHL tumor suppressor gene located on chromosome 3p. Within the central nervous system, pathologies that may be encountered include hemangioblastomas, WHO grade 1 tumors, or metastases from renal cell carcinomas. Management and treatment of these conditions is similar to those cases that arise outside this clinical setting.

References

[1] Shebata BM, Stockwell CA, Castellano-Sanchez AA, et al. Von Hippel-Lindau (VHL) disease: an update on the clinico-pathologic and genetic aspects. *Adv Anat Pathol.* 2008; 15: 165-171.

[2] Lindau A. Studien uber Kleinhirncysten. Bau. Pathogeneses and Beziehungen zur Angiomatosisi retinae [*Pathogenesis and relation to retinal angiomatosis*]. *Acta Pathol Microbiol Scand.* 1926; Suppl 1.1-128.

[3] Neumann HPH, Lips CJM, Hsia YE, et al. Von Hippel-Lindau syndrome. *Brain Pathol.* 1995; 5: 181-193.

[4] Solomon DA, Perry A. Familial tumor syndromes. In: *Practical Surgical Neuropathology.* 2nd Edition. Perry A and Brat DJ, editors. Elsevier. Philadelphia, PA 2018. pp. 520-524.

[5] Iliopoulos O, Ohh M, Kaelin Jr WG. pVHL19 is a biologically active product of the von Hippel-Lindau gene arising from internal translation initiation. *Proc Natl Acad Sci USA.* 1998; 95: 11661-11666.

[6] Varshney N, Kebede AA, Owusu-Dapaah H, et al. A review of von Hippel-Lindau syndrome. *J Kidney Cancer and VHL.* 2017; 4(3): 20-29.

[7] Lonser RR, Glenn GM, Walther M, et al. Von Hippel-Lindau disease. *Lancet.* 2003; 361(9374): 2059-2067.

[8] Singh AD, Shields CL, Shields JA, et al. Von Hippel-Lindau disease. *Surv Ophthalmol.* 2001; 46(2): 117-142.

[9] Richard S, Graff J, Lindau J, et al. Von Hippel-Lindau disease. *Lancet.* 2004; 363(9416): 1231-1234.

[10] Maher ER, Neuman HP, Richard S. Von Hippel-Lindau disease: A clinical and scientific review. *Eur J Hum Genet.* 2011; 19(6): 617-623.

[11] Wind JJ, Lonser RR. Management of von Hippel-Lindau disease-associated CNS lesions. *Expert Rev Neurother.* 2011; 11(10): 1433.

[12] Ang SO, Chen H, Hirota K, et al. Disruption of oxygen homeostasis underlies congenital Chuvash polycythemia. *Nat Genet.* 2002; 32: 614-621.

[13] Gordeuk VR, Sergueeva AI, Miasnikova GY, et al. Congenital disorder of oxygen-sensing: association of the homozygous Chuvash polycythemia VHL mutation with

thrombosis and vascular abnormalities but not tumors. *Blood.* 2004; 103: 3924-3932.

[14] Lamiell JM, Salazar FG, Hsia YE. Von Hippel-Lindau disease affecting 43 members of a single kindred. *Medicine.* 1989; 68: 1-29.

[15] Aiello LP, George DJ, Cahill T, et al. Rapid and durable recovery of visual function in a patient with von Hippel Lindau syndrome after systemic therapy with vascular endothelial growth factor receptor inhibitor SU5416. *Ophthalmol.* 2002; 109: 1745-1751.

[16] Girmens JF, Erginay A, Massin P, et al. Treatment of von Hippel-Lindau retinal hemangioblastoma by the vascular endothelial growth factor receptor inhibitor SU5416 is more effective for associated macular edema than for haemangioblastomas. *Am J Ophthalmol.* 2003; 136: 194-196.

[17] Maher ER, Yates JRW, Harries R, et al. Clinical features and natural history of von Hippel-Lindau disease. *Quart J Med.* 1990; 77: 1151-1163.

[18] Ong KR, Woodward ER, Killick P, et al. Genotype-phenotype correlations in von Hippel-Lindau disease. *Hum Mut.* 2007; 28: 143-149.

[19] Chittiboina P, Lonser RR. Von Hippel-Lindau disease. *Handb Clin Neurol.* 2015; 132: 139-156.

[20] Mandriota SJ, Turner KJ., Davies DR, et al. HIF activation identifies early lesions in VHL kidneys: evidence for site-specific tumor suppressor function in the nephron. *Cancer Cell.* 2002; 1: 459-468.

[21] Waither MM, Choyke PL, Glenn G, et al. Renal cancer in families with hereditary renal cancer: Prospective analysis of a tumor size threshold for renal parenchymal sparing surgery. *J Urol.* 1999; 161: 1475-1479.

[22] Cassol C, Mete O. Endocrine manifestations of von Hippel-Lindau disease. *Arch Pathol Lab Med.* 2015; 139(2): 263-268.

[23] Shanbhogue KP, Hoch M, Fatterpaker G, et al. Von Hippel-Lindau disease: Review of genetics and imaging. *Radiol Clin North Am.* 2016; 54(3): 409-422.

[24] Wanebo JE, Lonser RR, Glenn GM, et al. The natural history of central nervous system hemangioblastoma in patients with von Hippel-Lindau disease. *J Neurosurg.* 2003; 98: 82-94.

[25] Gläsker, Krüger MT, Klinger JH, et al. Hemangioblastomas and neurogenic polyglobulia. *Neurosurgery.* 2013; 72(6): 930-935.

[26] Böhling T, Mäenpää A, Timonen T, et al. Different expression of adhesion molecules on stromal cells and endothelial cells of capillary hemangioblastoma. *Acta Neuropathol.* 1996; 92(5): 461-466.

[27] Hoang MP, Amirkhan RH. Inhibin alpha distinguishes hemangioblastoma from clear cell renal cell carcinoma. *Am J Surg Pathol.* 2003; 27(8): 1152-1156.

[28] Roy S, Chu A, Trojanowski JQ, et al. D2-40, a novel monoclonal antibody against the M2A antigen as a marker to distinguish hemangioblastomas from renal cell carcinomas. *Acta Neuropathol.* 2005; 109(5): 497-502.

[29] Doyle LA, Fletcher CD. Peripheral hemangioblastoma: clinicopathologic characterization in a series of 22 cases. *Am J Surg Pathol.* 2014; 38(1): 119-127.

Chapter 4

Sturge-Weber Syndrome: Central Nervous System Pathology

Richard A. Prayson*, MD, MEd
Department of Anatomic Pathology, Cleveland Clinic, Cleveland, Ohio, USA

Abstract

Sturge-Weber syndrome or encephalofacial angiomatosis is a disorder marked by coexistence of cutaneous and central nervous system lesions. Classically, patients have a nevus flammeus or port-wine stain, typically in the trigeminal nerve distribution, combined with leptomeningeal angiomatosis. The brain parenchyma underlying the leptomeningeal angiomatosis is marked by cortical atrophy due to loss of neurons and microcalcifications, accounting for a characteristic radiographic appearance. Occasionally, other malformative lesions of the central nervous system including angiomatous and meningothelial proliferation of the choroid plexus, polymicrogyria and heterotopias may be seen. The disorder is due to somatic activating mutations in the GNAQ gene located on chromosome 9q21.2.

This chapter will review the clinicopathologic features of this disorder, with a primary focus on the central nervous system associated pathology.

Introduction

The neurocutaneous disorder known as Sturge-Weber syndrome was first described by William Allen Sturge in 1879 in a 6 ½-year-old girl [1, 2]. The

* Corresponding Author's Email: praysor@ccf.org.

In: Central Nervous System Pathologies in Hereditary Tumor Syndromes
Editor: Richard A. Prayson
ISBN: 979-8-88697-620-5

patient presented with twitching on the left side of her body at age 6 months. Over time, the twitching spread to the other side of the body and was accompanied by loss of consciousness. She had a "mother's mark" on the right side of the head and face. The right eye was larger and appeared to be affected by the vascular malformation. Sturge called the skin lesion a "port-wine" stain. It was not until 1901 that Siegfried Kalischer provided pathologic proof that the epilepsy and brain abnormality was somehow related to the cutaneous lesion [3]. In 1922, Parkes Weber first described the calcifications on x-ray imaging: "...a more or less calcified and apparently 'festooned' lesion on the surface of the left cerebral hemisphere..." [4].

This chapter will review the clinical and pathologic features of Sturge-Weber syndrome, focusing on the neuropathologic findings that have been described in this syndrome.

Genetics of Sturge-Weber Syndrome

In 2013, Shirley and colleagues identified a nonsynonymous single-nucleotide variant (c.548G->A, p.Arg183GLN) in GNAQ in samples from patients affected with Sturge-Weber syndrome [5]. The GNAQ gene is located on chromosome 9q21 [6]. The mutation in GNAQ increases activity in pathways transmitting signals from a subset of G protein coupled receptors (GCPR).

General Clinical Features

Port-wine stains are cutaneous venous capillary malformations that occur in about 3 out of every 1,000 newborns, usually involving the head and neck region of the body [7-9]. In Sturge-Weber, the port-wine stain classically affects the skin in the distribution of the ophthalmic branch of the trigeminal nerve. Similar lesions may arise in the leptomeninges and the eye [5]. The disorder has no definite gender predilection. It occurs in about 1 in 20,000 to 1 in 50,000 live births [7]. If a child is born with a port-wine stain on the face, that child has approximately a 6% chance of having Sturge-Weber syndrome [8] with the risk increasing to 26% when the port-wine stain is located in the distribution of the ophthalmic branch of the trigeminal nerve [9].

Many patients with a port-wine stain have increased ocular pressure or glaucoma in the eye adjacent to the birthmark [6]. Glaucoma is the most common ophthalmic complication of Surge-Weber syndrome, seen in between 30-70% of cases [10, 11]. The presentation of glaucoma in affected individuals appears to be bimodal with about 60% of patients developing it in infancy and the remaining patients later in the course of the disease [12].

Diagnosis of Sturge-Weber syndrome is based on having two out of three diagnostic criteria: facial port-wine stain, increased ocular pressure and leptomeningeal angiomatosis [6].

Neurologic Clinical Features

Clinically, patients with Sturge-Weber syndrome suffer from a variety of neurologic problems including epilepsy, learning disabilities, attention-deficit hyperactivity disorder, behavioral disturbances, stroke-like episodes, hemiparesis and migraine headaches [12]. Most patients who have brain involvement will develop seizure activity during infancy. Overall, 75-90% of children with Sturge-Weber will develop epilepsy [12]. In a subset of patients, a fever or infection precipitates the onset of the seizures. The seizures are thought to be due to cortical damage caused by hypoxia and circulatory stasis related to the overlying leptomeningeal lesion.

One study has suggested that patients who start having seizures before the age of two years or whose seizures are pharmacoresistent are more likely to suffer from mental retardation [10]. Ultimately, about half or slightly more than half of patients will have developmental delay or mental retardation. Headaches may be seen in 30-45% of Sturge-Weber patients [12]. The headaches may be related to abnormalities of the vasculature and to neuronal hyperexcitability which can result in alterations in cortical perfusion and oxygenation [13, 14]. Stroke-like episodes or transient focal deficits manifesting most commonly as episodes of hemiparesis or visual field defects are also not uncommonly seen. Because of the variety of neurologic manifestations and sequelae, the psychosocial aspects related to the physical and social disabilities of the disease also need to be considered in managing patients with Sturge-Weber syndrome [12].

Imaging Findings

Plain skull x-ray imaging studies highlight the tram-track or tram-line calcifications that often develop over tie in the cortex underlying the leptomeningeal vascular proliferation; this finding is often evident later in the disease course [12]. Angiography studies, which are currently not employed since the advent of magnetic resonance imaging (MRI), showed an overall paucity of superficial cortical veins, nonfilling of the dural sinuses and a tortuous course of veins toward the vein of Galen.

MRI studies highlight prominent leptomeningeal enhancement (on T1-weighted, gadolinium-enhanced studies). The calcifications seen in the underlying cortex are better visualized on computed tomographic (CT) studies. Ipsilateral atrophy is also common in affected patients, marked by widening of the subarachnoid space and ventriculomegaly. White matter alterations may also be evident and are thought to be secondary to the chronic ischemic damage in the overlying cortex. Areas of hypoperfusion can be seen on single-photon emission computed tomographic studies [12]. Positron emission tomography (PET) studies have demonstrated areas of hypometabolism in the cortex which have been correlated with seizures [15].

Neuropathologic Findings

The most common pathology seen in the central nervous system in Sturge-Weber is the presence of focal meningeal angiomatosis, marked by a proliferation of thin-walled venous and capillary blood vessels (Figure 1). The vessels appear benign and sometimes tortuous (Figure 2). The underlying cortex is marked by loss of neurons, which may result in grossly or microscopically evident atrophy, and gliosis. Microcalcifications are often present in many cases in the affected cortex and can be sometimes accompanied by focal hemosiderin deposition (Figure 3). Other pathologies that have been described in this setting have included angiomatosis in the choroid plexus and meningothelial hyperplasia. Associated malformations have included heterotopias and polymicrogyria in select cases [16]. A rare case of coexistent pleomorphic xanthoastrocytoma has been described, presenting in an 11-year-old male who presented with a long history of epilepsy and gradually progressive bilateral motor weakness [17].

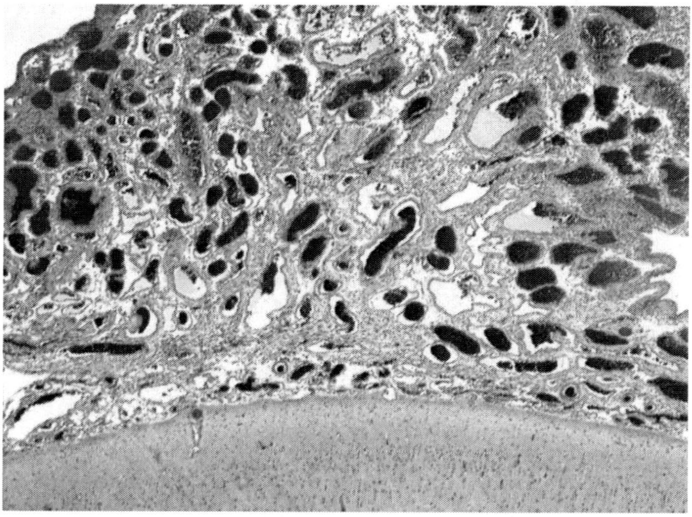

Figure 1. Sturge Weber is marked by a proliferation of meningeal blood vessels (top) (hematoxylin and eosin, original magnification 50X).

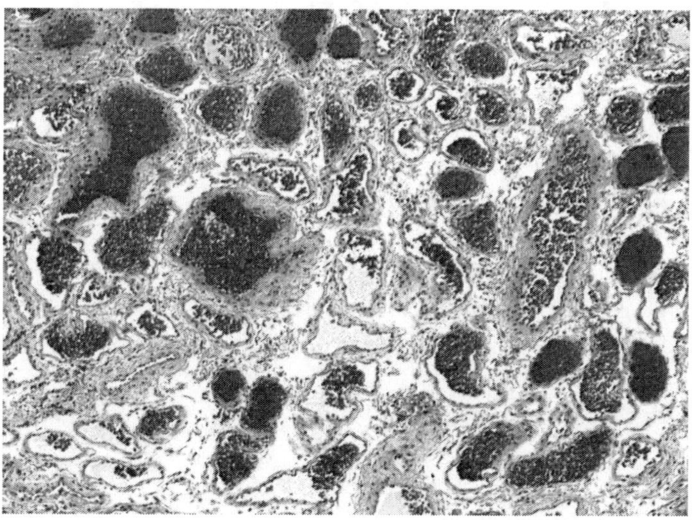

Figure 2. The meningeal vascular proliferation is marked by benign appearing vessels, mostly veins and capillaries with an occasional intermixed artery (hematoxylin and eosin, original magnification 100X).

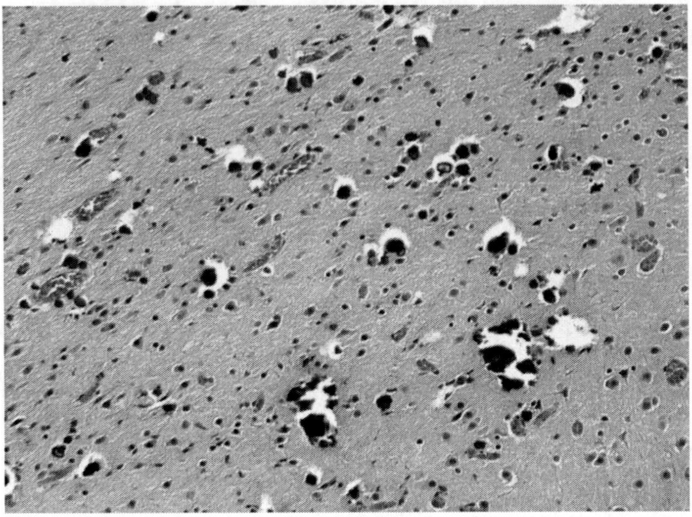

Figure 3. The cortex underlying the meningeal vascular proliferation is marked by calcifications, seen here, and loss of neurons (hematoxylin and eosin, original magnification 200X).

Special stains and immunostains are generally not required to make a pathologic diagnosis. A differential diagnostic consideration may include angiomatous meningioma for the leptomeningeal vascular proliferation. Most meningiomas would be marked by a more prominent meningothelial cell component, which could be highlighted on somatostatin receptor 2a (SSTR2a), epithelial membrane antigen (EMA) or progesterone receptor (PR) immunostains if needed.

Rare cases of meningioma arising in the setting of Sturge-Weber have been described: one case of an intraventricular angiomatous meningioma arising in a 3-year-old boy [18] and the other patient being a 30-year-old female with a right cerebellar mass [19].

Treatment and Prognosis

Treatment of patients with Sturge-Weber requires constant monitoring for the development of seizures glaucoma and other neurologic symptoms. Medical management of symptoms can be employed but at times, surgical intervention is necessary. In patients who have pharmacoresistent seizures, surgical intervention may be successful in diminishing or alleviating the epilepsy and may slow down further cognitive deterioration [20, 21].

The prognosis of patients with Sturge-Weber varies considerably. Patients with more extensive brain involvement (bilateral disease or hemispheral disease) tend to be at risk for the greatest complications but that is not always the case with this group. Conversely, a subset of patients who appear to have relatively little brain involvement can have an aggressive clinical course.

Conclusion

Sturge-Weber syndrome is a rare disorder caused by somatic activating mutations of the GNAQ gene situated on chromosome 9q. Neuropathologic features that may be encountered in the setting of Sturge Weber syndrome include most commonly leptomeningeal angiomatosis, often accompanied by underlying cortical neuron loss, microcalcifications and gliosis. Less frequently, meningothelial or angiomatous proliferations of the choroid plexus, polymicrogyria and heterotopias may be seen.

References

[1] Sturge W A. A case of partial epilepsy, apparently due to a lesion of one of the vasomotor centres of the brain. *Trans. Clin. Soc. Lond.* 1879; 12:162.

[2] Pearce J M S. Sturge-Weber syndrome (encephalotrigeminal or leptomeningeal angiomatosis). *J. Neurol. Neurosurg. Psychiatry.* 2006; 77(11): 1291-1292.

[3] Kalischer S. Ein Fall von Telangiektasie (Angiom) des Gesichts und der weichen Hirnhaute [*A case of telangiectasia (angioma) of the face and soft meninges*]. *Arch. Psychiatr. Nervenkrankheiten Berl.* 1901; 34: 171-180.

[4] Weber F P. Right-sides hemi-hypertrophy resulting from right-sided congenital spastic hemiplegia with a morbid condition of the left side of the brain revealed by radiograms. *J. Neurol. Psychopathol. (Lond).* 1922; 3: 134-139.

[5] Shirley M D, Tang H, Gallione C J, et al. Sturge-Weber syndrome and port-wine stains caused by somatic mutation in GNAQ. *N. Engl. J. Med.* 2013; 368(21): 1971-1979.

[6] Bachur CD, Comi AM. Sturge-Weber syndrome. *Curr. Treat. Options Neurol.* 2013: 15(5): 607-617.

[7] Comi A M. Update on Sturge-Weber syndrome: diagnosis, treatment, quantitative measures, and controversies. *Lymphat. Res. Biol.* 2007; 5: 257-264.

[8] Piram M, Lorette G, Sirinelli D, et al. A Sturge-Weber syndrome in patients with facial port-wine stain. *Pediatr. Dermatol.* 2021; 29: 32-37.

[9] Ch'ng S, Tan ST. Facial port-wine stains – clinical stratification and risks of neuro-ocular involvement. *J. Plast. Reconstr. Aesthet. Surg.* 2008; 61: 889-893.

[10] Sujansky E, Conradi S. Outcome of Sturge-Weber syndrome in 52 adults. *Am. J. Med. Genet.* 1995; 57: 35-45.

[11] Roach E S. Congenital cutaneovascular disorders. In: Bogouslavsky J, Caplan L R, editors. *Stroke Syndromes*. London: Cambridge University Press. 1995; 481-490.

[12] Thomas-Sohl K A, Vaslow D F, Maria B L. Sturge-Weber syndrome: A review. *Pediatr. Neurol.* 2004; 30: 303-310.

[13] Lauritzen M. Pathophysiology of the migraine aura: The spreading depression theory. *Brain.* 1994; 117 (pt 1): 199-210.

[14] Kaube H, Keay K A, Hoskin K L, et al. Expression of C-Fos-like immunoreactivity in the caudal medulla and upper cervical spinal cord following stimulation of the superior sagittal sinus in the cat. *Brain Res.* 1993; 629: 95-102.

[15] Lee J S, Asano E, Muzik O, et al. Sturge-Weber syndrome: Correlation between clinical course and FDG PET findings. *Neurology.* 2001; 57: 189-195.

[16] Solomon D A, Perry A. Familial tumor syndromes. In: *Perry A, Brat DJ, editors. Practical Surgical Neuropathology. A Diagnostic Approach*. Philadelphia. Elsevier. 2018; 540.

[17] Kilickesmez O, Sanal H T, Haholu A, et al. Coexistence of pleomorphic xanthoastrocytoma with Sturge Weber syndrome: MRI features. *Pediatr. Radiol.* 2005; 35: 910-913.

[18] Ahmed Z, Prayson R A. Angiomatous meningioma in Sturge-Weber syndrome. *J. Clin. Neurosci.* 2015; 22(6): 1066-1068.

[19] Gökalp H Z, Ozkal F, Erdogan A, et al. A giant meningioma of the fourth ventricle associated with Sturge-Weber disease. *Acta Neurochirugica (Wein).* 1981; 57: 115-120.

[20] Kramer U, Kahana E, Shorer Z, et al. Outcome of infants with unilateral Sturge-Weber syndrome and early onset seizures. *Dev. Med. Child Neurol.* 2000; 42: 756-759.

[21] Prayson R A. Clinicopathological findings in patients who have undergone epilepsy surgery in the first year of life. *Pathol. Int.* 2000; 50: 620-625.

Chapter 5

Neuropathologic Features of Cowden Disease

Richard A. Prayson[*,1], MD, MEd
and Brigid E. Prayson[2]
[1] Department of Anatomic Pathology, Cleveland Clinic, Cleveland, Ohio, USA
[2] Allegheny Health Network, Pittsburgh, PA

Abstract

Cowden disease is a hereditary tumor syndrome marked by an autosomal dominant pattern of inheritance and associated with mutations of the PTEN tumor-suppressor gene located on chromosome 10q23.3. The disorder is marked by the development of hamartomatous lesions derived from any of the three germ cell layers and mucocutaneous lesions. Patients are also at risk of developing cancers in the thyroid, breast, uterus, kidney and colon.

In the central nervous system, the classic pathologic manifestation is the dysplastic cerebellar gangliocytoma (Lhermitte-Duclos disease). Patients with this cerebellar tumor most commonly present with dysmetria, cerebellar signs, and symptoms related to obstructive hydrocephalus. Histologically, the lesion is marked by an increased number of large ganglion cells with a relative preservation of the cerebellar architecture. Calcifications and dilated vessels are not uncommon concomitant findings. The lesion is generally cured by surgical resection, although recurrent lesions have been reported.

This chapter will review the features of Cowden's syndrome with a focus on the dysplastic cerebellar gangliocytoma.

---

* Corresponding Author's Email: praysor@ccf.org.

In: Central Nervous System Pathologies in Hereditary Tumor Syndromes
Editor: Richard A. Prayson
ISBN: 979-8-88697-620-5

Introduction

In 1963, Lloyd and Dennis reported on a case of a 20-year-old female who presented with anomalies involving all three germ cells layers (mesodermal, ectodermal and endodermal) [1]. They designated the disease as Cowden's syndrome, named for the patient, Rachel Cowden, who they wrote about and who died of breast cancer at the age of 30 years. In 1972, Weary et al. suggested a name change to multiple hamartoma syndrome to be more descriptive [2]. Gorlin and colleagues designated the entity as multiple hamartoma and neoplasia syndrome [3]. The primary central nervous system lesion associated with Cowden disease, the dysplastic cerebellar gangliocytoma, was first described in 1920 by Lhermitte and Duclos and is sometimes referred to as Lhermitte-Duclos disease [4].

The goal of this chapter is to review the clinical and pathogenetic features of Cowden's syndrome and the clinicopathologic features of the primary central nervous system manifestation of the syndrome, the dysplastic cerebellar gangliocytoma.

Genetics of Cowden Syndrome

Cowden disease is an autosomal dominant condition, with about half of cases considered sporadic due to new mutations. The disease is caused by an inactivating germline mutation in the PTEN (MMAC1/TEP1) gene on chromosome 10q23, a finding that is seen in about 80% of individuals with the disease [5]. PTEN (*p*hosphatase and *t*ensin homologue, deleted on chromosome *ten*) is a tumor suppressor gene which encoded a lipid and protein phosphatase, homologous to tensin and auxilin, which is involved in the regulation of cell growth, cell spread, apoptosis, and cell cycle arrest [6]. PTEN is ubiquitously expressed [7, 8] and there are high levels of PTEN protein expression in the thyroid gland, skin, autonomic nervous system of the gastrointestinal tract, and central nervous system, all sites more frequently involved by the disease process. PIP3 is the major substrate of PTEN; PIP3 is part of the PI13 pathway [9-11]. PIP3 can be converted to PIP2, which facilitates AKT hypophosphorylation, a cell survival factor via apoptosis. Nuclear PTEN signals via protein phosphatase activity down the cyclin D1/MAPK pathway, resulting in G1 arrest in glial and breast cells [9, 12-14]. Cytoplasmic PTEN signals via its lipid phosphatase activity down the P13K/AKT pathway [14].

Bannayan-Riley-Ruvalcaba syndrome (BBRS), which is marked by lipomatosis, hemangiomatosis, macrocephaly and speckled penis, is considered an allelic variant of Cowden syndrome [15, 16]. The overlapping mutation spectrum, existence of true overlap between familial cases, and genotype-phenotype associations suggests that these two syndromes are allelic and part of a single spectrum at the molecular level. Marsh et al. suggested that an aggregate term PTEN hamartoma tumor syndrome be used to denote such entities [16]. Other entities that seem to be in this spectrum of PTEN related lesions includes Proteus syndrome, VATER/VACTERL, autism spectrum disorder with macrocephaly, and juvenile polyposis of infancy.

General Clinical Features

International Cowden Consortium (ICC) and National Comprehensive Cancer Network (NCCN) operational criteria for Cowden syndrome without known family history of PTEN mutation includes the following pathognomonic criteria: adult dysplastic cerebellar gangliocytoma, mucocutaneous lesions (facial trichilemmomas - at least two biopsy proven, acral keratoses and papillomatous papules), mucosal lesions and autism spectrum disorder with macrocephaly [6, 17-20].

Major criteria include breast carcinoma, thyroid carcinoma (nonmedullary, especially follicular carcinoma, rarely papillary carcinoma), macrocephaly (megalocephaly), endometrial cancer, mucocutaneous lesions (one biopsy-proven trichilemmoma, multiple palmar plantar keratoses, multifocal cutaneous facial papules, or macular pigmentation of the glans penis), and multiple gastrointestinal hamartomas or ganglioneuromas. In women with Cowden syndrome, one series reported a lifetime breast cancer risk of 85% [21]. The mean patient age at the time of diagnosis of breast cancer is about 10 years younger than the general population [22]. Most of the breast cancers are infiltrating ductal adenocarcinomas. Lifetime risk for the development of thyroid carcinoma in Cowden syndrome may be as high as 35% [21].

Minor criteria include benign thyroid lesions (adenoma, multinodular goiter), decreased IQ (75 or less), gastrointestinal hamartomas, fibrocystic breast disease, lipomas, fibromas, renal cell carcinoma, genitourinary malformations and uterine leiomyomas. In the absence of a family history, classic mucocutaneous lesions plus two major criteria, one major and three minor criteria, or four minor criteria are necessary for diagnosis. In the presence of a family history, a diagnosis requires typical mucocutaneous lesions, one major criterion, two minor criteria, or a history of BRRS (a related PTEN hamartoma tumor syndrome)

A molecular based estimate of the prevalence of the syndrome is about 1 case per 200,000 population [23]. Mester and Eng estimated the de novo PTEN mutation frequency to be approximately 11% at minimum and 48% at maximum in probands that were evaluated [24].

Neurologic Clinical Features

Adult-onset dysplastic cerebellar gangliocytoma is highly predictive of a germline pathogenic variant in PTEN and is considered pathognomonic of Cowden syndrome. Dysplastic cerebellar gangliocytoma is commonly referred to also as Lhermitte-Duclos disease. Other synonyms that have been variously used in reference to this pathology include Purkinjeoma, gangliomatosis of the cerebellum, granule cell hypertrophy of the cerebellum and diffuse hypertrophy of the cerebellar cortex.

Overall, the lesion is rare and typically presents in the third and fourth decades, although the age range of presentation has varied from congenital up to age 74 years [26, 27]. The lesion usually develops unilaterally; there is no preference regarding laterality. Rare cases of bilateral lesions have been reported [28, 29]. In one study of 211 patients with Cowden syndrome, 32% developed a cerebellar lesion [30].

The neurologic symptoms tend to be chronic in their evolution (mean preoperative duration of symptoms of about 40 months) and can include ataxia, dysmetria, seizures, or symptoms related to obstructive hydrocephalus or increased intracranial pressure [31]. Cranial nerve deficits, macrocephaly, orthostatic hypotension and acute subarachnoid hemorrhage have also been reported.

Imaging Findings

On imaging, the lesion presents as a nonenhancing hemispheric expansion of the cerebellum. The lesions are hypointense on T1-weighted magnetic resonance images (MRI) and hyperintense on T2-weighted images [32-34]. Parallel linear striations or tiger stripes, representing abnormally thickened folia, are often present on the surface of the lesion. Calcifications may be present in some lesions and are best seen on computed tomography (CT) studies.

Neuropathologic Findings

Grossly, the cerebellar folia appear thickened and appear to blend into adjacent unaltered cortex. The large folia have a pale appearance or yellow-white discoloration, resulting from the abnormal myelination in the region.

Microscopically, the dysplastic cerebellar gangliocytoma is marked by a proliferation of variably sized neuronal or ganglionic cells (Figure 1).

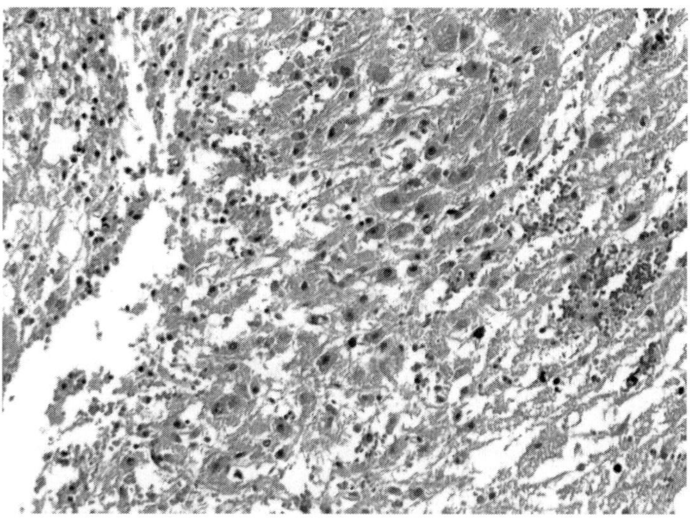

Figure 1. Dysplastic cerebellar gangliocytoma is marked by an abnormal collection of neuronal cells (hematoxylin and eosin, original magnification 200X).

Overall, there is a relative preservation of the cerebellar architecture with expansion of the folia. In some cases, a collection of granular type neurons and abnormal ganglion cells may be seen in the subpial region of the molecular layer. Abnormal myelination of the molecular layer may be seen due to the myelination of abnormal neurons that reside in the granule cell layer with extending axons into the molecular zone. Microcalcifications may be present in some cases (Figure 2). The number of Purkinje cells is often reduced in the affected area. Ectatic blood vessels and vacuolization of the cerebellar white matter have also been described in some cases.

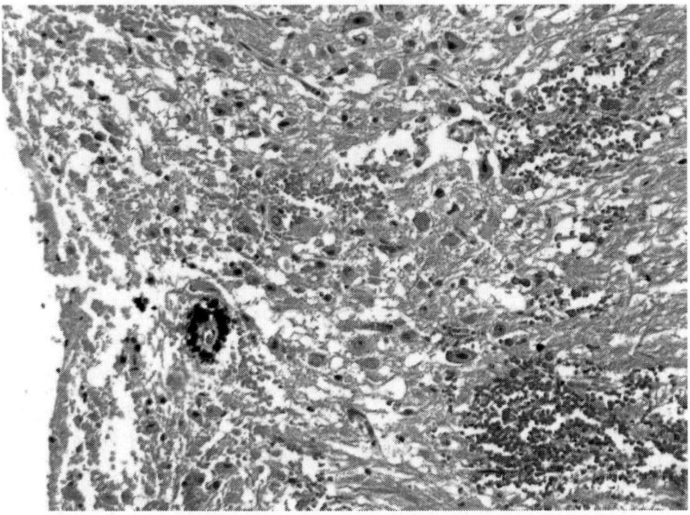

Figure 2. Angiocentric calcification is a dysplastic cerebellar gangliocytoma (hematoxylin and eosin, original magnification 200X).

The lesion typically demonstrates a low or absent rate of cell proliferation, as evidenced by low Ki-67 or MIB-1 labeling indices. The atypical neuronal or ganglion cells stain with markers of neuronal differentiation (synaptophysin, neurofilament, chromogranin and NeuN) and do not stain with antibody to glial fibrillary acidic protein (GFAP). Immunomarkers that normally stain Purkinje cells (CD3 PCP2, PCP4, and calbindin) do not stain the majority of the ganglionic cells, suggesting that most of them are not derived from a Purkinje cell source [35].

The main differential diagnostic consideration from a pathology perspective is with a ganglioglioma. The dysplastic cerebellar gangliocytoma lacks an atypical glioma component to the lesion which marks a ganglioglioma. Gangliogliomas often have BRAF V600E mutations and lack PTEN mutations, in contrast to the dysplastic cerebellar gangliocytoma.

Treatment and Prognosis

The dysplastic cerebellar gangliocytomas are considered curable by surgery, although occasional recurrences have been seen, if the lesion is incompletely excised [36]. There is no need for adjuvant radiation therapy or chemotherapy. Patients with Cowden syndrome may develop malignant tumors, as previously discussed, outside the central nervous system, that may metastasize to the brain and necessitate adjuvant therapy.

Conclusion

Cowden disease is a hereditary tumor syndrome marked by an autosomal dominant pattern of inheritance and associated with mutations of the PTEN tumor-suppressor gene located on chromosome 10q23.3. In the central nervous system, the classic pathologic manifestation is the dysplastic cerebellar gangliocytoma (Lhermitte-Duclos disease). Patients with this cerebellar tumor most commonly present with dysmetria, cerebellar signs, and symptoms related to obstructive hydrocephalus. Pathologically, the lesion is marked by a proliferation of large ganglion cells. In most instances, the lesion is cured by surgical resection, although occasionally recurrent lesions have been reported.

References

[1] Lloyd, K. M., and Dennis, M. (1963). Cowden's disease: a possible new symptom complex with multiple system involvement. *Ann Intern Med.*, 58, 136-142.

[2] Weary, P. E., Gorlin, R. J., Gentry, W. C., et al. (1972). Multiple hamartoma syndrome (Cowden's disease). *Arch Dermatol.*, 105, 682-690.

[3] Gorlin, R. J., Pindborg, J., and Cohen, M. (1976). *Syndromes of the Head and Neck.* 2nd edition. McGraw-Hill Book Company.

[4] Lhermitte, J., and Duclos, P. (1920). Sur un ganglioneuroma diffus du cortex du cervelet. *Bull Assoc Fr Etud Cancer.*, 9, 99-107.

[5] Robinsom, S., and Cohen, A. R. (2006). Cowden disease and Lhermitte-Duclos disease: an update. Case report and review of the literature. *Neurosurg Focus.*, 20, E6.

[6] Gustafson, S., Zbuk, K. M., Scacheri, C., et al. (2007). Cowden syndrome. *Semin Oncol.*, 34, 428-434.

[7] Steck, P. A., Pershouse, M. A., Jasser, S. A., et al. (1997). Identification of a candidate tumor suppressor gene, MMAC1, at chromosome 10q23.3 that is mutated in multiple advanced cancers. *Nat Genet.*, 15(4), 356-362.

[8] Gimm, O., Attie-Bitach, T., Lees, J. A., et al. (2000). Expression of the PTEN tumour suppressor protein during human development. *Hum Mol Genet.*, 9(11), 1633-1639.

[9] Fumari, F. B., Huang, H. J., and Cavenee, W. K. (1998). The phosphoinositol phosphatase activity of PTEN mediates a serum-sensitive G1 growth arrest in glioma cells. *Cancer Res.*, 58(22), 5002-5008.

[10] Stambolic, V., Suzuki, A., de la Pompa, J. L., et al. (1998). Negative regulation of PKB/Akt-dependent cell survival by the tumor suppressor PTEN. *Cell.*, 95(1), 29-39.

[11] Dahia, S., Aguiar, R. C., Alberta, J., et al. (1999). PTEN is inversely correlated with the cell survival factor Akt/PKB and is inactivated via multiple mechanisms in haematological malignancies. *Hum Mol Genet.*, 8(2), 185-193.

[12] Fumari, F. B., Lin, H., Huang, H. S., et al. (1997). Growth suppression of glioma cells by PTEN requires a functional phosphatase catalytic domain. *Proc Natl Acad Sci USA.*, 94(23), 12479-12484.

[13] Li, J., Simpson, L., Takahashi, M., et al. (1998). The PTEN/MMAC1 tumor suppressor induces cell death that is rescued by the AKT/protein kinase B oncogene. *Cancer Res.*, 58(24), 5667-5672.

[14] Minaguchi, T., Waite, K. A., and Eng, C. (2006). Nuclear localization of PTEN is regulated by Ca(2+) through a tyrosil phosphorylation-independent conformational modification in major vault protein. *Cancer Res.*, 66(24), 11677-11682.

[15] Marsh, D. J., Dahia, P. L., Zheng, Z., et al. (1997). Germline mutations in PTEN are present in Bannayan-Zonana syndrome. *Nat Genet.*, 16(4), 333-334.

[16] Marsh Jum, J. B., Lunetta, K. L., et al. (1999). PTEN mutation spectrum and genotype-phenotype considerations in Bannayan-Riley-Ruvalcaba syndrome suggest a single entity with Cowden syndrome. *Hum Mol Genet.*, 8(8), 1461-1472.

[17] Uppal, S., Mistry, D., and Coatesworth, A. P. (2007). Cowden disease: a review. *Int J Clin Pract.*, 61(4), 645-652.

[18] Pilarski, R., Burt, R., and Kohlman, W., et al. (2013). Cowden syndrome and the PTEN hamartoma tumor syndrome: systematic review and revised diagnostic criteria. *J Natl Cancer Inst.*, 105, 1607-1616.

[19] Tan, M. H., Mester, J., Peterson, C., et al. (2011). A clinical scoring system for selection of patients for PTEN mutation testing is proposed on the basis of prospective study of 3042 probands. *Am J Hum Genet.*, 88(1), 42-56.

[20] National Comprehensive Cancer Network (NCCN). (2010). NCCN clinical practice guidelines in oncology oncology (NCCN guidelines): genetic/familial high-risk assessment: breast and ovarian cancer. Version 1.2010. Fort Washington (PA):NCCN.

[21] Tan, M. H., Mester, J., Nigeow, J., et al. (2012). Life-time cancer risks in individuals with germline PTEN mutations. *Clin Cancer Res.*, 18(2), 400-407.

[22] Starink, T. M., van der Veen, J. P., Arwert, F., et al. (1986). The Cowden syndrome: a clinical and genetic study in 21 patients. *Clin Genet.*, 29(3), 222-233.

[23] Nelen, M. R., Kremer, H., Konings, I. B., et al. (1999). Novel PTEN mutations in patients with Cowden disease: absence of clear genotype-phenotype correlations. *Eur J Hum Genet.*, 7(3), 267-273.

[24] Mester, J., and Eng, C. (2012). Estimate of de novo mutation frequency in probands with PTEN hamartoma tumor syndrome. *Genet Med.*, 14(9), 819-822.

[25] Zhou, X. P., Marsh, D., Morrison, C. D., et al. Germline inactivation of PTEN and dysregulation of the phosphoinositol-3-kinase/Akt pathway cause human Lhermitte-Duclos disease in adults. *Am J Hum Genet.* 2003, 73(5), 1191-1198.

[26] Abel, T. W., Baker, S. J., Fraser, M. M., et al. (2005). Lhermitte-Duclos disease: a report of 31 cases with immunohistochemical analysis of the PTEN/AKT/mTOR pathway. *J Neuropathol Exp Neurol.*, 64($), 341-349.

[27] Albrecht, S., Haber, R. M., Goodman, J. C., et al. (1992). Cowden syndrome and Lhermitte-Duclos disease. *Cancer.*, 70(4), 869-876.

[28] Khandpur, U., Huntoon, K., Smith-Cohn, M., et al. (2019). Bilateral recurrent dysplastic cerebellar gangliocytoma (Lhermitte-Duclos disease) in Cowden syndrome, a case report and literature review. *World Neurosurg.*, 127, 319-325.

[29] Borni, M., Kammoun, B., Kolsi, F., et al. (2019). The Lhermitte-Duclos disease: a rare bilateral cerebellar location of a rare pathology. *Pan Afr Med J.*, 33, 118.

[30] Riegert-Johnson, D. L., Gleeson, F. C., Roberts, M., et al. (2010). Cancer and Lhermitte-Duclos disease are common in Cowden patients. *Hered Cancer Clin Pract.*, 8(1), 6

[31] Vinchon, M., Blond, S., Lejeune, J. P., et al. (1994). Association of Lhermitte-Duclos and Cowden disease: report of a new case and review of the literature. *J Neurol Neurosurg Psychiatry.*, 57(6), 699-704.

[32] Klisch, J., Juengling, F., Spreer, J., et al. (2001). Lhermitte-Duclos disease: assessment with MR imaging, positron emission tomography, single photon emission CT, and MR spectroscopy. *AJNR Am J Neuroradiol.*, 22(5), 824-830.

[33] Thomas, B., Krishnamoorthy, T., Radhakrishnan, V. V., et al. (2007). Advanced MR imaging in Lhermitte-Duclos disease: moving closer to pathology and pathophysiology. *Neuroradiology.*, 49(9), 733-738.

[34] Lok, C., Viseux, V., Avril, M. F., et al. (2005). Brain magnetic resonance imaging in patients with Cowden syndrome. *Medicine.*, 84, 129-136.

[35] Hair, L. S., Symmans, F., Powers, J. M., et al. (1992). Immunohistochemistry and proliferative activity in Lhermitte-Duclos disease. *Acta Neuropathol.*, 84(5), 570-572.

[36] Brat, D. J., and Perry, A. (2018). Neuronal and glioneuronal neoplasms. In: *Practical Surgical Neuropathology*. Perry A and Brat DJ, editors. Elsevier. Philadelphia, PA. 193-196.

Chapter 6

Schwannomatosis: Central Nervous System Pathology

Aiman J. Faruqi[1], BS
Mario S. Belfiglio[1], BS
and Richard A. Prayson[2,*], MD, MEd
[1] Cleveland Clinic Lerner College of Medicine, Cleveland, Ohio, USA
[2] Department of Anatomic Pathology, Cleveland Clinic, Cleveland, Ohio, USA

Abstract

Schwannomatosis is a hereditary tumor predisposition syndrome characterized by the development of multiple schwannomas in the absence of bilateral vestibular nerve involvement typical of neurofibromatosis type 2. With an estimated incidence of 1/40,000 to 1/70,000 births, its molecular pathogenesis is driven by a four-hit process that results in biallelic loss of function of either SMARCB1 or LZTR1 and NF2 on chromosome 22q.

The disease generally presents in the second to third decade of life with pain as the dominant symptom and may be diagnosed by a combination of clinical and molecular criteria. Magnetic resonance (MR) imaging with and without contrast is the preferred modality to identify schwannomas and exclude bilateral vestibular nerve involvement. Histologic morphology of schwannomas typically reveals Antoni A pattern with spindle-shaped cells and Verocay bodies and molecular characterization shows loss of SMARCB1 on immunohistochemistry for schwannomatosis-associated tumors.

* Corresponding Author's Email: praysor@ccf.org.

In: Central Nervous System Pathologies in Hereditary Tumor Syndromes
Editor: Richard A. Prayson
ISBN: 979-8-88697-620-5

Treatment is symptomatic and involves multimodal pharmacologic pain medication and surgical resection of tumors causing significant pain or neurologic deficits. Schwannomatosis is associated with significant diminished quality of life but has not been shown to reduce life expectancy.

Introduction

Initially identified in a small cohort of Japanese patients in the 1980s [1, 2], schwannomatosis is a hereditary tumor predisposition syndrome characterized by the development of multiple benign peripheral nerve sheath tumors of Schwann cell origin. Although this syndrome is closely related to neurofibromatosis type 2 (NF2), which also presents with schwannomas, schwannomatosis has been shown to be a distinct form of neurofibromatosis with later onset of presentation, the absence of bilateral vestibular schwannomas, and unique genetic drivers of disease. The epidemiology of schwannomatosis also differs from NF2, with an approximate incidence of 1 in every 40,000 to 70,000 births [3]. This chapter will review the genetic, clinical, and radiologic features of schwannomatosis with an emphasis on neuropathology.

Genetics of Schwannomatosis

The molecular pathogensis of schwannomatosis is principally driven by inactivating mutations (missense, splice site, frameshift) in SMARCB1 and leucin-zipper-like transcriptional regulator 1 (LZTR1) genes on the long arm (q) of chromosome 22 [4]. However, a simple two-hit hypothesis that underlies the molecular genetics of other autosomal dominant hereditary tumor syndromes does not adequately explain the pathogenesis of schwannomatosis. A four-hit hypothesis has been proposed: germline mutation of SMARCB1 or LZTR1 (hit 1), *trans* loss of wild-type SMARCB1 or LZTR1 and NF2 on chromosome 22q (hits 2 and 3), and somatic mutation of NF2 in *cis* with germline mutated SMARCB1 or LZTR1 (hit 4). The consequence of this cascade of genetic aberrations is biallelic loss of function of SMARCB1/LZTR1 and NF2 [5, 6]. However, a subset of tumors in schwannomatosis have been found to harbor mono-allelic loss of NF2 that is sufficient to drive tumorigenesis [7].

Clinical Features

Similar to NF2, schwannomatosis is characterized by the presence of multiple schwannomas, and more rarely, meningiomas in SMARCB1-driven disease [5, 7, 8]. The diagnosis can be made clinically or by a combination of clinical and molecular characteristics. Clinical diagnostic criteria include at least two non-intradermal schwannomas with at least one confirmed pathologically and the absence of bilateral vestibular schwannomas. Alternatively, one pathologically confirmed schwannoma or intracranial meningioma and an affected first-degree relative is sufficient for diagnosis. Combined molecular and clinical diagnostic criteria include at least two schwannomas with loss of heterozygosity on chromosome 22q with two different somatic NF2 mutations *and* at least two pathologically confirmed schwannomas or meningiomas. Alternatively, patients with germline pathogenic mutations in SMARCB1 or LZTR1 *and* one pathologically confirmed schwannoma or meningioma meet diagnostic criteria for the syndrome.

Key diagnostic exclusion criteria include germline pathogenic NF2 mutations, fulfilling the diagnostic criteria for NF2, first-degree relative with NF2, and the presence of schwannomas at sites of previous radiation therapy [7, 9]. Unlike NF1, schwannomatosis does not classically present with cutaneous findings such as café au lait spots [10]. Schwannomatosis generally presents later than NF2, between the ages of 30-60 years but most commonly in the second to third decade [8]. The dominant clinical symptom is significant, chronic pain secondary to neoplastic growth [11]. Depression and anxiety are common psychosocial complications that warrant appropriate vigilance and treatment. Beyond pain, additional neurologic symptoms are uncommon in schwannomatosis in the absence of surgical intervention that occasionally causes iatrogenic nerve injury in the process of schwannoma excision [8].

Imaging Findings

Magnetic resonance (MR) imaging is the preferred modality in the initial evaluation of peripheral nerve sheath tumors. High resolution MR imaging of the brain and spine with and without contrast is important in the diagnostic evaluation of schwannomatosis in particular to assess the internal auditory canals for the presence of bilateral schwannomas that are notably absent in this tumor syndrome but present in NF2. However, LRTZ1-driven schwannomatosis may be associated with unilateral vestibular schwannomas and schwannomas of non-vestibular cranial nerves. In the event imaging findings are congruent with features of both schwannomatosis and NF2, molecular evaluation is typically required to confirm the diagnosis. Beyond their anatomic distribution, the imaging features of schwannomas are indistinguishable in schwannomatosis and NF2, with well-defined, un-encapsulated fusiform or round soft-tissue masses on MR imaging. Whole body MR imaging and positron emission tomography have variable utility in assessing tumor burden and disease progression [12].

Neuropathologic Findings

The neuropathologic features of schwannomas are similar among tumor syndromes characterized by the presence of this tumor type. Schwannomas are derived from Schwann cells responsible for the myelination of axons in the peripheral nervous system and remain attached to the nerve as they grow. The histologic characteristics of schwannomas with hematoxylin and eosin staining include spindle-shaped hypercellular Antoni A patterning (Figure 1) with embedded areas of palisading nuclei alternating with areas without nuclei known as Verocay bodies (Figure 2) [10].

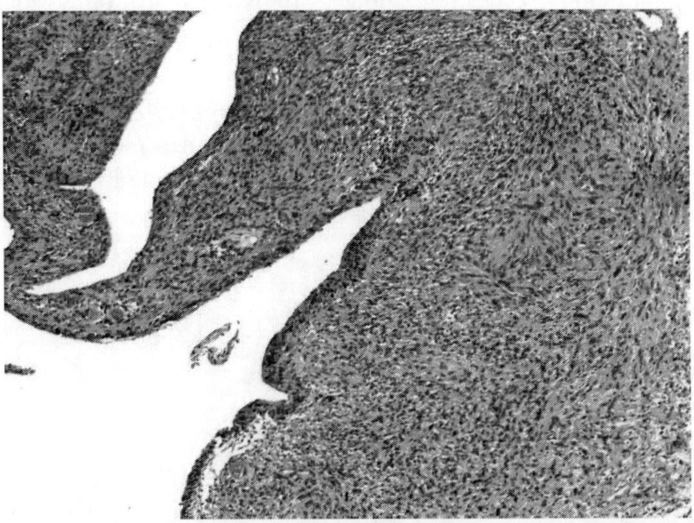

Figure 1. Cellular schwannoma marked by cystic areas and an Antoni A pattern (hematoxylin and eosin, original magnification 100X).

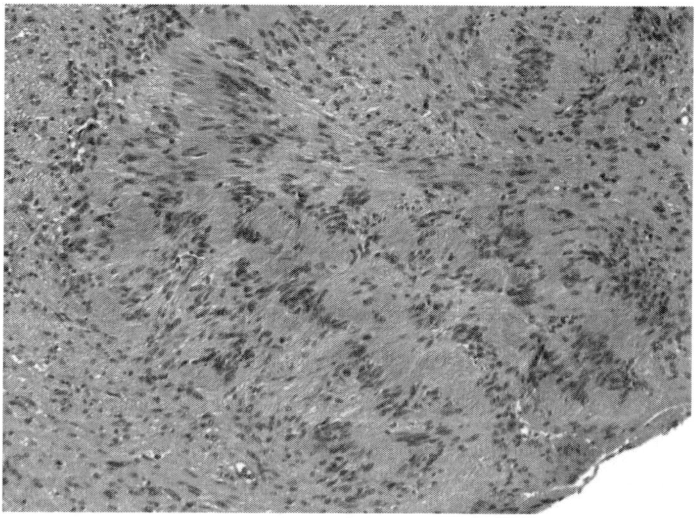

Figure 2. Palisaded Verocay bodies in a schwannoma (hematoxylin and eosin, original magnification 200X).

Tumor progression is also linked with histologic transitioning to hypocellular Antoni B patterning. Additional inflammatory cells such as macrophages and T cells may be prominent in a subset of tumors [13]. Schwannoma subtypes also exist, including plexiform schwannomas that encompass multiple nerve fascicles and are more common in schwannomatosis and NF2. As the morphologic features of isolated and syndromic schwannomas are typically indistinguishable, immunohistochemical loss of SMARCB1 is helpful in establishing a molecular diagnosis of schwannomatosis from appropriate specimens.

Malignant peripheral nerve sheath tumors (MPSNTs) have also been reported in patients with schwannomatosis, particularly with mutations in SMARCB1, though the strength of this association appears substantially weaker than NF1 [14]. These tumors may arise from normal peripheral nerves or from existing benign peripheral nerve sheath tumors; interestingly, in the latter case, most documented cases of MPSNTs appear to develop from neurofibromas rather than schwannomas, suggesting an independent process of tumorigenesis in patients with schwannomatosis including development of driver mutations such as loss of TP53 [15].

MPSNTs typically require microscopic evaluation to differentiate them from benign tumors and are histologically characterized by invasive spindle cells with prominent mitotic activity (Figure 3) [16]. However, low-grade MPSNTs may be challenging to distinguish from benign plexiform neurofibromas [15].

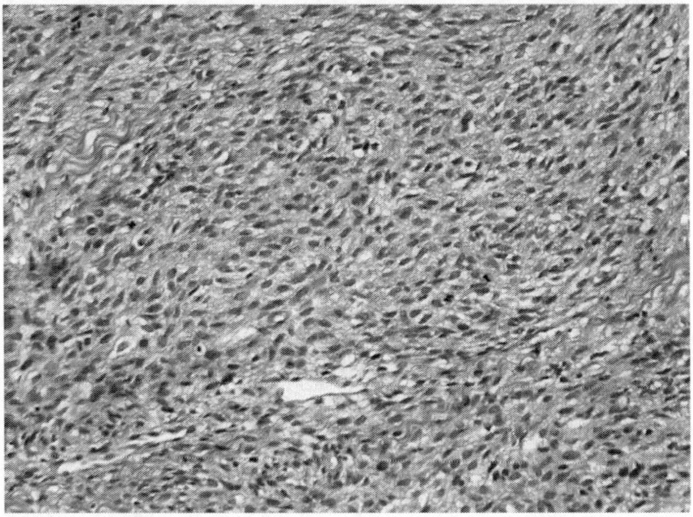

Figure 3. A malignant peripheral nerve sheath tumor marked by prominent mitotic activity (hematoxylin and eosin, original magnification 200X).

Schwannomatosis has also been linked to the development of meningiomas in less than ten percent of patients and appears to be linked to SMARCB1-driven disease. The histologic features of meningiomas typically include spindled cells in a whirling pattern and concentric lamellar calcifications known psammoma bodies (Figure 4). Immunohistochemical characterization with antibodies to epithelial membrane antigen (EMA), progesterone receptor and somatostatin receptor 2A (SST2A) may aid in histopathologic diagnosis. However, morphologic characteristics can vary substantially given the heterogenous array of tumor subtypes. The World Health Organization (WHO) currently recognizes 15 distinct meningioma variants across three grades of pathology. Whether specific variants are more commonly implicated in schwannomatosis is not well understood [17].

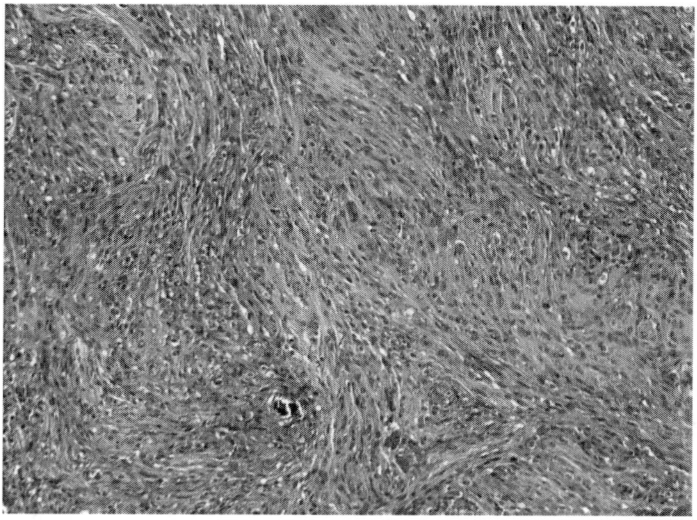

Figure 4. A fibrous meningioma, WHO grade 1, with spindled cells and a rare psammomatous calcification (hematoxylin and eosin, original magnification 200X).

Treatment and Prognosis

The management of schwannomatosis primarily involves symptom management. Multimodal pain management is the mainstay of treatment; gabapentin, tricyclic anti-depressants, and serotonin-norepinephrine reuptake inhibitors such as venlafaxine are typical first-line pharmacologic options [5]. Surgical resection is indicated for schwannomas causing neurologic deficits or localized pain but also carries the risk of iatrogenic nerve injury. The role of radiation therapy is not well established due to a paucity of robust evidence supporting its benefit, but has typically been avoided due to the theoretical risk of malignant transformation [4, 5]. With respect to prognosis, patients with schwannomatosis suffer from decreased quality of life due to pain, but the syndrome has not been linked to decreased life expectancy to date.

Conclusion

Schwannomatosis is associated with biallelic loss of function of either LZTR1 or SMARCB1 and the NF 2 genes. The neuropathologic finding that is most typically associated with the condition, as suggested by its name, is the development of multiple schwannomas in the absence of bilateral vestibular nerve schwannomas that are classically encountered in neurofibromatosis type 2.

References

[1] Shishiba T, Niimura M, Ohtsuka F, ET AL. Multiple cutaneous neurilemmomas as a skin manifestation of neurilemmomatosis. *J. Am. Acad. Dermatol.* 1984;10 (5 Pt 1):744-754.

[2] MacCollin M, Woodfin W, Kronn D, ET AL. Schwannomatosis: a clinical and pathologic study. *Neurology*. 1996;46(4):1072-1079.

[3] Schraepen C, Donkersloot P, Duyvendak W, ET AL. What to know about schwannomatosis: a literature review. *Br. J. Neurosurg*. 2022;36(2):171-174.

[4] Plotkin S R, Wick A. Neurofibromatosis and schwannomatosis. *Semin. Neurol.* 2018;38(1):73-85.

[5] Dhamija R, Plotkin S, Asthagiri A, et al. Schwannomatosis. In: Adam M P, Everman D B, Mirzaa G M, et al., eds. *GeneReviews®*. University of Washington, Seattle; 1993.

[6] Tamura R. Current understanding of neurofibromatosis type 1, 2, and schwannomatosis. *Int. J. Mol. Sci.* 2021;22(11):5850.

[7] Kehrer-Sawatzki H, Farschtschi S, Mautner V F, et al. The molecular pathogenesis of schwannomatosis, a paradigm for the co-involvement of multiple tumour suppressor genes in tumorigenesis. *Hum. Genet.* 2017;136(2):129-148.

[8] Blakeley J O, Plotkin S R. Therapeutic advances for the tumors associated with neurofibromatosis type 1, type 2, and schwannomatosis. *Neuro-Oncol*. 2016;18(5): 624-638.

[9] Plotkin S R, Blakeley J O, Evans D G, et al. Update from the 2011 International Schwannomatosis Workshop: from genetics to diagnostic criteria. *Am. J. Med. Genet. A*. 2013;0(3):405-416.

[10] Koontz N A, Wiens A L, Agarwal A, et al. Schwannomatosis: the overlooked neurofibromatosis? *Am. J. Roentgenol*. 2013; 200(6):W646-W653.

[11] Kresak J L, Walsh M. Neurofibromatosis: a review of NF1, NF2, and schwannomatosis. *J. Pediatr. Genet*. 2016;5(2):98-104.

[12] Ahlawat S, Blakeley J O, Langmead S, et al. Current status and recommendations for imaging in neurofibromatosis type 1, neurofibromatosis type 2, and schwannomatosis. *Skeletal Radiol*. 2020;49(2):199-219.

[13] Helbing D L, Schulz A, Morrison H. Pathomechanisms in schwannoma development and progression. *Oncogene*. 2020;39(32):5421-5429.

[14] Evans D G R, Huson S M, Birch J M. Malignant peripheral nerve sheath tumours in inherited disease. *Clin. Sarcoma Res*. 2012;2(1):17.

[15] Knight S W E, Knight T E, Santiago T, et al. Malignant peripheral nerve sheath tumors—a comprehensive review of pathophysiology, diagnosis, and multidisciplinary management. *Children*. 2022;9(1):38.

[16] Wippold F J, Lubner M, Perrin R J, et al. Neuropathology for the neuroradiologist: Antoni A and Antoni B tissue patterns. *AJNR Am. J. Neuroradiol.* 2007;28(9):1633-1638.

[17] Huntoon K, Toland AMS, Dahiya S. Meningioma: a review of clinicopathological and molecular aspects. *Front. Oncol.* 2020;10:579599.

Chapter 7

Clinical and Pathological Aspects of Li-Fraumeni Syndrome - Focus on the Central Nervous System

Georgi Galev, MD
and Richard A. Prayson*, MD, MEd
Department of Anatomic Pathology, Cleveland Clinic, Cleveland, Ohio, USA

Abstract

Li-Fraumeni syndrome (LFS) is an inherited disorder caused by various alterations in the TP53 gene located on chromosome 17p13.1. It has an autosomal dominant pattern of inheritance with variable penetrance and expressivity. The protein product of the TP53 gene (p53) serves as an important cell cycle regulator and its pathologic alteration leads to cell cycle dysregulation, and eventually, neoplastic transformation.

LFS manifests with a variety of neoplasms in all age groups, most commonly breast carcinoma, sarcomas, central nervous system (CNS) neoplasms and adrenocortical carcinomas. In the CNS, medulloblastomas (SHH-activated, TP53 mutated), astrocytic neoplasms and choroid plexus carcinomas are most commonly encountered. Several criteria for the clinical recognition of patients with possible LFS have been developed, with genetic testing for pathogenic variants of the TP53 gene being the gold standard for making the diagnosis.

This chapter will review the etiopathogenesis, the clinical and the pathologic features of LFS with emphasis on its CNS manifestations.

---

* Corresponding Author's Email: praysor@ccf.org.

In: Central Nervous System Pathologies in Hereditary Tumor Syndromes
Editor: Richard A. Prayson
ISBN: 979-8-88697-620-5

Introduction

The first report of what came to be known as Li-Fraumeni syndrome (LFS) was in the 1969 paper by Frederick Li and Joseph Fraumeni where they described four families with unusually high incidence of various malignant neoplasms, most commonly various sarcomas and breast carcinoma [1]. In the coming decades, LFS established itself as a hereditary cancer syndrome following additional reports of similar familial neoplasms among which were neoplasms of the central nervous system (CNS) [2-6]. Underlying hereditary genetics were suspected as causative of LFS, but it was not until 1990, when germline p53 mutations were discovered in families with LFS [7]. Today, LFS is a well-defined both clinically and pathologically, with CNS neoplasms being an established part of its tumor spectrum.

Etiology and Pathogenesis

LFS is caused by a germline mutation of the TP53 gene, located on chromosome 17p13.1 [7-9]. The physiologic role of the TP53 gene and its transcript p53 is well described in literature [10, 11]. Briefly, p53 is activated in cases of hypoxic or oncogenic stress, halting the cell cycle and initiating either repair, senescence or apoptosis, depending of the severity of the noxious effect. Thus, the role of p53 is to prevent further DNA damage in cases of injurious or oncogenic cellular stress. Consecutively, a mutant TP53 will produce a dysfunctional p53 protein that is unable to halt the cell cycle and thus creates an environment where DNA damage goes unchecked and mutations accumulate, culminating in neoplastic transformation. It is postulated that 50% of human neoplasia have a TP53 mutation [12], pointing to its central role in oncogenesis. Where in the vast majority of neoplasia there is a somatic TP53 mutation, in LFS the mutation is a germline one.

Clinical Features

LFS is inherited in autosomal-dominant fashion with variable penetrance depending on the type of mutation. For example, dominant-negative mutations have a higher penetrance compared to loss-of-function mutations [13]. The frequency of mutant TP53 has been estimated to be between 1 in 5,000 to 1 in

20,000 live births; however, the exact prevalence of pathogenic variants is unclear [14-16]. Patients with LFS develop neoplasms at a significantly earlier age compared with the general population. The carriers of a TP53 mutation almost inevitably develop a malignant neoplasm in their lifetime [7]. The signs and symptoms of a neoplasm in a patient with LFS do not differ from those of a sporadic malignancy. Although in LFS, the mutant TP53 is found throughout all tissues, certain neoplasms occur with higher frequency compared to others. In addition, the cancer profile differs in sporadic and germline TP53 mutations. The most common neoplasms in LFS are breast carcinoma, sarcomas, CNS neoplasms and adrenocortical carcinomas. Other malignancies may also be encountered, including leukemia, melanoma, prostate cancer, lung cancer, gastric cancer and pancreatic cancer.

The classical clinical criteria for LFS are summarized in Table 1. The criteria developed by Birch and Eels are also commonly used in the clinical practice in suspected LFS patients (those criteria are also known as Li-Fraumeni-like syndrome) [9, 11]. Clinically suspected LFS has to be confirmed by molecular testing and genetic counseling should be provided. Due to the extremely high lifetime risk of developing a malignancy, early detection and prevention are the main strategies in LFS patients. Various management guidelines have been published and focus rigorous follow-up [13, 17, 18].

Table 1. Classical clinical criteria for Li-Fraumeni syndrome [5]

Sarcoma diagnosed before the age of 45 years
First degree-relative with any cancer before the age of 45 years
First- or second-degree relative with any cancer before the age of 45 years or a sarcoma at any age

LFS does not have specific neurologic manifestations. In a patient that develop CNS neoplasms, the signs and symptoms do not differ from sporadic tumors. Depending on the location of the tumor, the most common presentations are headache, seizures, focal neurologic deficits, nausea and vomiting. In children, ataxia, developmental delay and macrocephaly (the latter mostly in infants) can also be encountered. Patients that are suspected to have a CNS neoplasm should undergo imaging studies. The radiologic appearance of CNS tumors in LFS is not unique and depends on the type of neoplasm. Further management requires pathologic examination of a tissue sample obtained either by stereotactic or open surgical approach.

Pathology

The gross and microscopic appearance of tumors occurring in LFS does not differ from sporadic ones. Immunohistochemical (IHC) staining for p53 can be used as a surrogate marker for a p53 mutant tumor with diffuse or completely absent nuclear staining indicating a missense or a truncating mutation respectively. IHC cannot discriminate between germline and sporadic mutation. This section will deal mainly with CNS tumors occurring in the setting of LFS.

The tumors occurring in the CNS of patients with LFS are (in decreasing order of frequency) diffuse astrocytomas, medulloblastomas and choroid plexus carcinomas and show a bimodal distribution (Figures 1-3). The first peak is in the pediatric age group and the second is in the third and fourth decades. The pediatric LFS patients develop IDH-wildtype glioblastomas, SHH-activated, TP53-mutant medulloblastomas as well as choroid plexus carcinomas. In the adult population, IDH-mutant astrocytomas are more common. Often, those tumors have a higher frequency of the noncanonical p.R132C IDH mutation and its discovery should prompt TP53 germline testing [19]. Other entities, amongst which are ependymomas and oligodendrogliomas, are encountered, although less frequently. With the exception of the IDH-mutant astrocytomas, all other CNS neoplasms in LFS have an aggressive behavior and poor prognosis [14]. The gross and histologic appearance of the CNS neoplasms in the context of LFS is not unique to the syndrome. As described above, p53 IHC can be used to screen for a p53 mutation, however molecular confirmation is warranted.

In the setting of LFS, the TP53 gene most commonly has a missense mutation. Abnormal variants can also be due to nonsense mutations, deletions, insertions and splice-site mutations. Testing for pathogenic variants can be done with various sequencing techniques. There are well recognized pathogenic sequences; however, results interpretation remains a challenge. There are resources such as societal guidelines and databases that can help with results interpretation [20].

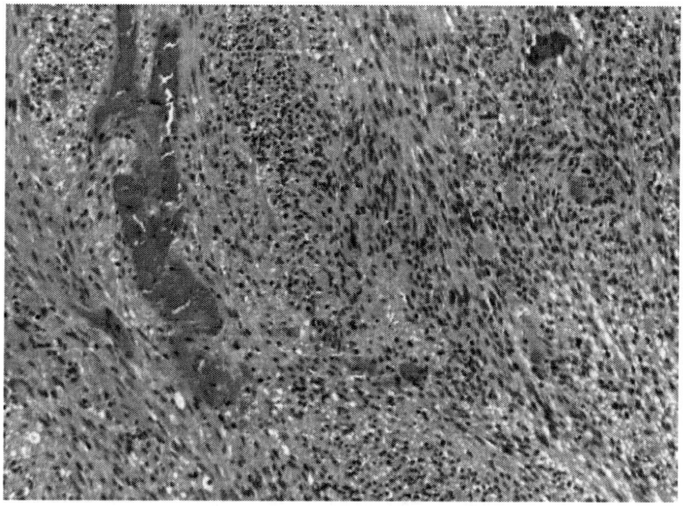

Figure 1. A World Health Organization (WHO) grade 3 astrocytoma marked by prominent cellularity and mitotic figures in a patient with Li-Fraumeni; the tumor was IDH-wildtype (hematoxylin and eosin, original magnification 200X).

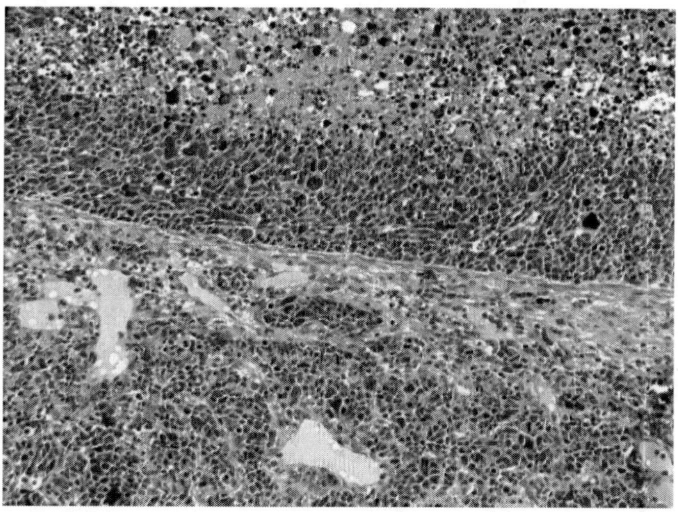

Figure 2. A large cell/anaplastic medulloblastoma (WHO grade 4) marked by pleomorphic cells and geographic necrosis (hematoxylin and eosin, original magnification 200X).

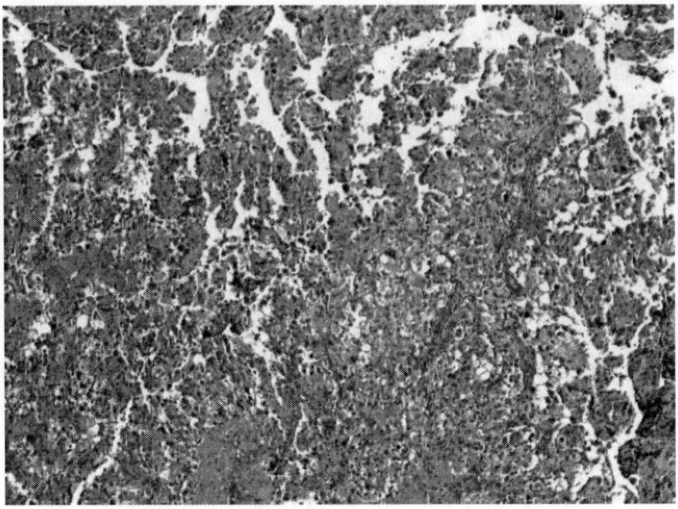

Figure 3. A lateral ventricular choroid plexus carcinoma (WHO grade 3) in a 1-year-old patient with Li-Fraumeni syndrome (hematoxylin and eosin, original magnification 100X).

Treatment and Prognosis

The treatment of neoplasms in the setting of LFS does not differ from sporadic ones. However, there is the caveat that LFS patients often develop secondary neoplasms due to radiation therapy and the risks and the benefits of this treatment modality should be discussed with the patient. The same holds true for CNS neoplasms where standard treatment protocols are followed. Various strategies to target a mutant p53 are being investigated [21] and some have reached the stage of clinical trials [22]. The extremely high lifetime risk of developing a malignant neoplasm drives the prognosis of LFS patients.

Conclusion

LFS is one of the most common tumor predispositions syndromes. Patients suspected to have the syndrome should be tested for TP53 variants, routinely and vigorously followed-up and genetic counseling should be provided for them and their relatives. The pathologist can contribute to identifying a LFS patient: p53- mutant choroid plexus carcinomas, diffuse astrocytomas with noncanonical IDH mutations are suggestive of the disorder and pediatric adrenocortical carcinoma is almost pathognomonic [23].

References

[1] Li F. P., Fraumeni J. F., Bethesda F. Soft-tissue sarcomas, breast cancer, and other neoplasms. A familial syndrome? *Ann Intern Med.* 1969;71(4):747–52.

[2] Duncan M. H. Another family with the Li-Fraumeni cancer syndrome. *JAMA J Am Med Assoc.* 1983 Jan 14;249(2):195–195.

[3] Birch J. M., Hartley A. L., Marsden H. B., et al., Excess risk of breast cancer in the mothers of children with soft tissue sarcomas. *Br J Cancer.* 1984;49(3):325–31.

[4] Pearson A. D. J., Craft A. W., Ratcliffe J. M., et al., Two families with the Li-Fraumeni cancer family syndrome. *J Med Genet.* 1982;19(5):362–5.

[5] Li F. P., Fraumeni J. F., Mulvihill J. J., et al., A cancer family syndrome in twenty-four kindreds. *Cancer Res.* 1988;48:5358–62.

[6] Lynch H. T., Mulcahy G. M., Harris R. E., et al., Genetic and pathologic findings in a kindred with hereditary sarcoma breast cancer, brain tumors, leukemia, lung, laryngeal, and adrenal cortical carcinoma. *Cancer.* 1978;41(5):2055–64.

[7] Malkin D., Li F. P., Strong L. C., et al., Germ line p53 mutations in a familial syndrome of breast cancer, sarcomas, and other neoplasms. *Science.* 1990;250.

[8] Srivastava S., Zou Z., Pirollo K., et al., Germ-line transmission of a mutated p53 gene in a cancer-prone family with Li-Fraumeni syndrome. *Nature.* 1990;348.

[9] Birch J. M., Hartley A. L., Tricker K. J., et al., Prevalence and diversity of constitutional mutations in the p53 gene among 21 Li-Fraumeni families. *Cancer Res.* 1994;54(March):1298–304.

[10] Lane D. P53, guardian of the genome. *Nature.* 1992;358(July):16.

[11] Eeles R. Germline mutations in the TP53 gene. *Cancer Surv.* 1995;25:101–24.

[12] Duffy M. J., Synnott N. C., Crown J. Mutant p53 as a target for cancer treatment. *Eur J Cancer.* 2017;83:258–65.

[13] Kratz C. P., Steinke-Lange V., Spier I., et al., Overview of the clinical features of Li-Fraumeni syndrome and the current European ERN GENTURIS Guideline. Vol. 82, *Geburtshilfe und Frauenheilkunde.* Georg Thieme Verlag; 2022. p. 42–9.

[14] Brat D. J. Solomon, D. A. Rosenblum, M. K. et al., WHO classification of tumours editorial board. Central nervous system tumours [Internet]. *WHO Classification of Tumours.* 5th ed. 2021.

[15] De Andrade K. C., Frone M. N., Wegman-Ostrosky T., et al., Variable population prevalence estimates of germline TP53 variants: A gnomAD-based analysis. *Hum Mutat.* 2019;40:97–105.

[16] César De Andrade K., Mirabello L., Stewart D. R., et al., Higher-than-expected population prevalence of potentially pathogenic germline TP53 variants in individuals unselected for cancer history. *Hum Mutat.* 2017;38(December):1723–30.

[17] Kumamoto T., Yamazaki F., Nakano Y., et al., Medical guidelines for Li-Fraumeni syndrome 2019, version 1.1. *Int J Clin Oncol*. 2021;26(12):2161–78.

[18] Frebourg T., Bajalica Lagercrantz S., Oliveira C., et al., Guidelines for the Li-Fraumeni and heritable TP53-related cancer syndromes. *Eur J Hum Genet*. 2020;28(10):1379–86.

[19] Watanabe T., Anne A. E., Ae V., et al., Selective acquisition of IDH1 R132C mutations in astrocytomas associated with Li-Fraumeni syndrome. *Acta Neuropathol*. 2009;117(June):653–6.

[20] Li M. M., Datto M., Duncavage E. J., et al., Standards and guidelines for the interpretation and reporting of sequence variants in cancer. *J Mol Diagnostics*. 2017;19(1):4–23.

[21] Hu J., Cao J., Topatana W., et al., Targeting mutant p53 for cancer therapy: direct and indirect strategies. *J Hematol Oncol* 2021 141. 2021 Sep 28;14(1):1–19.

[22] Levine A. J. Targeting The p53 protein for cancer therapies: the translational impact of p53 research. *Cancer Res*. 2022 Feb 2;82(3):362.

[23] Solomon D. A., Perry A. Familial tumor syndromes. In: Perry A, Brat DJ (editors) *Practical Surgical Neuropathology*. Elsevier. Philadelphia, PA. 2017. p. 531.

Chapter 8

Carney Complex: Nervous System Pathology

Maleeha F. Ahmad[1]
and Richard A. Prayson[2,*]**, MD, MEd**
[1] Cleveland Clinic Lerner College of Medicine, Cleveland, OH, USA
[2] Department of Anatomic Pathology, Cleveland Clinic, Cleveland, OH, USA

Abstract

Carney complex is a very rare multiple neoplasia and lentiginosis syndrome characterized primarily by cutaneous, endocrine, and cardiac manifestations. Although there is a high degree of phenotypic variability amongst patients, the most common features include spotty pigmentation, cutaneous myxomas, thyroid lesions, primary pigmented nodular adrenocortical disease, large cell-calcifying Sertoli cell tumors, and cardiac myxomas.

The main neuroclinical features of Carney complex are growth hormone (GH)-secreting pituitary neuroendocrine tumors (adenomas) and melanotic schwannomas. In the majority of cases, disease is caused by inactivating, heterozygous mutations of the *PRKAR1A* gene located on 17q24.2-24.3.

This chapter will review the genetics, clinical presentation, imaging findings, histopathologic features, treatment, and prognosis of Carney complex, with a primary focus on the nervous system-associated clinical and histopathologic findings.

---

* Corresponding Author's Email: praysor@ccf.org.

In: Central Nervous System Pathologies in Hereditary Tumor Syndromes
Editor: Richard A. Prayson
ISBN: 979-8-88697-620-5

Introduction

In 1985, Dr. J. Aiden Carney, a pathologist at the Mayo Clinic, and his team conducted a retrospective study to identify 40 patients with combinations of Cushing syndrome, cardiac myxoma, other myxoid tumors, and spotty skin pigmentation, a curious presentation of diverse lesions they believed could not be a coincidence- rather they must be pathogenetically related [1]. A year after the publication of their results, what they described as a "complex of myxomas, spotty pigmentation, and endocrine overactivity" came to be named "Carney Complex" (CNC) [2]. It should be noted that CNC is a distinct entity from two other diseases named after Dr. Carney: Carney triad and Carney-Stratakis syndrome. This chapter will review the clinical and pathologic features of CNC, with a particular focus on the neuropathologic findings.

Epidemiology

CNC is a rare disease with approximately 750 total patients of varying ethnicities described in the literature [3]. CNC has a female preponderance, as observed in the largest genotyped series of CNC patients to date, in which 221 of 353 total patients (63%) were female [4].

Genetics of Carney Complex

Approximately 70% of CNC cases are inherited in an autosomal-dominant manner ("familial") with virtually 100% penetrance, with the remainder occurring due to *de novo* gene mutations ("sporadic") [3, 5].

In the majority (73%) of CNC patients, disease is caused by inactivating, heterozygous mutations of the *PRKAR1A* gene, found at the CNC1 locus on chromosome 17q24.2-24.3 [3, 4, 6, 7]. The *PRKAR1A* gene codes for the cAMP-dependent protein kinase type I-alpha regulatory subunit, one of four regulatory subunits of protein kinase A, a cAMP-dependent protein kinase that plays a key role in many vital signal transduction pathways. Over 130 pathogenic mutations in *PRKAR1A* have been identified in 401 unrelated families with CNC, ranging from single-nucleotide substitutions, to small ($\leq$15 base pair) insertions and deletions, to large amplifications or deletions spanning the whole gene [3, 8].

Although the genetics underlying the majority of *PRKAR1A*-negative CNC cases remain unknown, linkage analysis studies have revealed the CNC2 locus to be associated with CNC in a subset of these patients. The particular gene within the CNC2 locus on chromosome 2p16 that underlies the CNC2 phenotype is yet unidentified [3]. Interestingly, Matyakhina et al. demonstrated that even in tumor samples from 26 CNC patients with *PRKAR1A* mutations, 21 (81%) also harbored amplifications or deletions in the CNC2 locus, suggesting a tumorigenic role for genes on 2p16 contributing to the CNC phenotype [9].

General Clinical Features

Clinical manifestations of CNC are numerous and typically develop over the course of many years. Therefore, diagnosis of CNC is rarely made at birth or during infancy, with a median age at diagnosis of 20 years [5]. Although the CNC phenotype varies greatly between patients and often even between individuals of the same kindred, the most common manifestations may be summarized as cutaneous, endocrine, and cardiac [10].

Skin lesions are typically the earliest presenting and most common feature of CNC. Lentigines (flat, small, brown to black macules) or "spotty pigmentation" typically appear during childhood, assume their characteristic density and distribution (lips, conjunctiva, inner or outer canthi, vaginal or penile mucosa) during the peripubertal period, and are present in up to 80% of CNC patients. Other frequently occurring cutaneous manifestations include blue nevi (40%), epithelioid blue nevi (20-50%), and cutaneous myxomas (30-50%), while café-au-lait spots, depigmented lesions, and Spitz nevi may occur rarely [3, 5, 8].

Endocrine pathologies observed in CNC patients include cystic or nodular thyroid disease (≤75%), thyroid adenomas (≤25%) and carcinomas (papillary or follicular type, ≤10%), large-cell calcifying Sertoli cell tumors (LCCSCT, 41%), ovarian cysts or tumors (20-67%), and pituitary neuroendocrine tumors (adenomas) (10-12%). Additionally, up to 75% of individuals with CNC may have asymptomatic elevations in growth hormone (GH), prolactin (PRL), or insulin-like growth factor 1 (IGF1) in the absence of a tumor detectable through imaging studies. Primary pigmented nodular adrenocortical disease (PPNAD) is diagnosed in 25-60% of CNC patients and may cause adrenocorticotrophic hormone (ACTH)-independent Cushing's syndrome if symptomatic (3).

Cardiac myxomas are benign tumors identified in 20-40% of CNC patients that can occur in any chamber and are often multiple and recurrent [3]. They may be complicated by systemic embolism, heart failure, and sudden death.

Given the highly variable clinical presentation amongst patients, diagnosis of CNC may be achieved based on several different diagnostic criteria. Diagnosis requires the presence of two *major* criteria, or one *major* criterion and one *supplementary* criterion [3, 8]. The major diagnostic criteria are: spotty skin pigmentation in the typical distribution; myxoma (cutaneous and mucosal); cardiac myxoma; breast myxomatosis or fat-suppressed magnetic resonance imaging (MRI) findings suggestive of this diagnosis; PPNAD or paradoxical positive response of urinary glucocorticoid excretion to dexamethasone administration during the Liddle test; acromegaly due to growth hormone-producing pituitary neuroendocrine tumor; LCCSCT or characteristic calcification on testicular ultrasound; thyroid carcinoma (at any age) or multiple, hypoechoic nodules on thyroid ultrasound (in a prepubertal patient); psammomatous melanotic schwannoma; blue nevus, epithelioid blue nevus (multiple); breast ductal adenoma (multiple); and osteochondromyxoma. The supplementary criteria are an affected first-degree relative, or inactivating mutation of the *PRKAR1A* gene. All the aforementioned tumors require histologic confirmation for diagnosis of CNC.

Neurologic Clinical Features

The principle neurologic manifestations that may be found in CNC patients are pituitary neuroendocrine tumors and melanotic schwannomas [11].

GH-secreting pituitary neuroendocrine tumors with associated, slow-progressing acromegaly develop in 10-12% of CNC patients, typically emerge starting in the third decade of life, and likely contribute to the growth of cardiac myxomas in these cases [3, 12, 13]. Prolactinomas [14, 15] and corticotropinomas [16, 17] have also been reported in rare instances.

Melanotic schwannoma, recently renamed "malignant melanotic nerve sheath tumor" (MMNST), is a rare pigmented neural tumor that occurs in 8-10% of CNC patients [3]. They develop at an earlier age in CNC patients (mean of 22.5 years) as compared to individuals without CNC (mean of 33.2 years) [18]. Although these tumors may occur anywhere in the central or peripheral nervous system, they most commonly appear in the gastrointestinal tract (esophagus, stomach, liver, rectum), followed by the paraspinal sympathetic chain, and then the chest wall [3, 19].

Symptoms relate to the specific location and growth rate of the tumor, potentially affecting autonomic or other neurologic functions or causing mass effect [20]. For example, spinal tumors tend to present themselves with pain and radiculopathy. Malignancy occurs in up to 10% of affected patients and metastases classically spread to the liver, lung, and brain with poor prognosis [3, 8, 18].

Imaging Findings

Although the majority of CNC patients (up to 75%) have asymptomatic elevations in GH, PRL, or IGF1, pituitary imaging in these cases is normal. GH-secreting pituitary neuroendocrine tumors (pituitary adenomas) only develop in 10-12% of patients [3, 21]. As is the case for acromegaly in general, most CNC patients with acromegaly have pituitary "*macro*adenomas" - although "*micro*adenomas" have also been reported- that do not differ appreciably from their sporadic counterparts in terms of MRI findings [11, 22].

Symptoms suggestive of MMNST may necessitate brain, spine, chest, abdominal (retroperitoneal), and/or pelvic imaging for tumor detection [3, 5, 20]. On computed tomography (CT) images, MMNST typically appear as a well-circumscribed, hyperdense mass that may contain calcifications. In general, MRI findings of MMNST are similar to those of conventional schwannomas, with the exception that MMNST typically exhibit T1-weighted hyperintensity and T2-weighted hypointensity due to intracellular storage of melanin, while conventional schwannomas appear hypointense on T1-weighted sequences and hyperintense on T2-weighted sequences [23, 24].

MMNST of the gastrointestinal tract often presents with non-specific abdominal symptoms or is discovered incidentally upon imaging and should be differentiated from gastrointestinal stromal tumor (GIST), the most common mesenchymal tumor. Contrary to MMNST, GIST rarely show calcification on CT and present with T1 hypointensity and T2 hyperintensity on MRI [25]. MMNST of the spine typically appear on CT or MRI as "dumbbell" shaped soft-tissue tumors with possible bone erosion, reactive osteosclerosis, and enlargement of intravertebral foramina. Spinal canal stenosis or cord displacement due to potential mass effect may be noted [26].

MMNST of the chest wall may involve adjacent ribs and appear on radiograph as calcified soft tissue masses with osteosclerotic or osteolytic lesions [26].

Neuropathologic Findings

The histopathologic findings of the CNC-associated neurologic tumors (pituitary neuroendocrine tumors and MMNST) are similar to those of their sporadic counterparts and are summarized here [11, 19].

Although very rare cases of prolactinomas and corticotropinomas have been described in CNC [14, 16, 17], almost all CNC-associated pituitary tumors are GH-producing neoplasms. Excised pituitary tissue often demonstrates the presence of multiple tumors in the gland, indicating multicentricity [27]. These tumors may involve a monomorphic (Figure 1) or pleomorphic proliferation of tumor cells [22, 28].

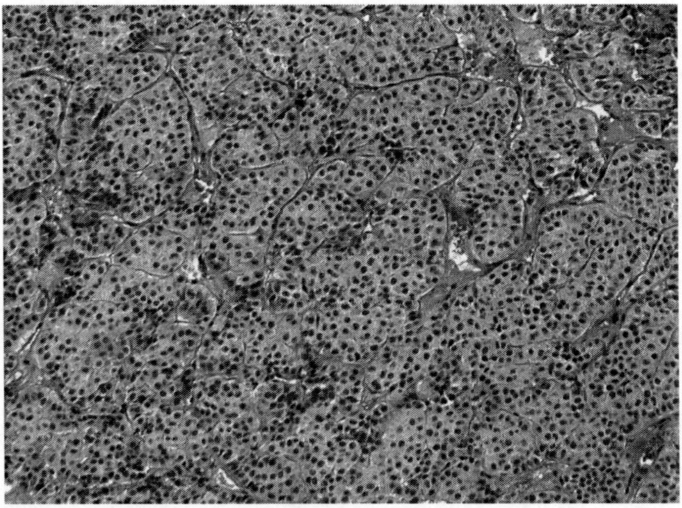

Figure 1. This pituitary neuroendocrine tumor (pituitary adenoma) is marked by a monomorphic proliferation of tumor cells. The tumor was associated with an elevated growth hormone level in the patient (hematoxylin and eosin, original magnification 200X).

Extratumoral pituitary parenchyma typically demonstrates somatomammotroph (GH- and PRL-producing cells) hyperplasia and has been conjectured by some to represent a precursor of frank tumor development that explains the biochemical abnormalities in GH and PRL secretion noted in many CNC patients without concurrent evidence of a pituitary tumor on imaging [21, 27]. Pituitary neuroendocrine tumor tissue and hyperplastic areas typically both stain positively for GH and PRL, while these regions may occasionally exhibit immunoreactivity for α-subunit, thyroid stimulating hormone (TSH) β-subunit, and luteinizing hormone (LH). Only non-tumoral cells entrapped within the tumor or hyperplastic areas have been shown to stain for ACTH and follicle-stimulating hormone (FSH) [21, 27]. Ultrastructural evaluation of the secretory granules within GH-producing adenomas from three CNC patients has revealed that these tumors can be phenotypically bi-hormonal (somatomammotrophic) and/or mono-hormonal (lactotrophic or somato-trophic), although they have similar clinical presentations and endocrine profiles [22, 29].

On gross examination, MMNSTs are typically solitary and ovoid, partially or completely encapsulated by a thin fibrous membrane, black-brown to gray-blue in appearance on their cut surfaces, and may contain areas of necrosis and hemorrhage [30]. The syncytial quality of the tumor derives from the fascicular or sheet-like growth pattern of the spindled or polygonal (epithelioid) cells and ill-defined cytoplasmic borders. MMNSTs are marked by abundant melanin pigment (Figure 2) that varies throughout the tumor, presenting either in coarse clumps or finely granular patterns.

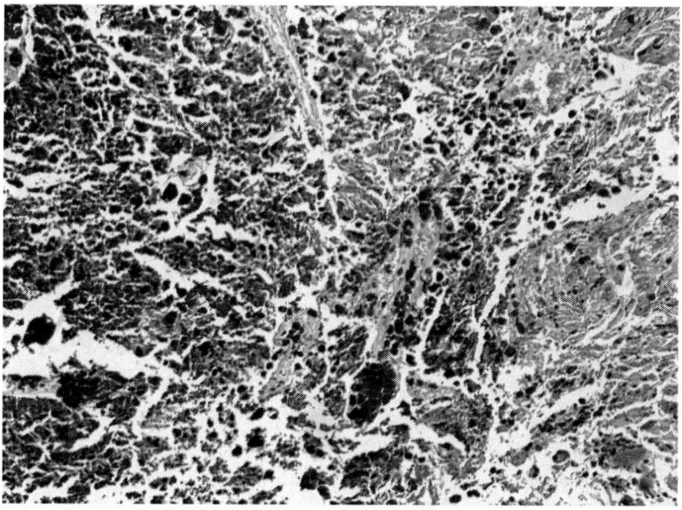

Figure 2. This 39-year-old woman with Carney complex presented with a sacral mass, seen here, marked by abundant melanin pigment in this schwannoma, diagnosed as an epithelioid MMNST (hematoxylin and eosin, original magnification 100X).

Nuclei may display intranuclear pseudoinclusions; the nuclear: cytoplasmic ratio of tumor cells is high, and nucleoli are often prominent [18, 31]. Two variants of MMNST have been identified- nonpsammomatous and psammomatous- and extensive sampling is sometimes needed to locate psammoma bodies [18]. Although both variants have been associated with CNC and their clinical behavior, histopathologic features (apart from presence or absence of psammoma bodies), immunohistochemical profile, and gene expression have been found to be essentially identical, psammomatous MMNST is the variant classically described in CNC [18, 32].

The main differential diagnostic considerations for MMNST include conventional schwannomas, metastatic melanoma, and melanocytomas. MMNST may be differentiated from conventional schwannomas based on the presence of psammoma bodies; adipose tissue; melanin pigment; positive staining for melanosome markers such as HMB-45, Melan-A, and tyrosinase; and premelanosomes and melanosomes seen in ultrastructural evaluation [11, 18]. Features of primary MMNST that aid in its differentiation from metastatic melanoma include: psammomatous calcifications, syncytial arrangement of cells, and lesser degree of nuclear atypia or mitotic activity than in metastatic melanoma [11, 18]. The presence of a pericellular basement membrane, which can be identified using collagen IV and laminin stains, differentiates MMNST from melanocytomas [11]. Finally, loss of expression of PRKAR1A is not a feature of melanoma, conventional schwannoma, nor melanocytoma, and may therefore be used to distinguish MMNST from these other tumors [18].

Treatment and Prognosis

Manifestations of CNC are each treated individually, given no systemic treatment exists. Cardiac myxomas are surgically removed and often require repeat operations due to tumor recurrence. Bilateral adrenalectomy is the preferred treatment for Cushing's syndrome due to PPNAD. Transsphenoidal surgical removal is preferred for pituitary neuroendocrine tumors, although medical treatment with somatostatin analogues or GH-receptor antagonists is offered if surgical treatment is insufficient or for patients without a detectable tumor. Removal of MMNST is ideal, but recurrence is common and those located in the paraspinal region are often inoperable due to entrapment of nerve roots. Once metastatic, there is no effective treatment [3, 8].

Complications of cardiac myxomas, including pulmonary and brain emboli, post-operative cardiomyopathy or arrhythmias, or sudden death due to valvular occlusion account for greater than half of the disease-associated mortality in CNC patients. Metastatic MMNST, other metastatic cancers (e.g., pancreatic), and non-cardiac post-operative complications are additional common causes of death in CNC patients [3, 11]. Although, historically, the average life span for CNC patients has been 50-55 years, normal life expectancy may be achieved with regular surveillance. Suggested routine studies include, but are not limited to, annual echocardiogram for detection of cardiac myxoma; regular skin exams; endocrine evaluations, as appropriate, including serum GH and PRL levels and urinary free cortisol; and appropriate imaging studies, which may include thyroid and testicular ultrasounds, computed tomography of the adrenals, and magnetic resonance imaging for detection of MMNST [3].

Conclusion

On gross examination, MMNSTs are typically solitary and ovoid, partially or completely encapsulated by a thin fibrous membrane, black-brown to gray-blue in appearance on their cut surfaces, and may contain areas of necrosis and hemorrhage [30]. The syncytial quality of the tumor derives from the fascicular or sheet-like growth pattern of the spindled or polygonal (epithelioid) cells and ill-defined cytoplasmic borders. MMNSTs are marked by abundant melanin pigment (Figure 2) that varies throughout the tumor, presenting either in coarse clumps or finely granular patterns.

References

[1] Carney JA, Gordon H, Carpenter PC, et al. The complex of myxomas, spotty pigmentation, and endocrine overactivity. *Medicine.* 1985; 64(4):270–283.

[2] Bain J. "Carney's Complex". *Mayo Clin Proc.* 1986. 61(6):508.

[3] Correa R, Salpea P, Stratakis CA. Carney complex: an update. *Eur J Endocrinol.* 2015; 173(4):M85-M97.

[4] Bertherat J, Horvath A, Groussin L, et al. Mutations in regulatory subunit type 1A of cyclic adenosine 5'-monophosphate-dependent protein kinase *(PRKAR1A)*: phenotype analysis in 353 patients and 80 different genotypes. *J Clin Endocrinol Metab.* 2009; 94(6):2085-2091.

[5] Stratakis CA, Kirschner LS, Carney JA. Clinical and molecular features of the Carney complex: diagnostic criteria and recommendations for patient evaluation. *J Clin Endocrinol Metab.* 2001; 86(9):4041-4046.

[6] Kirschner LS, Carney JA, Pack SD, et al. Mutations of the gene encoding the protein kinase A type 1-alpha regulatory subunit in patients with the Carney complex. *Nat Genet*. 2000; 26(1):89-92.

[7] Casey M, Vaughan CJ, He J, et al. Mutations in the protein kinase A R1alpha regulatory subunit cause familial cardiac myxomas and Carney complex. *J Clin Invest*. 2000; 106(5): R31-38. Erratum in: *J Clin Invest*. 2001; 107(2):235.

[8] Bouys L, Bertherat J. Management of endocrine disease: Carney complex: clinical and genetic update 20 years after the identification of the CNC1 (*PRKAR1A*) gene. *Eur J Endocrinol*. 2021; 184(3):R99-R109.

[9] Matyakhina L, Pack S, Kirschner LS, et al. Chromosome 2 (2p16) abnormalities in Carney complex tumours. *J Med Genet*. 2003; 40(4):268-277.

[10] Bertherat J. Carney complex (CNC). *Orphanet J Rare Dis*. 2006; 1(21).

[11] Solomon DA, Perry A. Familial Tumor Syndromes: Carney Complex. In: Perry A, Brat DJ, editors. *Practical Surgical Neuropathology: A Diagnostic Approach*. 2nd edition. Philadelphia, PA: Elsevier. 2018; 505-545.

[12] Marques P, Korbonits M. Pituitary Dysfunction in Systemic Disorders. In: Melmed S, editor. *The Pituitary*. 5th edition. Cambridge, MA: Academic Press. 2022; 385-412.

[13] Melmed S. Pituitary Masses and Tumors. In: Melmed S, Auchus RJ, Goldfine AB, Koenig RJ, & Rosen CJ. editors. *Williams Textbook of Endocrinology*. 14th edition. Philadelphia, PA: Elsevier. 2020; 236-302.

[14] Handley J, Carson D, Sloan J, et al. Multiple lentigines, myxoid tumors and endocrine overactivity; four cases of Carney's complex. *Br J Dermatol*. 1992; 126(4):367-371.

[15] Espiard S, Bertherat J. Carney complex. *Front Horm Res*. 2013; 41:50-62.

[16] Hernandez-Ramirez LC, Tatsi C, Lodish MB, et al. Corticotropinoma as a component of Carney complex. *J Endocr Soc*. 2017; 1(7): 918-925.

[17] Kiefer FW, Winhofer Y, Iacovazzo D, et al. *PRKAR1A* mutation causing pituitary-dependent Cushing disease in a patient with Carney complex. *Eur J Endocrinol*. 2017; 177(2):K7-K12.

[18] Goldblum JR, Folpe AL, Weiss SW. Soft Tissue Tumors Showing Melanocytic Differentiation. In: Goldblum JR, Folpe AL, Weiss SW, editors. *Enzinger and Weiss's Soft Tissue Tumors*. 7th edition. Philadelphia, PA: Elsevier. 2020;1009-1051.

[19] Legius E, Folpe AL, Jo VY, et al. Genetic tumour syndromes involving the CNS: Carney Complex. In: *WHO Classification of Tumours* Editors Board, editors. *WHO Classification of Tumours, Volume 6*: Central Nervous System Tumours. 5th edition. Lyon, France: International Agency for Research on Cancer. 2021;462-463.

[20] Stergiopoulos SG, Stratakis CA. Human tumors associated with Carney complex and germline *PRKAR1A* mutations: a protein kinase A disease! *FEBS Lett*. 2003; 546(1):59-64.

[21] Kirschner LS. *PRKAR1A* and the evolution of pituitary tumors. *Mol Cell Endocrinol*. 2010; 326(1-2):3-7.

[22] Stergiopoulos SG, Abu-Asab MS, Tsokos M, et al. Pituitary pathology in Carney complex patients. *Pituitary*. 2004; 7(2):73-82.

[23] Collart J, Vandeponseele M, Bosschaert P. Intracranial melanotic schwannomas: rare and distinctive tumors to know due to their risk of recurrence and metastases. *J Belg Soc Radiol*. 2018; 102(1):15.

[24] Solomou G, Silva AHD, Wong A, et al. Extramedullary malignant melanotic schwannoma of the spine: Case report and an up to date systematic review of the literature. *Ann Med Surg*. 2020; 59:217-223.

[25] Lin KY, Chen L, Hung SW, et al. A para-aortic malignant melanotic nerve sheath tumor mimicking a gastrointestinal tumor: a rare case report and review of literature. *BMC Surg*. 2022; 22(1):293.

[26] Courcoutsakis NA, Tatsi C, Patronas NJ, et al. The complex of myxomas, spotty skin pigmentation and endocrine overactivity (Carney complex): imaging findings with clinical and pathological correlation. 2013; 4(1):119-133.

[27] Pack SD, Kirschner LS, Pak E, et al. Genetic and histologic studies of somatomammotropic pituitary tumors in patients with the "complex of spotty skin pigmentation, myxomas, endocrine overactivity and schwannomas" (Carney complex). *J Clin Endocrinol Metab*. 2000; 85(10):3860-3865.

[28] Bossis I, Voutetakis A, Matyakhina L, et al. A pleomorphic GH pituitary adenoma from a Carney complex patient displays universal allelic loss at the protein kinase A regulatory subunit 1A (*PRKAR1A)* locus. *J Med Genet.* 2004; 41:596-600.

[29] Kurtkaya-Yapicier O, Scheithauer BW, Carney JA, et al. Pituitary adenoma in Carney complex: an immunohistochemical, ultrastructural, and immunoelectron microscopic study. *Ultrastruct Pathol.* 2002; 26(6):345-353.

[30] Shanmugam S, Ghosh M, Niamathullah S, et al. Psammomatous melanotic schwannoma as a component of Carney complex. *Ind J Pathol Microbiol.* 2015; 58(3):368-370.

[31] Ellison D, Love S, Chimelli L, et al. Peripheral nerve sheath neoplasms. In: Ellison D, Love S, Chimelli L, et al, editors. *Neuropathology: A Reference Text of CNS Pathology.* 3rd edition. Maryland Heights, MO: Mosby. 2013; 797-804.

[32] Torres-Mora J, Dry S, Li Xinmin, et al. Malignant melanotic schwannian tumor: a clinicopathologic, immunohistochemical, and gene expression profiling study of 40 cases, with a proposal for the reclassification of "melanotic schwannoma." *Am J Surg. Pathol.* 2014; 38(1):94-105.

Chapter 9

Lynch Syndrome: Central Nervous System Pathology

Surabhi Tewari[1]
and Richard A. Prayson[2,*], MD, MEd
[1] Cleveland Clinic Lerner College of Medicine, Cleveland, Ohio, USA
[2] Department of Anatomic Pathology, Cleveland Clinic, Cleveland, Ohio, USA

Abstract

Lynch syndrome, previously referred to as hereditary nonpolyposis colorectal cancer, is characterized primarily by colorectal and endometrial cancers. Germline mutations in mismatch repair proteins *MLH1*, *MSH2*, *MSH6*, and *PMS2* result in microsatellite instability and increased risk for malignancies, including several extra-colonic malignancies.

Lynch syndrome confers a four-fold increase in the lifetime risk for neurologic cancers, especially high-grade astrocytoma (glioblastoma). Similar to sporadic neurologic cancers, the prognosis for Lynch syndrome associated neurologic malignancies is poor. However, the true biologic behavior of Lynch syndrome associated glioblastoma is challenging to characterize and distinguish from sporadic cases given their overall low prevalence and high mortality.

This chapter will review the clinicopathologic features of Lynch syndrome, highlighting central nervous system associated pathology.

* Corresponding Author's Email: praysor@ccf.org.

In: Central Nervous System Pathologies in Hereditary Tumor Syndromes
Editor: Richard A. Prayson
ISBN: 979-8-88697-620-5

Introduction

Dr. Aldred Scott Warthin described the first cancer family in 1913, family G, by following the morbidity and mortality of his wife's seamstress's family; this seamstress disclosed her fear of dying from cancer due to her family history, and Warthin published the family's unique pedigree that demonstrated a disproportionate number of uterine and gastric cancers [1]. The natural history of family G was again updated in 1925 by Warthin, in 1936 by Weller and Hauser, and finally in 1971 by Dr. Henry T. Lynch [1, 2]. Lynch cataloged six generations of family G, gathering over 600 descendants of the family to highlight the apparent autosomal dominant inheritance within the family [3].

With limited knowledge about the biologic basis of this heterogenous cancer syndrome, challenges grew in both naming the disease and accurately identifying affected families [3]. The name "hereditary nonpolyposis colorectal cancer" (HNPCC) was coined by Lynch in 1985 to group these patients with young onset of colorectal cancer without the prolific polyposis seen in familial adenomatous polyposis (FAP) syndrome. However, the name HNPCC failed to represent the extracolonic manifestations of the disease. It was not until the discovery of microsatellite instability (MSI), the identification of DNA mismatch repair (MMR) complex genes, and the clarifying diagnostic criteria at the Bethesda conferences that Lynch syndrome was appropriately defined as the hereditary inactivation in the DNA MMR system that create a high risk for cancer [3].

In this chapter, the clinical and pathologic features of Lynch syndrome will be outlined with a special focus on the neuropathologic findings that have been described in this syndrome.

Genetics

Lynch syndrome is linked to mutations in MMR proteins *MLH1*, *MSH2*, *MSH6*, and *PMS2*. These mutations result in a significant increase in frequency of insertion or deletion mutations in simple repeat or microsatellite sequences [4, 5]. Lynch syndrome is caused by a heritable mutation in one copy of the MMR gene and a secondary, somatic loss of the corresponding normal allele [5]. This is distinct from constitutional mismatch repair deficiency syndrome (CMMRD), which is characterized by homozygous or compound heterozygous germline mutations in one of the four MMR genes, resulting in childhood neurologic and hematologic malignancies as well as gastrointestinal polyposis [6-8].

Much of Lynch syndrome is driven by mutations in *MLH1* and *MSH2*, both of which are essential MMR complex components. About 10-30% of the remaining cases are due to mutations in *MSH6* and *PMS2*, whereas CMMRD is predominantly due to mutations in *MSH6* and *PMS2* [4, 5, 9]. *MLH1/PMS2* and *MSH2/MSH6* form functional pairs, and loss of *MLH1* or *MSH2* will destabilize the respective partner proteins. However, the loss of *MSH6* or *PMS2* will not result in the loss of their respective partner proteins [10]. With regard to neurologic cancers, several reports suggest that *MSH2* mutations confer a higher risk than the other MMR genes, but the true genetic characteristics of Lynch related neurologic malignancies are likely limited by their rarity, young age of onset, and high mortality [11-15]. 3% of Lynch syndrome is also due to mutations in *EPCAM*, which is upstream of *MSH2* and is implicated in epithelial cell adhesion, cell signaling, and proliferation; mutations in the 3' end of *EPCAM* result in epigenetic hypermethylation of the *MSH2* promoter, resulting in Lynch syndrome [5, 16].

General Clinical Features

A diagnosis of Lynch syndrome requires proper knowledge of its associated tumors and a complete family history, especially with regard to early-onset cancers in first- and second-degree relatives. The current clinical criteria to identify patients with Lynch syndrome follow The Revised Bethesda Guidelines:

1) Colorectal cancer (CRC) in a patient under 50 years of age
2) Synchronous or metachronous CRC or other Lynch syndrome associated tumors (LASTs) regardless of age
3) CRC with MSI-high histology under 60 years of age
4) CRC or LSAT diagnosed at an age less than 50 years in a first degree relative
5) CRC or LSAT diagnosed in two first- or second-degree relatives at any age.

These LSATs include endometrial, stomach, ovarian, pancreas, ureter or renal pelvis, biliary tract, small bowel, and brain tumors [17, 18]. Those who develop cutaneous malignancies such as sebaceous gland adenomas and keratoacanthomas along with at least one visceral LSAT are considered to have Muir–Torre syndrome, a rare variant of Lynch syndrome that has been linked to mutations in *MLH1*, *MSH2*, and *MSH6* [19].

A definitive diagnosis of Lynch syndrome is made by the identification of a deleterious mutation in one of the MMR genes by evaluation of tumor tissue for deficient MMR proteins via immunohistochemistry or testing for MSI via polymerase chain reaction. Identification of MMR deficiency indicates need for germline testing [17, 20]. Lynch syndrome is classically associated with CRC, endometrial cancer, and ovarian cancer. The cumulative risk of CRC due to all MMR protein mutations is 42% by age 70 years, although this risk is markedly lower for those with MSH6 mutations (18%) in comparison to MLH1 (49%) or MSH2 (52%) mutations. As such, colonoscopy is recommended every 1 to 2 years starting at 20 to 25 years of age or 2 to 5 years before the earliest CRC diagnosis in a first- or second-degree relative. However, carriers of *MSH6* or *PMS2* mutations can begin colonoscopies at 30 and 35 years of age, respectively [20].

The lifetime risk of endometrial (40-60%) and ovarian cancers (10-12%) also varies by mutation type, but both carry a significantly elevated risk in comparison to the general population [21]. There is evidence to suggest that prophylactic hysterectomy and bilateral salpingo-oophorectomy (BSO) in patients with Lynch effectively reduces the risk of endometrial and ovarian cancer [22, 23]. Current National Comprehensive Cancer Network (NCCN) guidelines recommend individualized timing for hysterectomy based upon individual desires regarding childbearing, comorbidities, family history, and type of mutation. Similar recommendations exist for ovarian cancer risk reduction, but unlike recommendations for hysterectomy, BSO is not recommended for *MSH6* and *PMS2* mutant carriers given insufficient evidence of elevated cancer risk in comparison to the general population [21, 24].

With regard to other LSATs, there is insufficient evidence to suggest increased surveillance due to their relatively low lifetime risk of around 1-4% in spite of their elevated risks in comparison to the general population [18, 21].

Neurologic Clinical and Imaging Features

In the general population, the lifetime risk for primary brain cancers is relatively low at around 0.3-0.6% with a median age of diagnosis around 60 years [18]. The majority of these cases are glioblastoma and astrocytoma.

Patients with Lynch syndrome have a four-fold increase in primary brain cancer development in comparison to the general population with a much lower median age of diagnosis between 25-38 years of age, and the primary risk is development of glioblastoma, although lower grade astrocytoma, low grade glioma, meningioma, acoustic schwannoma, and neuroblastoma have also been reported [11, 14-15, 25-27]. Isolated case reports have also identified tumors of the sellar region associated with Lynch syndrome [26, 28-30]. CMMRD is also associated with glioblastoma formation but is differentiated from Lynch syndrome by both childhood onset of disease and concurrent café-au-lait macules, which are present in 90% of cases with CMMRD [9].

A study using the Danish HNPCC registry found that *MLH1* and MSH6 mutations confer a lower risk of brain tumors in comparison to *MSH2* mutations [26, 31]. The association between brain tumors and CRC is coined Turcot's syndrome. Turcot's syndrome type I is a subtype of Lynch syndrome, as it arises from MMR gene mutations and it is typically associated with gliomas and astrocytomas. Turcot's syndrome type II, on the other hand, is associated with *APC* gene mutations and generally results in medulloblastomas along with familial adenomatous polyposis [32]. Patients with Muir-Torre syndrome also have been shown to develop glioblastoma [33].

The clinical presentation of glioblastoma and other Lynch syndrome related neurologic cancers do not differ from their sporadic counterparts, including symptoms of increased intracranial pressure, seizures, or focal neurologic deficits [34]. There is no association between Lynch syndrome and other neurologic conditions such as epilepsy, learning disabilities, or cerebrovascular disease [15,26]. Neurologic imaging findings also do not differ between Lynch associated neurologic tumors and their sporadic counterparts, generally occurring in the supratentorial region with rim or heterogenous ring enhancement and perilesional edema [35].

Neuropathologic Findings

As seen in their sporadic counterparts, Lynch syndrome associated glioblastoma demonstrates hypercellularity and nuclear atypia (Figure 1); giant cells are more common in Lynch syndrome associated glioblastoma [36]. Necrosis as well as significant mitotic activity and microvascular proliferation are also classically seen on histopathology (Figure 2).

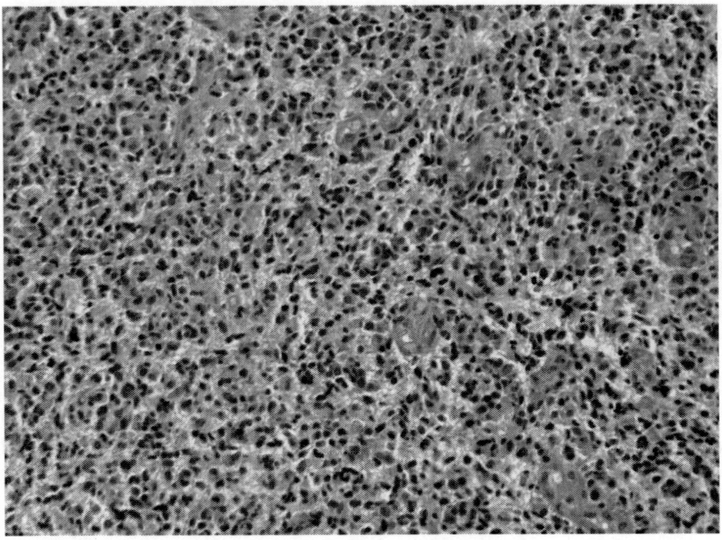

Figure 1. High grade astrocytoma marked by prominent cellularity in a patient with Lynch syndrome (hematoxylin and eosin, original magnification 200X).

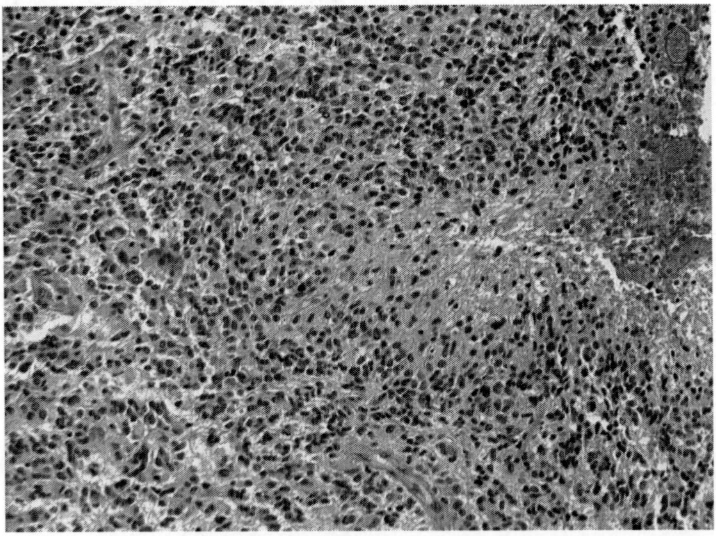

Figure 2. Same tumor as in Figure 1 with focal necrosis (right), consistent with a glioblastoma, WHO grade 4 (hematoxylin and eosin, original magnification 200X).

Malignant gliomas that arise in Lynch syndrome are more circumscribed than sporadic glioblastoma, which may lead to increased likelihood of surgical resection and debulking. In a study characterizing 13 Lynch syndrome associated neurologic tumors, 100% of tumors demonstrated loss of MMR proteins via immunohistochemistry and had correlating germline MMR gene mutations, indicating that immunohistochemistry is sufficient to identify MMR deficiency in brain tumors [10].

Treatment and Prognosis

The true prognosis of patients with Lynch syndrome associated astrocytomas and other is difficult to characterize given the relatively lower age of diagnosis and overall high mortality from glioblastoma, which many of the lesions end up being [15, 18]. Lynch associated glioblastoma may be vastly underreported as those with young-onset glioblastoma likely do not live long enough to develop additional LSATs, may not undergo genetic testing, and may not have children. The prognosis of Lynch syndrome associated glioblastoma and their sporadic counterparts do not differ significantly, but it is unknown if the biologic behavior of MMR deficient brain tumors confers differential survival [10]. Larger scale studies with robust, prospective data are needed to better characterize outcomes in this population.

There are interesting new insights in the treatment of Lynch associated glioblastoma. The treatment paradigm for glioblastoma often includes the alkylating agent temozolomide (TMZ), but some reports indicate that MMR deficiency results in TMZ-resistance [37, 38]. Given the association of Lynch syndrome with MSI-high and high tumor mutational burden, it is hypothesized that these tumors may be more responsive to immunotherapy due to a high production of neoantigens, but prospective studies are needed [10, 39].

Conclusion

Lynch syndrome is a rare disorder marked by germline mutations involving a variety of mismatch repair genes which result in microsatellite instability and an increased risk of developing colorectal and endometrial carcinomas. In the central nervous system, a subset of patients appear to be at risk for developing high grade astrocytomas, that morphotically resemble glioblastomas which arise outside this setting. The overall prognosis of such high grade gliomas in this setting is poor but more studies with more cases need to be done to get a better sense of the true biologic behavior of gliomas arising in this setting.

References

[1] Douglas, J. A., Gruber, S. B., Meister, K. A., et al. (2005). History and molecular genetics of Lynch syndrome in Family G: a century later. *JAMA.*, 294(17), 2195. doi: 10.1001/jama.294.17.2195.

[2] Boland, C. R., and Lynch, H. T. (2013). The history of Lynch syndrome. *Fam Cancer.*, 12(2), 145-157. doi: 10.1007/s10689-013-9637-8.

[3] Boland, C. R. (2005). Evolution of the nomenclature for the hereditary colorectal cancer syndromes. *Fam Cancer.*, 4(3), 211-218. doi:10.1007/s10689-004-4489-x.

[4] Li, G. M. (2008). Mechanisms and functions of DNA mismatch repair. *Cell Research.*, 18(1), 85-98. doi: 10.1038/cr.2007.115.

[5] Cohen, S. A., and Leininger, A. (2014). The genetic basis of Lynch syndrome and its implications for clinical practice and risk management. *Appl Clin Genet.*, 7, 147-158. doi: 10.2147/TACG.S51483.

[6] Hegde, M. R., Chong, B., Blazo, M. E., et al. (2005). A homozygous mutation in MSH6 causes Turcot syndrome. *Clin Cancer Res.*, 11(13), 4689-4693. doi: 10.1158/1078-0432.CCR-04-2025.

[7] Tan, T. Y., Orme, L. M., Lynch, E., et al. (2008). Biallelic PMS2 mutations and a distinctive childhood cancer syndrome. *J Pediatr Hematol Oncol.*, 30(3), 254-257. doi: 10.1097/MPH.0b013e318161aa20.

[8] Krüger, S., Kinzel, M., Walldorf, C., et al. (2008). Homozygous PMS2 germline mutations in two families with early-onset haematological malignancy, brain tumours, HNPCC-associated tumours, and signs of neurofibromatosis type 1. *Eur J Hum Genet.*, 16(1), 62-72. doi: 10.1038/sj.ejhg.5201923.

[9] Aronson, M., Colas, C., Shuen, A., et al. (2022). Diagnostic criteria for constitutional mismatch repair deficiency (CMMRD): recommendations from the international consensus working group. *J Med Genet.*, 59(4), 318-327. doi: 10.1136/jmedgenet-2020-107627.

[10] Kim, H., Lim, K. Y., Park, J. W., et al. (2022). Sporadic and Lynch syndrome-associated mismatch repair-deficient brain tumors. *Lab Invest.*, 102(2), 160-171. doi: 10.1038/s41374-021-00694-3.

[11] Gylling, A. H. S., Nieminen, T. T., Abdel-Rahman, W. M., et al. (2008). Differential cancer predisposition in Lynch syndrome: insights from molecular analysis of brain and urinary tract tumors. *Carcinogenesis.*, 29(7), 1351-1359. doi: 10.1093/carcin/bgn133.

[12] Barrow, E., Robinson, L., Alduaij, W., et al. (2009). Cumulative lifetime incidence of extracolonic cancers in Lynch syndrome: a report of 121 families with proven mutations. *Clin Genet.*, 75(2), 141-149. doi: 10.1111/j.1399-0004.2008.01125.x.

[13] Vasen, H. F., Stormorken, A., Menko, F. H., et al. (2001). MSH2 mutation carriers are at higher risk of cancer than MLH1 mutation carriers: a study of hereditary nonpolyposis colorectal cancer families. *J Clin Oncol.*, 19(20), 4074-4080. doi: 10.1200/JCO.2001.19.20.4074.

[14] Watson, P., and Lynch, H. T. (1993). Extracolonic cancer in hereditary nonpolyposis colorectal cancer. *Cancer.*, 71(3), 677-685. doi: 10.1002/1097-0142(19930201)71: 3<677::aid-cncr2820710305>3.0.co; 2-#.

[15] Watson, P., Vasen, H. F. A., Mecklin, J. P., et al. (2008). The risk of extra-colonic, extra-endometrial cancer in the Lynch syndrome. *Int J Cancer.*, 123(2), 444-449. doi: 10.1002/ijc.23508.

[16] Ligtenberg, M. J. L., Kuiper, R. P., Chan, T. L., et al. (2009). Heritable somatic methylation and inactivation of MSH2 in families with Lynch syndrome due to deletion of the 3′ exons of TACSTD1. *Nat Genet.*, 41(1), 112-117. doi: 10.1038/ng.283.

[17] Lynch, H. T., Snyder, C. L., Shaw, T. G, et al. (2015). Milestones of Lynch syndrome: 1895-2015. *Nat Rev Cancer.*, 15(3), 181-194. doi: 10.1038/nrc3878.

[18] Bansidhar, B. J. (2012). Extracolonic manifestations of Lynch syndrome. *Clin Colon Rectal Surg.*, 25(2), 103-110. doi: 10.1055/s-0032-1313781.

[19] South, C. D., Hampel, H., Comeras, I., et al. (2008). The frequency of Muir-Torre syndrome among Lynch syndrome families. *J Natl Cancer Inst.*, 100(4), 277-281. doi: 10.1093/jnci/djm291.

[20] Sinicrope, F. A. (2018). Lynch syndrome-associated colorectal cancer. *N Engl J Med.*, 379(8), 764-773. doi: 10.1056/NEJMcp1714533.

[21] Bonadona, V., Bonaïti, B., Olschwang, S., et al. (2011). Cancer risks associated with germline mutations in MLH1, MSH2, and MSH6 genes in Lynch syndrome. *JAMA.*, 305(22), 2304-2310. doi: 10.1001/jama.2011.743.

[22] Schmeler, K. M., Lynch, H. T., Chen, L., et al. (2006). Prophylactic surgery to reduce the risk of gynecologic cancers in the Lynch syndrome. *N Engl J Med.*, 354(3), 261-269. doi: 10.1056/NEJMoa052627.

[23] Chen, L., Yang, K. Y., Little, S. E., et al. (2007). Gynecologic cancer prevention in Lynch syndrome/hereditary nonpolyposis colorectal cancer families. *Obstet Gynecol.*, 110(1), 18-25. doi: 10.1097/01.AOG.0000267500.27329.85.

[24] Genetic/familial high-risk assessment: colorectal. Published online June 8, 2022. Accessed September 29, 2022. https://www.nccn.org/professionals/physician_gls/pdf/genetics_colon.pdf.

[25] Vasen, H. F., Sanders, E. A., Taal, B. G., et al. (1996). The risk of brain tumours in hereditary non-polyposis colorectal cancer (HNPCC). *Int J Cancer.*, 65(4), 422-425. doi: 10.1002/(SICI)1097-0215(19960208)65: 4<422::AID-IJC4>3.0.CO; 2-Z.

[26] Therkildsen, C., Ladelund, S., Rambech, E., et al. (2015). Glioblastomas, astrocytomas and oligodendrogliomas linked to Lynch syndrome. *Eur J Neurol.*, 22(4), 717-724. doi: 10.1111/ene.12647.

[27] Aarnio, M., Sankila, R., Pukkala, E., et al. (1999). Cancer risk in mutation carriers of DNA-mismatch-repair genes. *Int J Cancer.*, 81(2), 214-218. doi: 10.1002/(sici)1097-0215(19990412)81: 2<214::aid-ijc8>3.0.co; 2-l.

[28] Teuber, J., Reinhardt, A., Reuss, D., et al. (2021). Aggressive pituitary adenoma in the context of Lynch syndrome: a case report and literature review on this rare coincidence. *Br J Neurosurg*. Published online August 25, 1-6. doi: 10.1080/02688697.2021.1967881.

[29] Bengtsson, D., Joost, P., Aravidis, C., et al. (2017). Corticotroph pituitary carcinoma in a patient with Lynch syndrome (LS) and pituitary tumors in a nationwide LS cohort. *J Clin Endocrinol. Metab*., 102(11), 3928-3932. doi: 10.1210/jc.2017-01401.

[30] Voisin, M. R., Almeida, J. P., Perez-Ordonez, B., et al. (2019). Recurrent undifferentiated carcinoma of the sella in a patient with Lynch syndrome. *World Neurosurg*., 132, 219-222. doi: 10.1016/j.wneu.2019.08.180.

[31] Lucci-Cordisco, E., Zito, I., Gensini, F., et al. (2003). Hereditary nonpolyposis colorectal cancer and related conditions. *Am J Med Genet A*., 122A(4), 325-334. doi: 10.1002/ajmg.a.20475.

[32] Galiatsatos, P., and Foulkes, W. D. (2006). Familial adenomatous polyposis. *Am J Gastroenterol*., 101(2), 385-398. doi: 10.1111/j.1572-0241.2006.00375.x.

[33] Binder, Z. A., Johnson, M. W., Joshi, A., et al. (2011). Glioblastoma multiforme in the Muir-Torre syndrome. *Clin Neurol Neurosurg*., 113(5), 411-415. doi: 10.1016/j.clineuro.2010.12.011.

[34] McKinnon, C., Nandhabalan, M., and Murray, S. A., et al. (2021). Glioblastoma: clinical presentation, diagnosis, and management. *BMJ*., 374, n1560. doi: 10.1136/bmj.n1560.

[35] Ideguchi, M., Kajiwara, K., Goto, H., et al. (2015). MRI findings and pathological features in early-stage glioblastoma. *J Neurooncol*., 123(2), 289-297. doi: 10.1007/s11060-015-1797-y.

[36] Lusis, E. A., Travers, S., Jost, S. C., et al. (2010). Glioblastomas with giant cell and sarcomatous features in patients with Turcot syndrome type 1: a clinicopathological study of 3 cases. *Neurosurgery*., 67(3), 811-817, discussion 817. doi: 10.1227/01.NEU.0000375513.12925.5C.

[37] Higuchi, F., Nagashima, H., Ning, J., et al. (2020). Restoration of temozolomide sensitivity by PARP Inhibitors in mismatch repair deficient glioblastoma is independent of base excision repair. *Clin Cancer Res*., 26(7), 1690-1699. doi: 10.1158/1078-0432.CCR-19-2000.

[38] Goenka, A., Tiek, D., Song, X., et al. (2021). The many facets of therapy resistance and tumor recurrence in glioblastoma. *Cells*., 10(3), 484. doi: 10.3390/cells10030484.

[39] Le, D. T., Uram, J. N., Wang, H., et al. (2015). PD-1 blockade in tumors with mismatch-repair deficiency. *N Engl J Med*., 372(26), 2509-2520. doi: 10.1056/NEJMoa1500596.

Chapter 10

Familial Retinoblastoma: Central Nervous System Pathology

Suzie Kim[1], BS
and Richard A. Prayson[2,*], MD, MEd

[1] Cleveland Clinic Lerner College of Medicine, Cleveland, Ohio, USA
[2] Department of Anatomic Pathology, Cleveland Clinic, Cleveland, Ohio, USA

Abstract

Retinoblastoma is a malignancy that arises from the retina and is the most common childhood eye cancer. Patients generally present in infancy with leukocoria. Some hereditary cases may be characterized as trilateral retinoblastoma, in which retinoblastoma is accompanied by a primary neuroectodermal tumor that is most commonly a pineoblastoma. The study of retinoblastoma led to the first discovered tumor suppressor gene, *RB1*, and thus paved the way for development of Knudson's two-hit hypothesis. Germline mutations of *RB1* result in familial retinoblastoma which is inherited in an autosomal dominant fashion. Imaging and histopathology will characteristically demonstrate an intraocular tumor with calcifications. While it is generally a curable malignancy in the setting of early screening and detection, trilateral disease is often fatal.

This chapter will review the presentation and diagnosis of familial retinoblastoma and trilateral retinoblastoma with an emphasis on neuropathologic findings common in these conditions.

---

* Corresponding Author's Email: praysor@ccf.org.

In: Central Nervous System Pathologies in Hereditary Tumor Syndromes
Editor: Richard A. Prayson
ISBN: 979-8-88697-620-5

Introduction

Retinoblastoma is a rare intraocular malignancy that arises from retinal tissue and commonly presents during childhood [1–3]. Similar tumors have been described since the 16th century, with the first description of leukocoria as "cat's eyes in the dark" being recorded by Hayes in 1767. The term "retinoblastoma" was first developed in 1922 by Verhoeff due to its resemblance with the embryologic retina on pathology, and this was soon adopted by the American Ophthalmological Society in 1926 [4]. A hereditary mechanism for retinoblastoma, or familial retinoblastoma, was observed in 1971 by Alfred Knudson, who found that these patients developed intraocular tumors bilaterally rather than unilaterally [1, 4]. Hereditary cases are estimated to make up approximately 55% of cases of retinoblastoma and are more commonly bilateral [1].

Trilateral retinoblastoma was first characterized in 1971 in a case report by Meur et al., that described a syndrome consisting of familial retinoblastoma and a brain tumor composed of neuroectodermal tissue [5]. This was then distinguished from metastatic malignancy in 1977 by Jakobiec et al., who determined that these tumors were histologically distinct, establishing the cerebral tumor to be of primary origin [6, 7].

This chapter will provide a general overview of the genetics, clinical features, and histologic findings of familial retinoblastoma and trilateral retinoblastoma.

Genetics of Familial Retinoblastoma

Retinoblastoma results from the loss or mutation of both alleles of the tumor suppressor gene *RB1* which is found on chromosome 13q1.4. This was the first tumor suppressor gene–and the first genetic etiology for malignancy–that was identified [1]. Understanding of this gene resulted in Knudson's two-hit hypothesis, which proposed that the cancer must be caused by mutation of both tumor suppressor genes [8]. *RB1* encodes the protein RB, which serves its role as a tumor suppressor by regulating the G1-S transition of the cell cycle and inhibiting uncontrolled cellular differentiation [9].

Patients with familial retinoblastoma are more likely to develop retinoblastoma and other associated malignancies due to germinal inactivations of an *RB1* allele, necessitating only one additional somatic mutation in order for the cancer to develop. This is inherited in an autosomal dominant fashion with a high degree of penetrance at approximately 90% [1, 3, 10], and these children will develop the tumor bilaterally in 85% of cases [11].

Clinical Features

Retinoblastoma is a childhood cancer, with a median age of diagnosis of two years. It may initially present with leukocoria, which is a white pupillary reflex in contrast to a normal red reflex. Retinoblastoma may also present with strabismus, or misalignment of the eyes. More rarely, retinoblastoma may present with other ocular signs such as hypopyon, glaucoma, exophthalmia, and iris rubeosis, while other cases may be completely asymptomatic [1, 3].

Familial retinoblastoma may present with extra-ocular manifestations and other primary tumors, such as osteosarcomas, melanomas, and soft tissue sarcomas, for which risk may be increased due to not only genetic predisposition but from radiotherapy treatment as well [3].

Trilateral retinoblastoma additionally presents with tumors derived from the primitive neuroectoderm, most commonly with a pineoblastoma or another tumor located in the supra, and parasellar regions of the brain [3, 7, 12]. According to a 2014 meta-analysis, age of diagnosis for pineal trilateral retinoblastoma is generally much later than cases with non-pineal trilateral retinoblastoma, with a mean age of 31 months compared to ten months [12]. The cerebral tumors of trilateral retinoblastoma may present with signs of intracranial hypertension such as headache, lethargy and vomiting, with some cases potentially causing upward gaze palsy. Symptoms related to spinal cord metastasis may subsequently develop, resulting in various defects in sensation and/or motor control [13, 14].

Imaging Findings

Retinoblastoma may be diagnosed and monitored with a wide array of ophthalmic and neuroradiologic imaging. It is generally diagnosed initially on fundoscopy and ocular ultrasonography (US), which can determine numerous important characteristics of the retinoblastoma such as tumor size, location, and extent of seeding into other compartments of the eye [15].

The imaging modality that can best evaluate the extent of local tumor growth is magnetic resonance imaging (MRI) [1, 16]. On high-resolution contrast-enhanced MRI, retinoblastomas will appear irregular in contour and on T1-weighted images are hyperintense in signal relative to the vitreous. They enhance heterogeneously with gadolinium and may demonstrate calcifications, which are present in 95% of cases. Evaluation of retinoblastoma with computed tomography (CT) has fallen out of favor due to the high sensitivity and specificity of utilizing US and MRI for diagnosis [16].

MRI is also useful for evaluation of trilateral retinoblastoma, especially in cases of familial retinoblastoma where suspicion may be higher for an additional cerebral tumor [15, 17]. Baseline brain imaging upon initial diagnosis of retinoblastoma to assess for a primitive neuroectodermal tumor, particularly in the pineal gland, may facilitate earlier detection and potentially increase chance of survival. Such tumors frequently present similarly to retinoblastoma on MRI as enhancing, predominantly solid masses [16, 17].

Neuropathologic Findings

Gross pathology after eye enucleation will demonstrate a white tumor with an encephaloid appearance with chalky areas of calcification and yellow areas of necrosis [18–20]. On histopathologic evaluation, retinoblastoma demonstrates sheets and nests of small, round hyperchromatic cells (Figure 1).

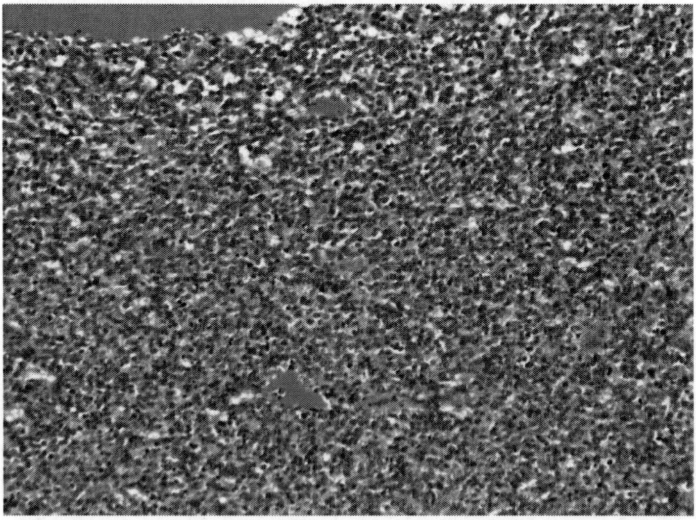

Figure 1. A retinoblastoma marked by a sheet of small embryonal-like cells with scattered apoptotic cells (hematoxylin and eosin, original magnification 200X).

These cells generally have a high nuclear to cytoplasm ratio with irregular basophilic nuclei and prominent mitotic activity [18, 19]. Dystrophic calcification is a common finding in retinoblastoma and areas of necrosis are also frequently seen (Figure 2 [20]).

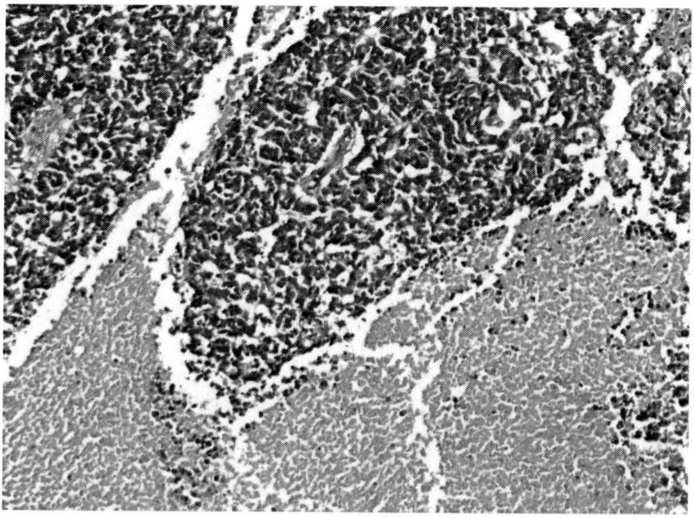

Figure 2. Geographic area of necrosis in retinoblastoma (hematoxylin and eosin, original magnification 200X).

The level of retinal differentiation in retinoblastomas may be distinguished by the category of rosette encountered: Homer Wright rosettes represent primitive neuroblastic cells, Flexner-Wintersteiner rosettes represent early retinal differentiation (Figure 3), and fleurettes are indicative of photoreceptor differentiation and the most advanced stage (Figure 4). High-risk features on histology include invasion of the optic nerve, choroid, or anterior segment or extension of the tumor beyond the sclera [19].

Retinoblastomas may have either endophytic or exophytic growth patterns. They are more commonly endophytic, in which the tumor remains attached to the inner retinal layers and grows into the vitreous [16, 19]. In contrast, tumors with exophytic growth originate from the outer retinal layers and grow posteriorly into the subretinal space, potentially resulting in retinal detachment [16, 19, 20].

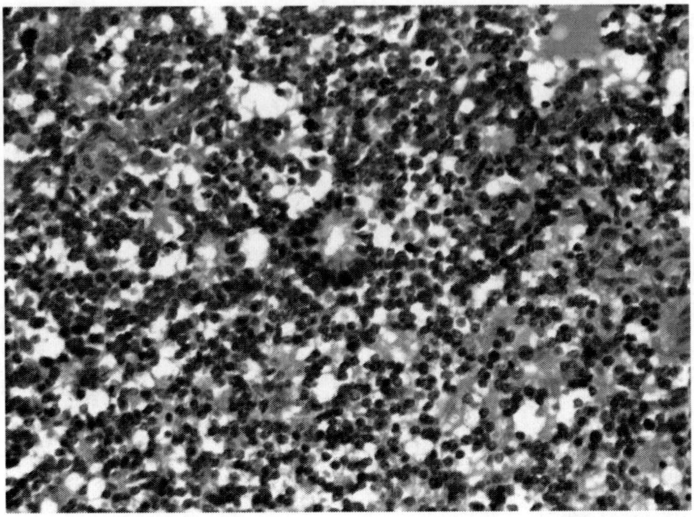

Figure 3. Flexner-Wintersteiner rosette marked by tumor cells arranged around a central space (true rosette) (hematoxylin and eosin, original magnification 400X).

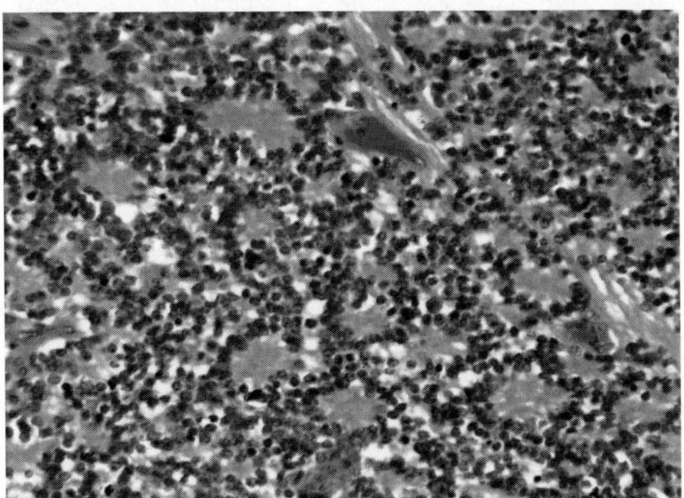

Figure 4. Several fleurettes, evidence of photoreceptor differentiation, are seen here and are marked by central cytoplasmic projections surrounded by tumor cell nuclei (hematoxylin and eosin, original magnification 400X).

Trilateral retinoblastomas will resemble retinoblastomas on histologic findings but do not represent metastasis [6, 7, 12]. Meta-analysis by Marcus and colleagues found that the majority (61.5%) of cases were undifferentiated primitive neuroectodermal tumors on central nervous system histopathology while the remaining had varying degrees of either photoreceptor or neuronal differentiation [21].

Diagnostic Criteria and Differential Diagnosis

A diagnosis of retinoblastoma is made via fundoscopic exam, which reveals one or more intraocular tumors, and ultrasound, which will classically show calcifications as described above [15]. Genetic counseling is recommended for patients with a confirmed diagnosis of retinoblastoma to evaluate for germline RB1 mutations, especially if features suggestive of genetic predisposition are present (e.g., young age of diagnosis, syndromic presentation) [1].

Further evaluation after diagnosis will determine the tumor stage and thus guide clinical management. The first classification scheme for retinoblastoma was the Reese-Ellsworth classification system, which aimed to predict success of external beam radiotherapy in salvaging the eye. However, due to the introduction of chemotherapy as a new treatment for this malignancy, this has since been replaced by the International Intraocular Retinoblastoma Classification (IIRC) system and the Intraocular Classification of Retinoblastoma (ICRB) [22, 23]. These systems categorize retinoblastoma into five groups from A to E which describe increasing high risk features such as increasing tumor size and increased extent of tumor seeding. Classification according to the ICRB may predict the probability of saving the eye with intravenous chemotherapy: while Group E eyes must be enucleated, Group D retinoblastoma can be treated with successful salvage in approximately half of cases while Groups A through C may result in successful salvage in over 90% of cases [22].

The differential diagnosis for retinoblastoma includes Coats disease, a disorder of retinal vascularization; infection such as that of *Toxocara canis*; persistent hyperplastic primary vitreous; and other hereditary disorders such as tuberous sclerosis and von Hippel-Lindau syndrome. Such conditions may resemble atypical retinoblastoma due to the presence of abnormal retinal vascularization or exudates [1, 3]. Additionally, trilateral retinoblastoma must be differentiated from a pineal cyst, a benign finding that may be incidental on MRI in children [16].

Treatment and Prognosis

If retinoblastoma is detected early and is contained within the eye, it is largely a curable malignancy. After staging, potential treatment options include a wide range of modalities including cryotherapy, local intra-arterial chemotherapy, systemic intravenous chemotherapy, enucleation of the eye, and in cases of microscopically incomplete resection, external beam radiation [1, 3, 24]. Bilateral retinoblastoma may be managed initially with neoadjuvant chemotherapy with a combination of cytotoxic drugs (e.g., carboplatin, etoposide) to better enable conservative treatment thereafter. Such treatment with local and systemic chemotherapy has been demonstrated to be highly effective in salvaging the eye and preventing the need for enucleation [1, 25]. Close follow-up with monthly fundoscopy under anesthesia is recommended after treatment, and MRI is recommended for detection of trilateral retinoblastoma in bilateral cases [1].

Though retinoblastoma will result in death if left untreated, the prognosis of retinoblastoma in developed countries is excellent, as the cure rate is approximately 95% [1, 2]. In contrast, trilateral retinoblastoma is often fatal with a median survival after diagnosis of less than 12 months despite treatment and a 5-year survival of 22% [12, 14, 26]. Rate of survival may increase with earlier detection and intensive treatment with chemotherapy prior to dissemination of the disease [7, 27].

Conclusion

Familial retinoblastoma syndrome is an autosomal dominant condition marked by germline mutations in the RB1 gene on chromosome 13q. In addition to the development of retinoblastomas of the eye, a subset of patients with trilateral retinoblastoma may additionally develop a pineoblastoma.

References

[1] Aerts I. Retinoblastoma. *Orphanet Journal of Rare Diseases*. 2006; 1:31.

[2] Dimaras H. Retinoblastoma. *Nature Reviews Disease Primers*. 2015; 1(1): 1–23.

[3] Lohmann D R. Retinoblastoma. In: Adam MP, Mirzaa G M, Pagon R A, Wallace S E, Bean L J, Gripp K W, Amemiya A, editors. *GeneReviews®*. Seattle (WA): University of Washington, Seattle. 1993.

[4] Alzahem T. History and Genetics of Retinoblastoma. In: *Alkatan H, editors. Retinoblastoma - Past, Present, and Future*. London: IntechOpen. 2019; 3-16.

[5] Meur G. Retinal tumor and cerebral tumor: a case. *Bulletin De La Societe Belge D'ophtalmologie*. 1971; 159: 661–670.

[6] Jakobiec FA. Retinoblastoma and intracranial malignancy. *Cancer*. 1977; 39(5): 2048–2058.

[7] Kivelä T. Trilateral retinoblastoma: a meta-analysis of hereditary retinoblastoma associated with primary ectopic intracranial retinoblastoma. *J. Clin. Oncol.* 1999; 17(6): 1829–1829.

[8] Knudson AG. Mutation and cancer: statistical study of retinoblastoma. *Proc. Nat. Acad. Sci. USA*. 1971; 68(4): 820–823.

[9] Otterson G A. Incomplete penetrance of familial retinoblastoma linked to germ-line mutations that result in partial loss of RB function. *Proc. Nat. Acad. Sci. USA*. 1997; 94(22): 12036–12040.

[10] Naumova A. The genetics of retinoblastoma, revisited. *Am. J. Hum. Genetics*. 1994; 54(2): 264–273.

[11] Abramson D H. Familial retinoblastoma, where and when? *Acta Ophthalmol. Scand.* 1998; 76(3): 334–338.

[12] de Jong M C. Trilateral retinoblastoma: a systematic review and meta-analysis. *Lancet Oncol.* 2014; 15(10): 1157–1167.

[13] De Potter P. Clinical variations of trilateral retinoblastoma: a report of 13 cases. *J. Pediatr. Ophthalmol. Strabismus*. 1994; 31(1): 26–31.

[14] Holladay D A. Clinical presentation, treatment, and outcome of trilateral retinoblastoma. *Cancer*. 1991; 67(3): 710–715.

[15] de Graaf P. Guidelines for imaging retinoblastoma: imaging principles and MRI standardization. *Pediatr. Radiol.* 2012; 42(1): 2–14.

[16] Silvera V M. Retinoblastoma: What the neuroradiologist needs to know. *Am. J. Neuroradiol.* 2021; 42(4): 618-626.

[17] Rodjan F. Trilateral retinoblastoma: neuroimaging characteristics and value of routine brain screening on admission. *J. Neuro-Oncol.* 2012; 109(3): 535–544.

[18] Singh L. Update on pathology of retinoblastoma. *Int. J. Ophthalmol.* 2018; 11(12): 2011–2016.

[19] Alsharif H. Histopathological Characteristics and Classification for Prognostic Indicators. In: Alkatan H, editor. *Retinoblastoma - Past, Present, and Future.* London: IntechOpen. 2019; 89-106.

[20] Eagle R C. The pathology of ocular cancer. *Eye*. 2013; 27(2): 128–136.

[21] Marcus D M. Trilateral retinoblastoma: insights into histogenesis and management. *Surv. Ophthalmol.* 1998; 43(1): 59–70.

[22] Fabian I D. The management of retinoblastoma. *Oncogene*. 2018; 37(12): 1551–1560.

[23] Shields C L. Diagnosis and management of retinoblastoma. *Cancer Cont.* 2004; 11(5): 317–327.

[24] Wyse E. A review of the literature for intra-arterial chemotherapy used to treat retinoblastoma. *Pediatr. Radiol.* 2016; 46(9): 1223–1233.

[25] Francis J H. Current treatment of bilateral retinoblastoma: the impact of intraarterial and intravitreous chemotherapy. *Neoplasia*. 2018; 20(8): 757–763.

[26] Provenzale JM. Trilateral retinoblastoma: clinical and radiologic progression. *Am. J. Roentgenol.* 2004; 183(2): 505–511.

[27] Wright K D. Successful treatment of early detected trilateral retinoblastoma using standard infant brain tumor therapy. *Pediatr Blood Cancer*. 2010; 55(3): 570–572.

Chapter 11

Fanconi Anemia: A Neuropathologic Perspective

Joshua L. Tidd[1]
Samantha J. Stallkamp Tidd[2]
and Richard A. Prayson[3], MD, MEd

[1] Northeast Ohio Medical University, Rootstown, OH, USA
[2] Cleveland Clinic Lerner College of Medicine, Cleveland, OH, USA
[3] Department of Anatomic Pathology, Cleveland Clinic, USA

Abstract

Fanconi anemia is a clinically heterogeneous disorder which results in clinical manifestations in all organ systems due to genetic instability. Patients with Fanconi anemia have deficits in homologous recombination and repair of DNA crosslinking due to germline mutations in the FANC genes. Clinical features include growth retardation, abnormal thumbs, absent radii, café-au-lait spots, progressive bone marrow failure, increased cancer risk, triangular facies, microcephaly, abnormal kidneys, and decreased fertility. Fanconi anemia can occur in patients without these diagnostic clues, resulting in remarkable phenotypic variability, partially explained by genetic heterogeneity.

Genetic instability in Fanconi anemia contributes to tumorigenesis, including medulloblastoma. Biallelic variants of BRCA2 or PALB2 most significantly predispose to medulloblastoma. Anaplastic/large cell subtypes of medulloblastoma are frequently found in Fanconi anemia.

This chapter presents a review of Fanconi anemia's clinical presentation, genetics, neural manifestations, and histopathology.

In: Central Nervous System Pathologies in Hereditary Tumor Syndromes
Editor: Richard A. Prayson
ISBN: 979-8-88697-620-5

Introduction

Guido Fanconi was first to describe Fanconi anemia (FA); in 1927, he published a case report in which he discovered that a trio of siblings had aplastic anemia and other congenital defects such as brown skin pigmentation and microcephaly [1–4]. As other scientists described similar cases, they were puzzled by the great variety in presentation. Fanconi realized that these patients had a singular disease which presented with a wide range of hematologic and physical abnormalities [4]. By 1964, as others at the time suggested that these patients had an autosomal recessive disorder due to a single gene, Guido Fanconi published a hypothesis, suggesting that FA was caused by chromosomal translocation [2, 5]. Shortly thereafter, scientists were able to uncover the true etiology of the FA: chromosomal instability [2, 6–8]. In this chapter, we will review FA and its broad clinical presentation, genetic etiology and consequences, and neuropathologic manifestations.

Genetics of Fanconi Anemia

FA occurs in approximately 1 in 100,000 to 360,0000 births [9, 10]. Patients with FA have deficits in homologous recombination repair of double-strand breaks and DNA crosslinking due to germline mutations in at least 22 FANC genes, named FANCA to FANCW [11, 12]. FA is usually inherited in an autosomal recessive pattern, although exceptions exist, depending on the underlying gene. Patients with complementation group B (FANCB) and complementation group R (RAD51) demonstrate X-linked and autosomal dominant inheritance patterns, respectively [13, 14].

Fanconi syndrome is diagnosed with chromosome breakage analysis, a test where defective homologous recombination results in hypersensitivity to alkylating agents such as diepoxybutane (DEB) and mitomycin c (MMC) [15–17]. Patients should also undergo next-generation sequencing to identify the specific mutations to ensure adequate genetic counseling [18].

General Clinical Features

Classic clinical features of FA include bone marrow failure, acute myelocytic leukemia, myelodysplasia, solid tumors, growth retardation, abnormal thumbs, absent radii, café-au-lait spots, increased cancer risk, triangular facies, microcephaly, abnormal kidneys, and decreased fertility [19–22]. The risk of cancer development increases with age, as damage to DNA accumulates [23]. In patients with FANCD1/BRCA2, a severe mutation, the cumulative risk of cancer is as high as 97% by the age of 7 years [22].

FA can occur in patients without these diagnostic clues, resulting in remarkable phenotypic variability, partially explained by genetic heterogeneity [24]. The presence of unilateral congenital abnormalities, such as absent radii, suggests that FANC gene mutations do not directly result in developmental defects but rather the mutation greatly increases the odds of defects occurring [24]. Mutations in FANCA, FANCC, and FANCG make up 90% of the mutations of FA and are more associated with the classic presentation [25].

As many as one third of FA patients lack congenital malformations, adding to the difficulty in making an early diagnosis. Of these patients without congenital abnormities, most are diagnosed after they develop hematologic manifestations, or a sibling is affected [26]. Patients who have heterozygous FA mutations are usually considered asymptomatic carriers. However, FANCS (BRCA1) and FANCD1 (BRCA2) heterozygous mutations will increase the risk of ovarian, breast and other cancers in the family members of FA patients [27].

Neurologic Clinical Manifestations

The great variability in presentation of FA extends to the central nervous system. Medulloblastoma makes up 25% of pediatric central nervous system (CNS) tumors in general and is the predominant CNS tumor arising in the setting of FA [20, 28–34]. Medulloblastoma is more likely to occur in patients with two inherited copies of BRCA2 or PALB2, which consequentially also results in a greatly increased risk of childhood malignancy [29, 35, 36]. In one study, 25 cases of brain tumor were found in 71 patients with the FANCD1 (BRCA2) and 7 cases of brain tumor were found in 16 patients with the FANCN (PALB2) mutation. Medulloblastoma was the most common brain tumor, accounting for 21 of the cases [37]. Occasionally, FA patients may present with clinical sequalae of medulloblastoma, as the first recognized symptoms [38]. Patients with FA are also susceptible to other CNS tumors, including astrocytoma [25, 39, 40].

Besides symptoms associated with a space-occupying brain lesion, patients can have other neurologic findings including Arnold Chiari malformation, absent corpus callosum, pituitary abnormalities, Bell's palsy, hearing loss, and hyperreflexia [24, 41, 42].

Patients with FA are associated with unique features on imaging. On imaging, patients are more likely to have pituitary, corpus callosum and posterior fossa abnormalities [42, 43]. Pituitary height may possibly vary between different complementation groups [42]. Ectopic neurohypophysis is also a unique feature seen on magnetic resonance imaging (MRI) in FA [42].

Neuropathologic Findings

Medulloblastoma can be classified on a molecular or histopathologic basis. The World Health Organization (WHO) classification currently divides molecularly defined medulloblastomas (grade 4) into four groups:

(1) WNT-activated
(2) SHH-activated and TP53-wildtype
(3) SHH-activated and TP53-mutant
(4) Non-WNT/non-SHH (44).

A number of histopathologic variants of medulloblastoma can be encountered, including classic, desmoplastic/nodular, medulloblastoma with extensive nodularity (MBEN), and anaplastic/large cell types. (Figure 1) [44]. Medulloblastomas due to mutations in PALB2 and BRCA2 are more commonly seen into molecular groups 2, 3 and 4 [31]. Anaplastic/large cell, desmoplastic, and classic, subtypes of medulloblastoma have all been reported on as well [34, 35].

As previously mentioned, FA are also susceptible to other CNS tumors, including astrocytoma [25, 39, 40]. Morphologically, there is nothing different in the fibrillary astrocytomas encountered in this setting versus those encountered outside the setting of FA (Figures 2 and 3). In patients without FA, there is increased expression of the FA pathway in patients with high grade astrocytoma, and FANCD2 is more likely to be expressed in higher grade tumors [45].

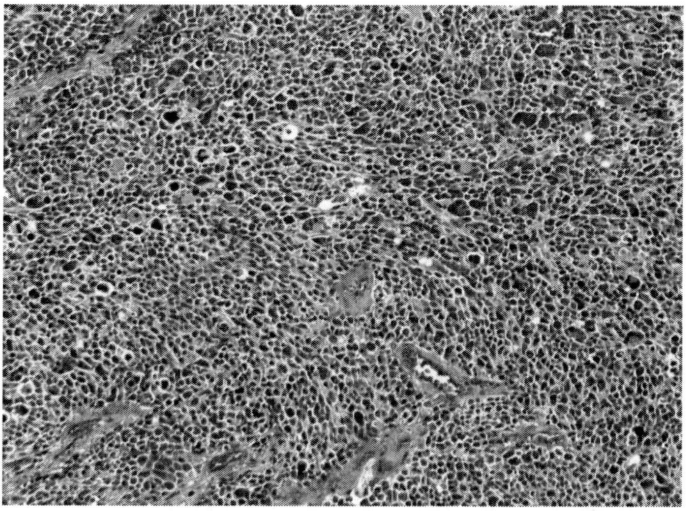

Figure 1. Fanconi anemia patient with a large cell/anaplastic medulloblastoma marked by prominent cellularity, mitotic figures and nuclear pleomorphism (hematoxylin and eosin, original magnification 200X).

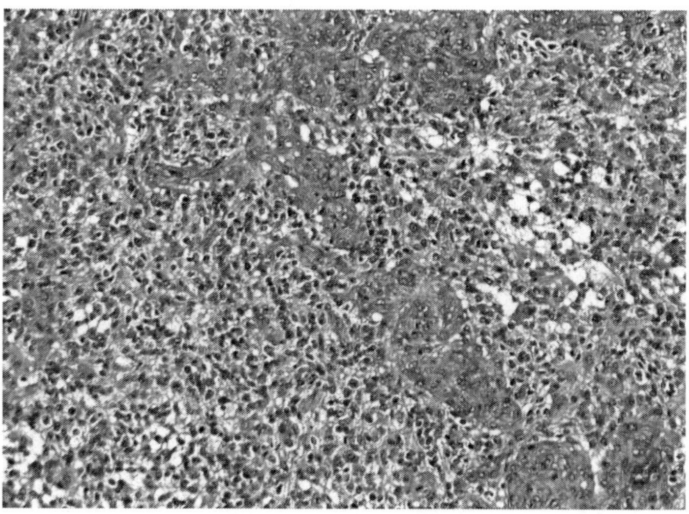

Figure 2. Patient with Fanconi anemia and a glioblastoma (IDH-1 wild-type) marked by prominent cellularity, mitotic figures and vascular proliferation (hematoxylin and eosin, original magnification 200X).

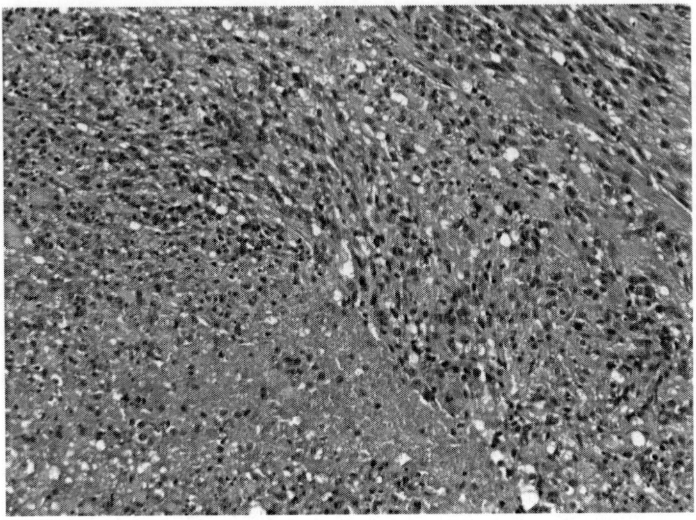

Figure 3. Same tumor (glioblastoma) as in Figure 1 with focal necrosis (lower left corner of the field) (hematoxylin and eosin, original magnification 200X).

Treatment and Prognosis

In general, treatment of FA is difficult due to the variable clinical manifestations and therefore, treatment is focused to the patient's unique symptomology. It is commonly focused on bone marrow failure, transplantation, and androgen supplementation. Patients should undergo routine cancer surveillance and prevention, including regular full skin examinations and human papillomavirus (HPV) vaccination. Due to increased sensitivity to chemotherapy, and radiation, patients may require a dose reduction when treating malignancy. All patients with congenital malformations characteristic of FA or myelodysplastic syndrome with complex cytogenetic changes should have their blood tested for cross-linking hypersensitivity. In addition, all siblings of FA patients should be screened [24].

Medulloblastoma in the setting of FA involves treatment with resection of the tumor when possible, radiation therapy, and chemotherapy [28, 30, 34, 38]. Although patients with FANCD1 may have hypersensitivity to DNA crosslinking agents, such as platinum-based drugs, cyclophosphamide, and anthracyclines, some patients may be treated without dose reduction.

Furthermore, toxicity to chemotherapy may vary among patients with FA, even within the same family [34].

For medulloblastoma patients in general, patients with desmoplastic/ nodular histology appear to have a slightly better prognosis than those with classic morphology and patients with large cell/anaplastic histology have a worse prognosis [46]. In regard to molecular classification, medulloblastomas in molecular subgroups 1 and 2 have better prognosis compared to groups 3 and 4 [47].

Conclusion

Fanconi anemia is marked by abnormalities in homologous recombination and repair of DNA crosslinking due to germline mutations in the FANC gene. Most cases have an autosomal recessive pattern of inheritance. Patients with Fanconi anemia are predisposed to the development of medulloblastomas (WHO grade 4) in the brain, particularly anaplastic and large cell variants.

References

[1] Akkari Y, Olson S. Fanconi anemia: a decade of discoveries. *J Assoc Genet Technol.* 2004;30(2):48–53.

[2] Lobitz S, Velleuer E. Guido Fanconi (1892-1979): a jack of all trades. *Nat Rev Cancer.* 2006 Nov;6(11):893–8.

[3] Che R, Zhang J, Nepal M, Han B, & Fei P. Multifaceted Fanconi anemia signaling. *Trends Genet.* 2018 Mar;34(3):171–83.

[4] Lichtman MA, Spivak JL, Boxer LA, Shattil E. editors. - Commentary on and reprint of Fanconi G, Familiäre infantile perniziosaartige Anämie (perniziöses Blutbild und Konstitution) [*Familial infantile pernicious-like anemia (pernicious blood picture and constitution)*], in *Jahrbuch für Kinderheilkunde.* (1927) 117:257–280. In: *Hematology* [Internet]. San Diego: Academic Press; 2000 [cited 2022 Sep 25]. p. 127–66. Available from: https://www.sciencedirect.com/science/article/pii/B9780 124485105501060.

[5] Fanconi G. Hypothesis of chromosomal translocation as a genetic interpretation of Fanconi's familial constitutional panmyelopathy. *Helv Paediatr Acta.* 1964 Jun;19: 29–33.

[6] Schroeder TM, Anschütz F, Knopp A. Spontaneous chromosome aberrations in familial panmyelopathy. *Humangenetik.* 1964;1(2):194–6.

[7] Schmid W, Schärer K, Baumann T, Fanconi G. Chromosal fragility in familial panmyelopathy (Fanconi type). *Schweiz Med Wochenschr*. 1965 Oct 23;95(43): 1461–4.

[8] Schroeder TM. Cytogenetic finding and etiology of Fanconi's anemia. A case of Fanconi's anemia without hexokinase deficiency. *Humangenetik*. 1966;3(1):76–81.

[9] Rosenberg PS, Tamary H, Alter BP. How high are carrier frequencies of rare recessive syndromes? Contemporary estimates for Fanconi anemia in the United States and Israel. *Am J Med Genet A*. 2011 Aug;155A(8):1877–83.

[10] Swift M. Fanconi's anaemia in the genetics of neoplasia. *Nature*. 1971 Apr 9;230(5293):370–3.

[11] Kimble DC, Lach FP, Gregg SQ, et al. A comprehensive approach to identification of pathogenic FANCA variants in Fanconi anemia patients and their families. *Hum Mutat*. 2018 Feb;39(2):237–54.

[12] García-de-Teresa B, Rodríguez A, Frias S. Chromosome instability in Fanconi anemia: from breaks to phenotypic consequences. *Genes (Basel)*. 2020 Dec 21;11 (12):1528.

[13] Meetei AR, Levitus M, Xue Y, et al. X-linked inheritance of Fanconi anemia complementation group B. *Nat Genet*. 2004 Nov;36(11):1219–24.

[14] Wang W. Emergence of a DNA-damage response network consisting of Fanconi anaemia and BRCA proteins. *Nat Rev Genet*. 2007 Oct;8(10):735–48.

[15] Auerbach AD. Fanconi anemia diagnosis and the diepoxybutane (DEB) test. *Exp Hematol*. 1993 Jun;21(6):731–3.

[16] Chirnomas SD, Kupfer GM. The inherited bone marrow failure syndromes. *Pediatr Clin North Am*. 2013 Dec;60(6):10.1016/j.pcl.2013.09.007.

[17] Alter BP. Fanconi's anemia, transplantation, and cancer. *Pediatr Transplant*. 2005 Dec;9 Suppl 7:81–6.

[18] Ameziane N, Sie D, Dentro S, et al. Diagnosis of Fanconi anemia: mutation analysis by next-generation sequencing. *Anemia*. 2012;2012:132856.

[19] Bagby GC, Lipton JM, Sloand EM, et al. Marrow failure. *Hematology Am Soc Hematol Educ Program*. 2004;318–36.

[20] de Chadarévian JP, Vekemans M, Bernstein M. Fanconi's anemia, medulloblastoma, Wilms' tumor, horseshoe kidney, and gonadal dysgenesis. *Arch Pathol Lab Med*. 1985 Apr;109(4):367–9.

[21] Alter BP, Caruso JP, Drachtman RA, et al. Fanconi anemia: myelodysplasia as a predictor of outcome. *Cancer Genet Cytogenet*. 2000 Mar;117(2):125–31.

[22] Alter BP. Fanconi anemia and the development of leukemia. *Best Pract Res Clin Haematol*. 2014 Dec;27(3–4):214–21.

[23] Alter BP. Fanconi's anemia and malignancies. *Am J Hematol*. 1996 Oct;53(2):99–110.

[24] Auerbach AD. Fanconi anemia and its diagnosis. *Mutat Res*. 2009 Jul 31;668(1–2):4–10.

[25] Kutler DI, Singh B, Satagopan J, et al. A 20-year perspective on the international fanconi anemia registry (IFAR). *Blood*. 2003 Feb 15;101(4):1249–56.

[26] Giampietro PF, Verlander PC, Davis JG, et al. Diagnosis of Fanconi anemia in patients without congenital malformations: An international Fanconi anemia registry study. *Am J Med Genet.* 1997 Jan 10;68(1):58–61.

[27] Ramus SJ, Song H, Dicks E, et al. Germline mutations in the BRIP1, BARD1, PALB2, and NBN genes in women with ovarian cancer. *J Natl Cancer Inst.* 2015 Aug 27;107(11):djv214.

[28] Hirsch B, Shimamura A, Moreau L, et al. Association of biallelic BRCA2/FANCD1 mutations with spontaneous chromosomal instability and solid tumors of childhood. *Blood.* 2004 Apr 1;103(7):2554–9.

[29] Reid S, Schindler D, Hanenberg H, et al. Biallelic mutations in PALB2 cause Fanconi anemia subtype FA-N and predispose to childhood cancer. *Nat Genet.* 2007 Feb;39(2):162–4.

[30] Rizk T, Taslakian B, Torbey PH et al. Sequential development of wilms tumor and medulloblastoma in a child: an unusual presentation of fanconi anemia. *Pediatric Hematology and Oncology.* 2013 Aug;30(5):400–2.

[31] Waszak SM, Northcott PA, Buchhalter I, et al. Spectrum and prevalence of genetic predisposition in medulloblastoma: a retrospective genetic study and prospective validation in a clinical trial cohort. *The Lancet Oncology.* 2018 Jun;19(6):785–98.

[32] Cacciotti C, Fleming A, Ramaswamy V. Advances in the molecular classification of pediatric brain tumors: a guide to the galaxy. *J Pathol.* 2020 Jul;251(3):249–61.

[33] Sari N, Akyuz C, Aktas D, et al. Wilms tumor, AML and medulloblastoma in a child with cancer prone syndrome of total premature chromatid separation and Fanconi anemia: triple malignancy, total PCS and Fanconi anemia. *Pediatr Blood Cancer.* 2009 Aug;53(2):208–10.

[34] Svojgr K, Sumerauer D, Puchmajerova A, et al. Fanconi anemia with biallelic FANCD1/BRCA2 mutations – Case report of a family with three affected children. *Eur J Med Genet.* 2016 Mar;59(3):152–7.

[35] Miele E, Mastronuzzi A, Po A, et al. Characterization of medulloblastoma in Fanconi Anemia: a novel mutation in the BRCA2 gene and SHH molecular subgroup. *Biomark Res.* 2015 Dec;3(1):13.

[36] Alter BP, Rosenberg PS, Brody LC. Clinical and molecular features associated with biallelic mutations in FANCD1/BRCA2. *J Med Genet.* 2006 Jul 6;44(1):1–9.

[37] McReynolds LJ, Biswas K, Giri N, et al. Genotype-cancer association in patients with Fanconi anemia due to pathogenic variants in FANCD1 (BRCA2) or FANCN (PALB2). *Cancer Genet.* 2021 Nov;258–259:101–9.

[38] Tischkowitz MD, Chisholm J, Gaze M, et al. Medulloblastoma as a first presentation of fanconi anemia. *J Pediatr Hematol Oncol.* 2004 Jan;26(1):52–5.

[39] Alter BP, Tenner MS. Brain tumors in patients with Fanconi's anemia. *Arch Pediatr Adolescent Med.* 1994 Jun 1;148(6):661–3.

[40] Sjarif DR, Révész T, de Koning TJ et al. Isolated glycerol kinase deficiency and Fanconi anemia. *Am J Med Genet.* 2001 Mar 1;99(2):159–60.

[41] Verheij E, Oomen KPQ, Smetsers SE et al. Hearing loss and speech perception in noise difficulties in Fanconi anemia. *Laryngoscope.* 2017 Oct;127(10):2358–61.

[42] Johnson-Tesch BA, Gawande RS, Zhang L, et al. Fanconi anemia: correlating central nervous system malformations and genetic complementation groups. *Pediatr Radiol*. 2017 Jun;47(7):868–76.

[43] Stivaros SM, Alston R, Wright NB, et al. Central nervous system abnormalities in Fanconi anaemia: patterns and frequency on magnetic resonance imaging. *Br J Radiol.* 2015 Dec;88(1056):20150088.

[44] Louis DN, Perry A, Wesseling P, et al. The 2021 WHO classification of tumors of the central nervous system: a summary. *Neuro Oncol.* 2021 Jun 29;23(8):1231–51.

[45] Patil AA, Sayal P, Depondt ML, et al. FANCD2 re-expression is associated with glioma grade and chemical inhibition of the Fanconi Anaemia pathway sensitises gliomas to chemotherapeutic agents. *Oncotarget*. 2014 Aug 15;5(15):6414–24.

[46] Packer RJ, Vezina G. Management of and prognosis with medulloblastoma: therapy at a crossroads. *Arch Neurol.* 2008 Nov;65(11):1419–24.

[47] Xu J, Margol AS, Shukla A, et al. Disseminated medulloblastoma in a child with germline BRCA2 6174delT mutation and without Fanconi anemia. *Front Oncol.* 2015;5:191.

Chapter 12

Clinicopathologic Review of the Familial Paraganglioma Syndromes

Samantha J. Stallkamp Tidd[1], BS
Joshua L. Tidd[2], BS
and Richard A. Prayson[3,*], MD, MEd

[1] Cleveland Clinic Lerner College of Medicine, Cleveland, OH, USA
[2] Northeast Ohio Medical University, Rootstown, OH, USA
[3] Department of Anatomic Pathology, Cleveland Clinic, Cleveland, OH, USA

Abstract

Paragangliomas are neuroendocrine tumors of the autonomic nervous system. Familial paraganglioma syndromes are a group of genetic conditions in which the development of paragangliomas is one of the possible tumor manifestations. There have been over 20 identified susceptibility genes associated with the development of these tumors. The most common of these syndromes are Neurofibromatosis Type 1, von Hippel-Lindau and Multiple Endocrine Neoplasia Type II. Pheochromocytomas arise from the adrenal medulla, and are the most common subtype of paragangliomas, accounting for 80-85% of all paragangliomas. The remaining 15-20% of paragangliomas occur outside of the adrenal medulla in the spine, head, neck, chest, heart, abdomen, pelvis, or bladder.

The classic presentation of a paraganglioma involves signs and symptoms of catecholamine excess including hypertension, tachycardia, palpitations, sweating and anxiety. Not all paragangliomas actively secrete catecholamines, and in this case the tumors are usually discovered incidentally or secondary to symptoms of mass effect. Though all

* Corresponding Author's Email: praysor@ccf.org.

In: Central Nervous System Pathologies in Hereditary Tumor Syndromes
Editor: Richard A. Prayson
ISBN: 979-8-88697-620-5

familial paraganglioma syndromes share the possibility of paraganglioma development, features of the tumors differ depending on the molecular consequences of the mutations causing them.

The goal of this chapter is to review the spectrum of familial paraganglioma syndromes, focusing on the clinical picture, genetics and histopathology of the paraganglioma tumors that arise in these syndromes.

Introduction

In the winter of 1883, the then 18-year-old Minna Roll was suddenly struck with attacks of palpitations, anxiety, headaches, dizziness, vomiting, weakness and constipation. She was hospitalized on December 11, 1884, and died just ten days later following repeated attacks and severe chest pain. On autopsy, she was found to have had bilateral renal tumors [1]. These tumors later became known as pheochromocytomas. Her case was the first to be described extensively in the literature and was shocking due to her young age [1]. Many years later, a group of scientists traced Minna's family history and found ancestors of her brother still living. Many of the family members had suffered from various tumors in the many years since Minna's death, including pheochromocytomas [1]. Scientists were able to isolate a family specific *RET* mutation, which came to be understood as the hallmark of multiple endocrine neoplasia type 2 (MEN-2). This syndrome was likely the cause of Minna's untimely death and represents one of the many genetic syndromes that have been linked to the development of pheochromocytomas and paragangliomas [1]. Since then, over 20 inherited genetic mutations have been discovered to lead to the development of these tumors (Table 1) [2]. In this chapter, we will describe the genetics, clinical presentation, diagnosis, histopathology and briefly the treatment of these syndromes in the context of classic features of sporadic cases.

General Features of Paragangliomas and Pheochromocytomas

Paragangliomas and pheochromocytomas are tumors of the autonomic nervous system. Paragangliomas are tumors of the autonomic nervous system, arising from cells of the embryonic nervous system, located around the adrenal glands, blood vessels and nerves called paraganglia. Pheochromocytomas are intra-adrenal paragangliomas arising from the chromaffin cells of the adrenal medulla [3, 4]. For the remainder of the chapter, unless talking about a feature specific to pheochromocytomas, we will use the larger encompassing term paraganglioma.

Table 1. Familial paraganglioma syndromes and germline mutations [2, 4, 10, 13, 26, 27]

Mutated gene	Name of syndrome	Frequency [2]	Cluster	Other findings
NF1	NF1	3%	2	Cafe-au-lait spots, neurofibromas, Lisch nodules, optic gliomas, meningiomas, sphenoid dysplasia, neuroendocrine and gastrointestinal stromal tumors
VHL	VHL	7%	1B	Hemangioblastomas, retinal angiomas, clear cell renal cell carcinoma, neuroendocrine tumors, and pancreatic tumors
RET	MEN-2	6%	2	Medullary thyroid carcinoma, Parathyroid hyperplasia, Mucosal neuromas, and Marfanoid habitus
EPAS1	Pacak-Zhuang syndrome	1%	1B	Polycythemia and duodenal somatostatinoma
EGLN1	no name	2 patients	1B	Polycythemia
SDHA	PGL5	<5%	1A	Gastrointestinal stromal tumors, renal cell carcinoma, and pituitary neuroendocrine tumors
SDHB	PGL4	10%	1A	Gastrointestinal stromal tumors, renal cell carcinoma, and pituitary neuroendocrine tumors
SDHC	PGL3	1%	1A	Gastrointestinal stromal tumors, and renal cell carcinoma
SDHD	PGL1	9%	1A	Gastrointestinal stromal tumors, renal cell carcinoma, and pituitary neuroendocrine tumors
SDHAF2	PGL2	<1%	1A	Insufficient data
FH	Reed syndrome/ HLRCC	1%	1A	Leiomyomas of the skin and uterus
TMEM127	no name	1-2%	2	Clear cell renal cell carcinoma
MAX	no name	1%	2	Insufficient data
MDH2	no name	5 patients	1A	Insufficient data
GOT2	no name	1 patient	1A	Insufficient data
SLC25A11	no name	8 patients	1A	Insufficient data
DLST	no name	4 patients	1A	Insufficient data
DNMT3A	no name	2 patients	N/A	Insufficient data
MET	no name	1 family	2	Type 1 papillary renal cell carcinoma
MERTK	no name	2 patients	2	Insufficient data
SUCLG2	no name	15 patients	1A	Insufficient data

PGL = Paraganglioma syndrome.

Paragangliomas often secrete one or more catecholamines into circulation resulting in clinical manifestations. The "classic triad" of presenting symptoms of this tumor are headaches, palpitations and sweating. However, the presentation tends to be variable depending on the location of the tumor and its functional status [5]. With the increased use of computed tomography (CT) imaging, more cases of paragangliomas are incidental findings in largely asymptomatic patients with relatively vague complaints [6]. In general, paragangliomas that secrete norepinephrine or epinephrine cause episodes of hypertension, sweating, heart palpitations, and anxiety [5]. Tumors that secrete dopamine are more likely to be asymptomatic, present with non-specific symptoms, or show signs and symptoms related to mass effect [7]. Lastly, those tumors that are non-secretory tend to be found incidentally or secondary to symptoms due to mass effect [5].

Genetics of Pheochromocytomas and Paragangliomas

Over the last two decades, the research into the genetics of paragangliomas has exponentially increased, with more than 20 susceptibility genes identified. In this chapter, we focus on germline mutations. Nevertheless, somatic mutations and their implications in treatment cannot be overemphasized [2, 8].

In 2017, the Cancer Genome Atlas divided genetic mutations in paraganglioma into three disease clusters based on shared molecular, clinical and imaging findings shared between them. Investigations are underway to examine if these clusters can be used to determine targeted therapy [9, 10]. We will briefly describe these clusters here, as to provide a framework for describing shared features of the tumor characteristics in these syndromes in the rest of the chapter. Further discussion of each specific mutations molecular impact is beyond the scope of this chapter.

Cluster 1: Pseudohypoxia

This group of mutations leads to an inappropriate hypoxic response resulting in tumorigenesis. This cluster can be subdivided into mutations that cause the accumulation of toxic TCA cycle metabolites (1A, Table 1) and those mutations that cause a disturbance in hypoxia-inducible factor (HIF) turnover (1B, Table 1) [9, 10].

Cluster 2: Kinase Signaling

This group of patients carry either somatic or germline mutations in genes involved in Kinase signaling pathways (Table 1) [9, 10].

Cluster 3: Wnt Signaling

This group of patients have mutations impacting the Wnt signaling pathway. All of these mutations are somatic, and thus not heritable (*CSDE1* and *MAML3*). Those patients solely in this cluster do not have a familial paraganglioma syndrome thus will not be discussed further [9, 10].

Defining Clinical Features of Paraganglioma Syndromes

Paragangliomas will present similarly in the paraganglioma syndromes as they do in sporadic cases. However, cases due to germline mutations occur more frequently in young patients with multiple tumors, extra-renal tumors, or in patients with a family history of tumors [11]. In addition, syndromes within the same cluster have shown shared characteristics [9, 10]. For example, several of the syndromes within each molecular cluster (Cluster 1) and 2) have co-occurring tumors or other unique clinical features that separate them clinically from cases arising from somatic mutations. The most common syndromes will be described further below. A list of important clinical features in less common syndromes is also contained in Table 1. Some newly identified mutations are excluded due to a scarcity of research [2].

Clinical Characteristics of Cluster 1: Pseudohypoxia

Functional paragangliomas in Cluster 1 syndromes tend to secrete dopamine and or norepinephrine. Cluster 1A tumors (TCA cycle related) can be silent or express this secretory phenotype. Cluster 1B tumors tend to be secretory and largely produce norepinephrine. The Cluster 1A tumors have the highest rate of metastatic disease, and overall the Cluster 1 tumors tend to be more aggressive and more likely to recur. Cluster 1 tumors tend to be extraadrenal, and when functional, secrete norepinephrine, presenting as sustained hypertension rather than episodic hypertension. These tumors develop at a relatively younger age [8, 10, 12, 13].

VHL

von Hippel-Lindau syndrome (VHL) is an autosomal dominant familial neoplastic syndrome caused by mutation of the tumor suppressor gene *VHL*. The common features of this disease includes the development of hemangioblastomas in the central nervous system and retina, renal cell carcinoma, pancreatic cysts, neuroendocrine tumors, and, of course, paragangliomas [2, 14]. It is important to note that not all mutations of *VHL* result in an increased risk of paragangliomas. VHL can be classified into two types depending on this risk. Type 1 VHL has low risk of paraganglioma development and is the result of a truncating mutation. Type 2 VHL has a high risk of the development of paraganglioma. Type 2 VHL is further divided into subtypes based on the risk of other tumors. It is frequently caused by missense mutations. Type 2A has a high risk of clear cell renal cell carcinoma, Type 2B has a low risk of kidney cancers and finally Type 2C patients tend to only develop paragangliomas. The location of the tumor is often bilateral in the adrenal medulla or in the abdomen. Two thirds of the time, patients with VHL who present with paragangliomas have positive family histories for syndromic tumors or VHL diagnosis [2]. Paragangliomas in this population tend to develop before the age of 20 years and thus may be the first presentation of VHL in a patient [2, 15].

Succinate Dehydrogenase Deficient Tumor Syndromes

The succinate dehydrogenase deficient tumor syndromes arise due to mutations in the genes coding for the protein subunits of succinate dehydrogenase. Mutations in any one of these subunit genes result in decreased activity of the enzyme, decreased energy production and accumulation of metabolites. Common among succinate dehydrogenase syndromes is the development of pheochromocytomas; hence, they also bare the names paraganglioma syndrome 1-5 [13, 16]. Other tumors seen in this syndrome include gastrointestinal stromal tumors, renal carcinomas, and pituitary adenomas. Paraganglioma syndrome 4 results from a mutation in *SDHB* and carries the highest malignant potential, is seen in younger individuals, and is associated with the largest tumor size at diagnosis [17].

Clinical Characteristics of Cluster 2: Kinase Signaling

Tumors in the Cluster 2 syndromes tend to be functional and secrete either a mixture of norepinephrine and epinephrine or epinephrine alone. These tumors tend to be located within the adrenal gland and are much less likely compared to Cluster 1 tumors to be aggressive or malignant. The presenting symptoms are episodic rather than persistent [8, 10, 12, 13].

RET

Gain of function mutations in the *RET* proto-oncogene results in multiple endocrine neoplasia type 2 (MEN2). There are two subtypes of MEN2, MEN2A and MEN2B. Both subtypes result in increased risk for the development of pheochromocytoma, occurring in 50% of patients. The average age of pheochromocytoma diagnosis is 30 years [2, 4, 18]. MEN2A is classically associated with pheochromocytoma, medullary thyroid carcinoma and hyperparathyroidism. MEN2B is classically associated with pheochromocytoma, medullary thyroid carcinoma, mucosal neuromas and a marfanoid habitus. The diagnosis of MEN2 in a family member should lead to intensive screening in families due to the nearly 100% likelihood of developing medullary thyroid carcinoma in mutation carriers [18, 19]. Family members found to be mutation carriers are recommended to undergo prophylactic thyroidectomy. With the increased use of this procedure in mutation carriers, pheochromocytomas are becoming the most common tumor type to be present in this population, underscoring the importance of routine screening [18, 19].

NF1

Neurofibromatosis type 1 (NF1), also known as von Recklinghausen disease is caused by a mutation in the NF1 gene coding for neurofibromin. Classic features of NF1 include café au lait spots, neurofibromas, axillary freckling, Lisch nodules, bony dysplasia, optic pathway gliomas, neuroendocrine tumors and gastrointestinal stromal tumors [2, 20]. NF 1 tends to be diagnosed earlier in life, with symptoms often manifesting during early childhood [20]. It should be noted, however, that NF1 cannot be excluded in patients only presenting with pheochromocytoma. Recently, several patients with pheochromocytoma without the classic clinical phenotype of NF1 were found to have the mutation. It is therefore reasonable to screen for this mutation in patients with no other obvious phenotypic features [21].

Diagnosis and Imaging in Paraganglioma and Paraganglioma Syndromes

The diagnosis of paraganglioma is a multi-step process and the recommended diagnostic approach can vary between societies. Here, we briefly discuss the diagnostic process. In a patient with signs and symptoms of catecholamine excess, the first step is to review their medications as these symptoms could be side effects. Next, patients undergo biochemical testing, usually through plasma free metanephrines (MN) and normetanephrine (NMN), or urine fractionated metanephrines and normetanephrine. Another biochemical test that may be ordered at this point is chromogranin A. However, this test is nonspecific and thus should be reserved for when there is high clinical suspicion for a non-functional tumor. This initial step of biomedical testing is also done for patients who are undergoing evaluation for an incidental mass or those with a strong family history. If biochemical testing is normal, but suspicion is still high, the test can be redone when the patient is more symptomatic. If there is a significant elevation in MN or NMN, imagining studies such as computed tomography (CT) or magnetic resonance imaging (MRI) are completed. In cases where the mass found is quite large, is extra adrenal, or no mass is found, further testing with functional imaging is warranted [12, 22].

Functional imaging choices for patients with unknown DNA mutations include somatostatin receptor imaging (68Ga-DOTA-SSA, 68 gallium labeled somatostatin analogues), 123-metaiodobenzylguanidine (123-MIBG) and 18F-fluorodeoxyglucose (18F-FDG) [10, 12, 22]. However, if the patient has a known DNA mutation, functional imaging may be personalized to maximize sensitivity. For those who have a cluster 1A mutation, the most sensitive functional imaging is 68Ga-DOTA-SSA. For those with Cluster 1B or Cluster 2 mutations, 18F-FDOPA is the most sensitive modality [8, 12].

All patients with paragangliomas should undergo genetic testing either before or after tumor resection for germline mutations, as this information can help guide treatment strategies and surveillance recommendations. All first degree relatives of a germline mutation carrier should be offered genetic testing. Management and surveillance strategies for asymptomatic carriers depends on the affected gene [4, 22].

Histopathological Features of Paraganglioma and Paraganglioma Syndromes

Most paragangliomas histopathologically display the prototypical "zellballen" pattern; zellballen consist of nests of round or elongated cells with granular amphophilic, basophilic or acidophilic cytoplasm, with a background of vascular stroma (Figure 1).

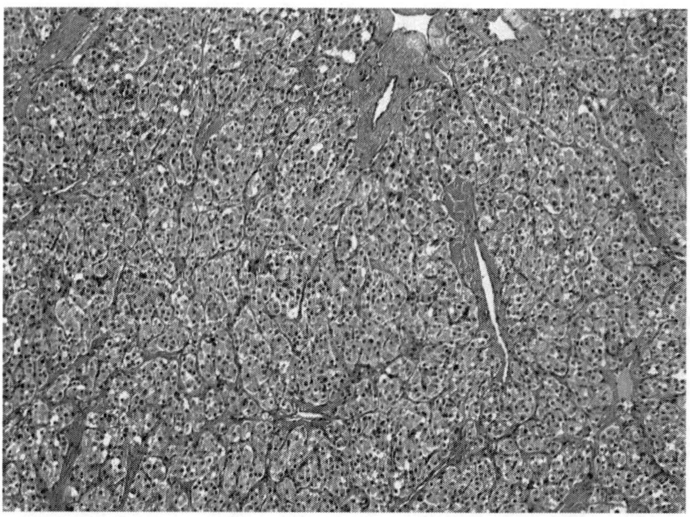

Figure 1. This paraganglioma arose in the lumbar paraspinal region of a person with neurofibromatosis type 1. The tumor is marked by clustered arrangement of epithelioid tumor cells (zellballen) (hematoxylin and eosin, original magnification 100X).

At the edges of the nests, there is a second cell population that is usually S-100 protein positive. These peripheral cells are known as "sustentacular cells" (Figure 2). The tumor is rarely necrotic and most often only has rare mitoses [12, 23].

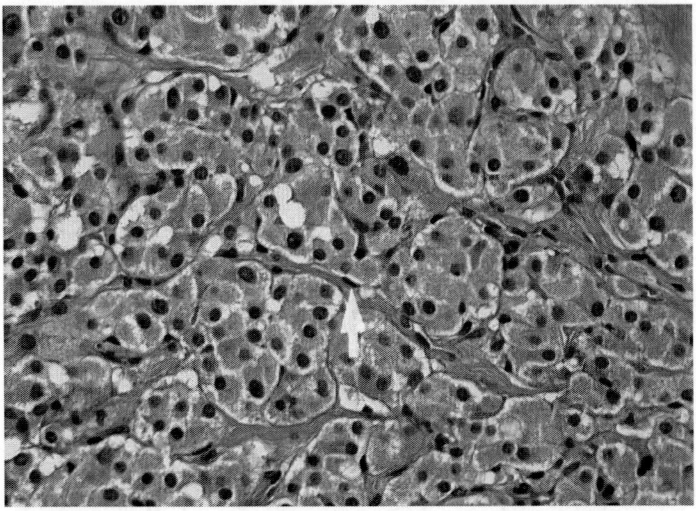

Figure 2. The clusters of cells in paraganglioma are delimited by thin bipolar sustentacular cells (arrow) which partially encircle the tumor nests (hematoxylin and eosin, original magnification 400X).

Tumor architecture may vary and given the fact that these tumors can arise in relatively unusual locations they present a diagnostic challenge. Immunohistochemistry is invaluable when attempting to diagnose unusual cases. Paragangliomas are most often positive for neuroendocrine immunohistochemistry markers such as synaptophysin and chromogranin (Figure 3). Paragangliomas are usually keratin negative, which is different from other neuroendocrine tumor types. A more specific stain is tyrosine hydroxylase [12, 23]. It is important to note that there are exceptions to these generalizations when it comes to staining. Non-functioning paragangliomas can be especially tricky, as they tend to not express or only be focally positive for chromogranin A and have absent tyrosine hydroxylase staining. However, non-functioning head and neck paragangliomas have been shown to almost universally express choline acetyltransferase [12, 23]. Another test that may be used for the diagnostic workup of these tumors is GATA3 reactivity [3].

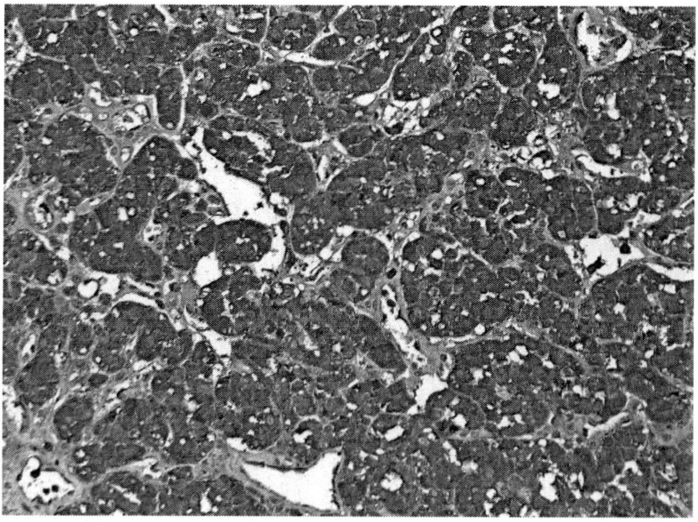

Figure 3. Paragangliomas typically stain with neuroendocrine markers such as chromogranin (seen in this image) or synaptophysin (original magnification 200X).

Several of the familial paraganglioma syndromes have unique histopathological manifestations. For example, tumors in patients with VHL tend to have a thick vascular capsule with amphophilic clear cells, but these findings can be variable [3, 23]. It is thought that the clear appearance of these cells is due to lipid or glycogen accumulation and can mimic an adrenal cortical tumor [3, 23]. Due to this possibility of a misdiagnosis, testing with other immunomarkers such as carbonic anhydrase IX, or PAX8 are encouraged to rule out a clear cell renal cell carcinoma. Loss of immunostaining for SDHB is found in all of the paraganglioma syndromes caused by mutations in the succinate dehydrogenase complex [3, 23]. Tumors with succinate hydrogenase complex mutations often have cells with variable intracytoplasmic vacuoles and eosinophilic cytoplasm [3].

Treatment and Prognosis

Management of patients with paraganglioma often require a multidisciplinary team. In general, the treatment for paraganglioma is tumor resection if the location is accessible and the cancer is not widely metastatic. Secondary therapy approaches include chemotherapy, targeted therapies and radionuclide therapy. Mutation and cluster specific therapy for paraganglioma is likely to become mainstream clinical practice in the coming years [3, 8, 24].

All patients with a history of paraganglioma, and all carriers of germline mutations require lifetime follow-up and screening. The type of screening and frequency is dependent on the specific mutation identified [8].

According to the 2022 World Health Organization (WHO) classification, all paragangliomas should be considered malignant neoplasms with variable metastatic potential [3]. There are currently no widely accepted risk stratification scores for prognostic use in paraganglioma, although a few are used in clinical practice. In general, location, cellular morphology and genetic mutations are factors used in these scores. More work has to be done to provide a widely accepted and validated risk score for this patient population [3]. Those with metastatic disease have widely variable survival with median overall survival of 24.6 years and disease specific survival of 33.7 years in one large longitudinal study [25]. In other studies, 5-year survival rates vary between 40 and 85% [24].

Over the last few decades, the research into the genetics and treatment of paragangliomas has exploded. For this patient population, effective personalized medicine is becoming a reality and we are excited to see what this era of medicine will bring [8].

Conclusion

Paragangliomas are neuroendocrine neoplasms derived form the autonomic nervous system. There are over 20 susceptibility genes that have been identified that are associated with the development of paragangliomas, hence their association with a variety of hereditary tumor syndromes including neurofibromatosis type 1, von Hippel-Lindau syndrome and multiple endocrine neoplasia type II.

References

[1] Neumann, HPH, Vortmeyer, A, Schmidt, D, et al. Evidence of MEN-2 in the original description of classic pheochromocytoma. *N Engl J Med*. 2007;357(13): 1311-1315. doi:10.1056/NEJMoa071407.

[2] Buffet A, Burnichon N, Favier J, et al. An overview of 20 years of genetic studies in pheochromocytoma and paraganglioma. *Best Pract Res Clin Endocrinol Metab.* 2020;34(2):101416. doi:10.1016/j.beem.2020.101416.

[3] Mete O, Asa SL, Gill AJ, et al. Overview of the 2022 WHO classification of paragangliomas and pheochromocytomas. *Endocr Pathol.* 2022;33(1):90-114. doi:10.1007/s12022-022-09704-6.

[4] Neumann HPH, Young WF, Eng C. Pheochromocytoma and paraganglioma. *N Engl J Med.* 2019;381(6):552-565. doi:10.1056/NEJMra1806651.

[5] Gunawardane PTK, Grossman A. Phaeochromocytoma and paraganglioma. *Adv Exp Med Biol.* 2017;956:239-259. doi:10.1007/5584_2016_76.

[6] Gruber LM, Hartman RP, Thompson GB, et al. Pheochromocytoma characteristics and behavior differ depending on method of discovery. *J Clin Endocrinol Metab.* 2019;104(5):1386-1393. doi:10.1210/jc.2018-01707.

[7] Foo SH, Chan SP, Ananda V, et al. Dopamine-secreting phaeo-chromocytomas and paragangliomas: clinical features and management. *Singapore Med J.* 2010;51(5): e89-93.

[8] Nölting S, Bechmann N, Taieb D, et al. Personalized management of pheochromocytoma and paraganglioma. *Endocr Rev.* 2022;43(2):199-239. doi:10. 1210/endrev/bnab019.

[9] Fishbein L, Leshchiner I, Walter V, et al. Comprehensive molecular characterization of pheochromocytoma and paraganglioma. *Cancer Cell.* 2017;31(2):181-193. doi: 10.1016/j.ccell.2017.01.001.

[10] Crona J, Taïeb D, Pacak K. New perspectives on pheochromocytoma and paraganglioma: toward a molecular classification. *Endocr Rev.* 2017;38(6):489-515. doi:10.1210/er.2017-00062.

[11] Neumann HPH, Bausch B, McWhinney SR, et al. Germ-line mutations in nonsyndromic pheochromocytoma. *N Engl J Med.* 2002;346(19):1459-1466. doi:10.1056/NEJMoa020152.

[12] Asa SL, Ezzat S, Mete O. The diagnosis and clinical significance of paragangliomas in unusual locations. *J Clin Med.* 2018;7(9). doi:10.3390/jcm7090280.

[13] Jhawar S, Arakawa Y, Kumar S, et al. New insights on the genetics of pheochromocytoma and paraganglioma and its clinical implications. *Cancers (Basel).* 2022;14(3). doi:10.3390/cancers14030594.

[14] Varshney N, Kebede AA, Owusu-Dapaah H, et al. A review of von Hippel-Lindau Syndrome. *J Kidney Cancer VHL.* 2017;4(3):20-29. doi:10.15586/jkcvhl.2017.88.

[15] Maher ER, Yates JR, Harries R, et al. Clinical features and natural history of von Hippel-Lindau disease. *Q J Med.* 1990;77(283):1151-1163. doi:10.1093/qjmed/77. 2.1151.

[16] Gill AJ. Succinate dehydrogenase (SDH)-deficient neoplasia. *Histopathology.* 2018;72(1):106-116. doi:10.1111/his.13277.

[17] Rednam SP, Erez A, Druker H, et al. Von Hippel-Lindau and hereditary pheochromocytoma/paraganglioma syndromes: clinical features, genetics, and surveillance recommendations in childhood. *Clin Cancer Res.* 2017;23(12):e68-e75. doi:10.1158/1078-0432.CCR-17-0547.

[18] Brandi ML, Gagel RF, Angeli A, et al. Guidelines for diagnosis and therapy of MEN type 1 and type 2. *J Clin Endocrinol Metab*. 2001;86(12):5658-5671. doi:10.1210/jcem.86.12.8070.

[19] Amodru V, Taieb D, Guerin C, et al. MEN2-related pheochromocytoma: current state of knowledge, specific characteristics in MEN2B, and perspectives. *Endocrine*. 2020;69(3):496-503. doi:10.1007/s12020-020-02332-2.

[20] Ferner RE, Huson SM, Thomas N, et al. Guidelines for the diagnosis and management of individuals with neurofibromatosis 1. *J Med Genet*. 2007;44(2):81-88. doi:10.1136/jmg.2006.045906.

[21] Gieldon L, Masjkur JR, Richter S, et al. Next-generation panel sequencing identifies NF1 germline mutations in three patients with pheochromocytoma but no clinical diagnosis of neurofibromatosis type 1. *Eur J Endocrinol*. 2018;178(2):K1-K9. doi:10.1530/EJE-17-0714.

[22] Garcia-Carbonero R, Matute Teresa F, Mercader-Cidoncha E, et al. Multidisciplinary practice guidelines for the diagnosis, genetic counseling and treatment of pheochromocytomas and paragangliomas. *Clin Transl Oncol Off Publ Fed Spanish Oncol Soc Natl Cancer Inst Mex*. 2021;23(10):1995-2019. doi:10.1007/s12094-021-02622-9.

[23] Tischler AS, deKrijger RR. 15 years of paraganglioma: Pathology of pheochromocytoma and paraganglioma. *Endocr Relat Cancer*. 2015;22(4):T123-T133. doi:10.1530/ERC-15-0261.

[24] Corssmit EPM, Snel M, Kapiteijn E. Malignant pheochromocytoma and paraganglioma: management options. *Curr Opin Oncol*. 2020;32(1):20-26. doi:10.1097/CCO.0000000000000589.

[25] Hamidi O, Young WFJ, Iñiguez-Ariza NM, et al. Malignant pheochromocytoma and paraganglioma: 272 patients over 55 years. *J Clin Endocrinol Metab*. 2017;102(9):3296-3305. doi:10.1210/jc.2017-00992.

[26] Hadrava Vanova K, Pang Y, Krobova L, et al. Germline SUCLG2 variants in patients with pheochromocytoma and paraganglioma. *J Natl Cancer Inst*. 2022;114(1):130-138. doi:10.1093/jnci/djab158.

[27] Vicha A, Mercado-Asis LB. Pacak-Zhuang syndrome: A new kid on the block. *Endocr Pract.* 2014;20(11):1234-1235. doi:10.4158/endp.20.11.g37v757188j41v24.

Chapter 13

Familial Melanoma-Astrocytoma Syndrome

Narendra Bhattarai, MD
and Richard A. Prayson*, MD, MEd
Department of Anatomic Pathology, Cleveland Clinic, Clevelend, Ohio, USA

Abstract

Melanoma-astrocytoma syndrome is a rare tumor predisposition syndrome caused by a germline mutation of the CDKN2A gene. People who carry the mutation are more likely to develop cutaneous melanoma, nervous system tumors, pancreatic cancer, nerve sheath tumors, and oropharyngeal squamous cell carcinoma. Astrocytoma is the most frequent nervous system tumor arising in this syndrome. The neoplastic risk of this syndrome has not been determined due to the small number of families reported. Early detection of melanoma improves outcomes. Nervous system tumors arising in this setting typically have a dismal prognosis depending on type, location, and stage.

This chapter will review the clinicopathologic features of this rare syndrome, with a focus on the central nervous system pathology.

Introduction

In a small percentage of patients with primary glial neoplasms of the central nervous system, a family history of brain tumors is an important risk factor [1, 2]. Melanoma-astrocytoma syndrome is an exceedingly rare form of inherited tumor predisposition syndrome. It is caused by a germline mutation that affects the CDKN2A tumor suppressor gene, which is located on chromosome

In: Central Nervous System Pathologies in Hereditary Tumor Syndromes
Editor: Richard A. Prayson
ISBN: 979-8-88697-620-5

9p21.3. The gene encodes regulators of the cell cycle, including p16INK4a and p14ARF [3-6].

In 1993, Kaufman and colleagues [5] were the first to identify it as a probable novel genetic condition seen in a family where eight individuals had both cutaneous malignant melanoma and cerebral astrocytoma. Azizi et al., [6] described a similar condition in 1995, as did Bahuau and coworkers [7] in 1997. This chapter will review the clinicopathologic features of this rare hereditary tumor syndrome.

Clinical Features

The syndrome is characterized by the appearance of cutaneous dysplastic nevi, melanomas and astrocytoma. Nerve sheath tumors, pancreatic cancer, and oropharyngeal squamous cell carcinoma are also common in patients [3]. Other central nervous system tumors that have been encountered in this syndrome include medulloblastomas, glioblastoma, ependymoma, meningioma, neuroblastomas, schwannoma, and acoustic neurilemmoma. All of these tumors are derived from the neural crest, mesenchyme, and/or neuroepithelium [8]. The nerve sheath tumors include paraspinal schwannoma like neoplasms and cutaneous neurofibroma-like neoplasms [7-10].

Histopathology

Patients with melanoma-astrocytoma syndrome develop dysplastic nevi, melanomas (Figure 1), and astrocytomas with comparable histologic features to sporadic occurrences. Diffuse astrocytic gliomas and pleomorphic xanthoastrocytomas are the two most common types of astrocytoma that develop [8-10]. Diffuse gliomas can be either low- or high-grade tumors (Figure 2). The histological features of astrocytomas that arises as part of this syndrome are not well described but appear to resemble those that arise outside of this setting [8]. Schwannoma (Figure 3) and neurofibroma are the two primary tumor types that develop in the nerve sheath when this condition is present [3]; similarly, their appearance resembles the tumors that arise outside the setting of this syndrome.

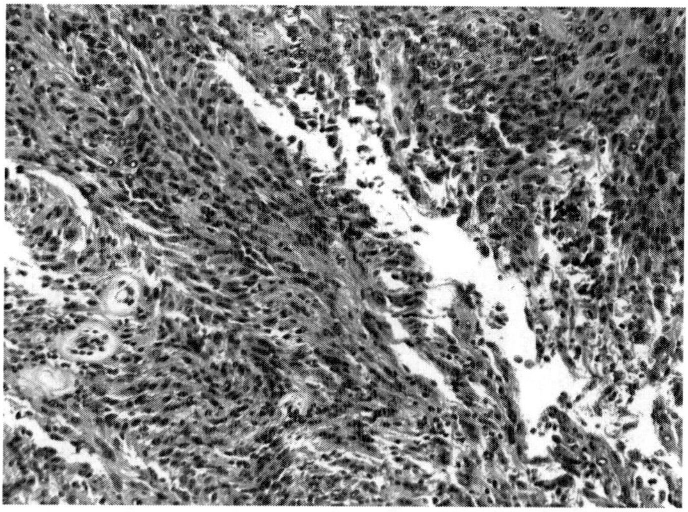

Figure 1. This prominently cellular tumor was excised from the right parietal lobe in a patent with melanoma-astrocytoma syndrome. The tumor stained with antibodies to SOX10 and melan A and did not stain with antibody to glial fibrillary acidic protein (GFAP), consistent with metastatic melanoma (hematoxylin and eosin, original magnification 200X).

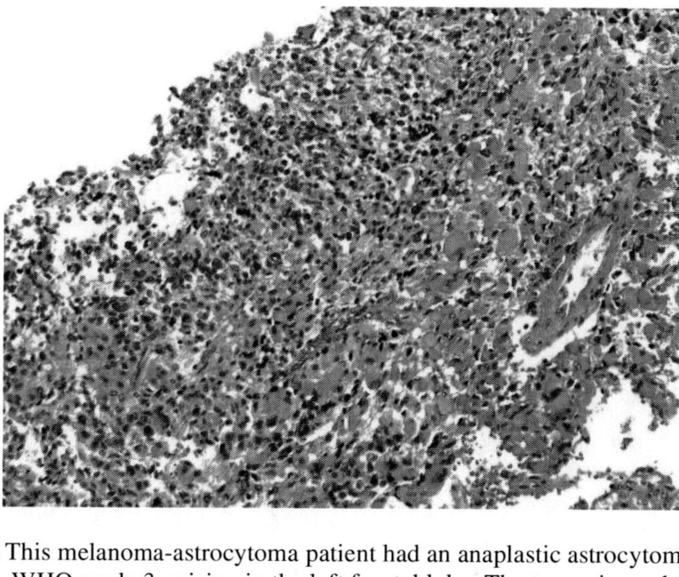

Figure 2. This melanoma-astrocytoma patient had an anaplastic astrocytoma, IDH-1 wild-type, WHO grade 3, arising in the left frontal lobe. The tumor is marked by focally prominent hypercellularity and increased gemistocytes (hematoxylin and eosin, original magnification 200X).

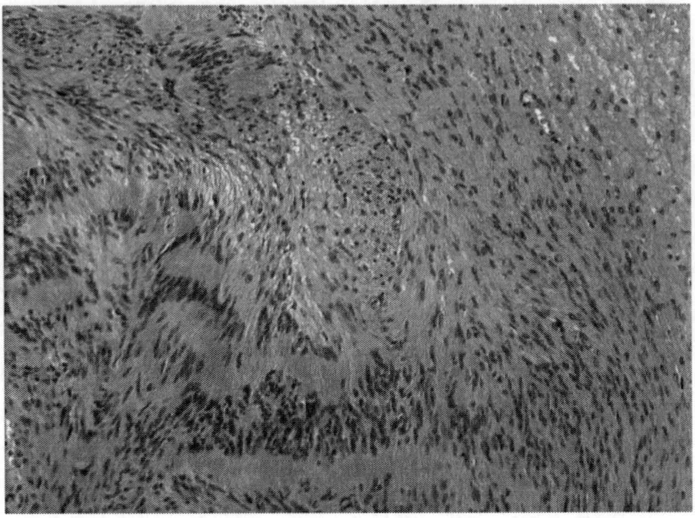

Figure 3. This thoracic paraspinal schwannoma, WHO grade 1, was excised in a patient with melanoma-astrocytoma syndrome. The tumor showed Verocay body formation (hematoxylin and eosin, original magnification 200X).

Dysplastic nevi are unique melanocytic lesions within the broader category of atypical nevi. They are frequently numerous and sporadic, having intermediate genetic characteristics between common acquired nevi and melanoma. Multiple, dysplastic nevi may be seen in people with familial melanoma syndrome. Even if their behavior is benign, they are infrequently precursors to melanoma [11]. CDKN2A mutations are often found in familial cases, a finding that is much less common in melanoma [12]. The lesions show architectural atypia including shouldering, bridging, lentiginous hyperplasia and irregular nesting along with cytological atypia including increased nuclear size, irregular nuclear membrane, prominent nucleoli and pleomorphism [11].

Melanomas can occur anywhere in the body and can rarely arise in association with the central nervous system in the meninges, spinal cord and posterior fossa region [13, 14]. Microscopically, the tumor is composed of hypercellular nests or sheets of spindled or epithelioid cells (Figure 1). The tumor cells show significant pleomorphism with prominent nucleoli and atypical mitosis. Necrosis along with invasion of adjacent structures are often seen. The tumor cells are positive staining with antibodies to Melan A, S -100 protein, SOX 10 and HMB45 but are negative for glial fibrillary acidic protein (GFAP) [13, 14].

Astrocytoma is a diffusely infiltrating glioma which may show mutations in isocitrate dehydrogenase (IDH)-1- or IDH-2, ATRX and/or TP53 but no chromosome 1p/19q co-deletion. Astrocytomas can occur anywhere in the brain, but are typically encountered within the frontal lobes. Diffusely infiltrating astrocytoma can range from World Health Organization (WHO) grade 2 to WHO grade 4 lesions. WHO grade 2 tumors are well differentiated with mild to moderately increased cellularity, mild nuclear atypia and very low mitotic activity. WHO grade 3 astrocytoma have significant mitotic activity with focal or dispersed anaplasia (Figure 2). Microvascular proliferation or necrosis are seen in WHO grade 4 astrocytomas. Homozygous deletion of CDKN2A and/or CDKN2B, when present in IDH mutated tumors, also puts astrocytomas into the WHO grade 4 category [15]. The tumor cells are positive for GFAP, OLIG2 and IDH-1. There is loss of nuclear expression of ATRX in most cases, corresponding to a mutation in ATRX. Strong nuclear expression of p53 is observed in cases with TP53 mutation [16-18].

Pleomorphic xanthoastrocytoma is a rare primary central nervous system tumor that is hypothesized to originate from subpial astrocytes or their progenitors [19]. Grossly, the tumor is solid and cystic and usually involves temporal lobe. Microscopically, the tumor cells are highly pleomorphic with occasional bizarre-looking nuclei and multinucleation. The cytoplasm is eosinophilic and contains varying amounts of hyaline protein and lipid droplets. The tumor cells are positive for GFAP on immunohistochemistry [20-22], often demonstrate increased reticulin staining between tumor cells and may demonstrate evidence of BRAF V600E staining. Most represent WHO grade 2 tumors; although, a subset of cases demonstrate increased mitotic activity and/or necrosis, warranting an anaplastic or grade 3 designation.

Schwannomas are benign nerve sheath tumors arising from differentiated Schwann cells. They may arise sporadically, or in the context of a familial tumor syndrome. Schwannomas have many morphological appearances, but generally behave as WHO grade 1 tumors and undergo malignant transformation relatively infrequently [23, 24]. Grossly, the lesion is well confined, and microscopically, it is made up of areas that are compact hypercellular Antoni A and myxoid/hypocellular Antoni B (Figure 3) [25, 26]. Verocay bodies with nuclear palisades are sometimes seen in the Antoni A areas of a schwannoma. The tumor cells are strongly and diffusely positive for S-100 protein [27].

Genetic and Molecular Features

Germline pathogenic mutations in the CDKN2A (cyclin dependent kinase inhibitor 2A) tumor suppressor gene spanning 27.5 kb on chromosome 9p21.3 are the underlying etiology of melanoma-astrocytoma syndrome [3, 28]. CDKN2A is a well know susceptibility gene for familial cutaneous melanoma, which is caused by point mutations and gene deletions [29]. It is now understood that familial melanoma-astrocytoma syndrome is an autosomal-dominant variant of familial melanoma syndrome [8].

CDKN2A uses an alternative first exon in combination with alternate reading frames to encode the two functionally separate cell cycle proteins p16 and p14ARF. p16 is a 156 amino acid protein translated from a transcript of three exons 1a, 2 and 3 [28, 30]. p14ARF is a 132 amino acid protein, encoded via an alternative open-reading frame and first exon (exon 1β) [31]. p16 blocks the progression from the G1 phase to the S phase by preventing the phosphorylation of RB, the release of E2F, and the transcription of genes involved in the S phase. This is accomplished by blocking the binding of Cyclin D to CDK4 and CDK6. By sequestering MDM2 and blocking it from targeting p53 for ubiquitination, P14ARF is able to suppress both the G1 to S transition as well as the G2 to M transition [3, 8, 10, 32]. Manifestations of nervous system-related malignancies such as astrocytoma and schwannoma were frequently observed in families with a CDKN2A locus deletion and/or lack of an intact p14ARF [28].

Diagnostic Criteria

- *Essential:* A pathogenic germline mutation of the CDKN2A gene (heterozygous) in an astrocytoma patient.
- *Desirable:* An individual or family history of dysplastic nevi and corresponding neoplasms.
- Somatic inactivation of the remaining wild-type CDKN2A allele in a resected tumor, accompanied with somatic changes (e.g., BRAF p.V600E mutation, IDH1 or IDH2 mutation) that aid in subtyping the tumor.

Management and Prognosis

There is no proven optimal treatment strategy for patients with familial melanoma-astrocytoma syndrome. The prognosis for nervous system tumors depends on kind, location, grade and stage. Although there are no particular recommendations for surveillance, routine brain imaging to track the growth of brain tumors is advised. Similarly regular dermatologic, ophthalmic and dental evaluation along with body imaging is required. Current recommendations for treating patients with CDKN2A germline pathogenic/likely pathogenic mutations focus on monitoring for melanoma and pancreatic cancer [33]. Genetic counseling for the patient's family and for the patient is also crucial [8]. Early detection of melanoma improves outcomes. Thus, precursor lesions must be carefully monitored. Clinical outcomes for the gliomas ad nerve sheath tumors that arise in the setting of melanoma-astrocytoma syndrome in comparison with their sporadic counterparts have not been well described.

Conclusion

Familial melanoma-astrocytoma syndrome is a rare disorder associated with germline mutations of the CDKN2A gene. Patients with this disorder are prone to the development of astrocytomas in the central nervous system as well as melanomas and rare cases of pleomorphic xanthoastrocytoma. Schwannomas may also be encountered in this condition.

References

[1] Wrensch M, Lee M, Miike R, et al. Familial and personal medical history of cancer and nervous system conditions among adults with glioma and controls. *Am. J. Epidemiol.* 1997;145(7):581-93.

[2] Malmer B, Grönberg H, Bergenheim A T, et al. Familial aggregation of astrocytoma in northern Sweden: an epidemiological cohort study. *Int. J. Cancer.* 1999;81 (3):366-70.

[3] Solomon D A, Reuss D E. Central Nervous System Tumors. In: Cree IA, Lokuhetty D, Peferoen L A N, White V A, eds. 5th ed. Lyon, France: *International Agency for Research on Cancer*; 2021:471-72.

[4] Perry A, Brat D J. *Practical Surgical Neuropathology.* 2nd ed. Philadelphia: Elsevier; 2017:538.

[5] Kaufman D K, Kimmel D W, Parisi J E, et al. A familial syndrome with cutaneous malignant melanoma and cerebral astrocytoma. *Neurology.* 1993;43(9):1728-31.
[6] Azizi E, Friedman J, Pavlotsky F, et al. Familial cutaneous malignant melanoma and tumors of the nervous system. A hereditary cancer syndrome. *Cancer.* 1995;76 (9):1571-8.
[7] Bahuau M, Vidaud D, Kujas M, et al. Familial aggregation of malignant melanoma/dysplastic naevi and tumours of the nervous system: an original syndrome of tumour proneness. *Ann. Genet.* 1997;40(2):78-91.
[8] Chan A K, Han S J, Choy W, et al. Familial melanoma-astrocytoma syndrome: synchronous diffuse astrocytoma and pleomorphic xanthoastrocytoma in a patient with germline CDKN2A/B deletion and a significant family history. *Clin. Neuropathol.* 2017;36(5):213-21.
[9] Vanneste R, Smith E, Graham G. Multiple neurofibromas as the presenting feature of familial atypical multiple malignant melanoma (FAMMM) syndrome. *Am. J. Med. Genet. A.* 2013;161a(6):1425-31.
[10] Sargen MR, Merrill SL, Chu EY, et al. CDKN2A mutations with p14 loss predisposing to multiple nerve sheath tumours, melanoma, dysplastic naevi and internal malignancies: a case series and review of the literature. *Br. J. Dermatol.* 2016;175(4):785-9.
[11] Wiedemeyer K, Hartschuh W, Brenn T. Dysplastic nevi: morphology and molecular and the controversies In-between. *Surg. Pathol. Clin.* 2021;14(2):341-57.
[12] Goldstein A M, Tucker M A, Crutcher W A, et al. The inheritance pattern of dysplastic naevi in families of dysplastic naevus patients. *Melanoma Res.* 1993;3(1):15-22.
[13] Bobos M. Histopathologic classification and prognostic factors of melanoma: a 2021 update. *Ita.l J. Dermatol. Venerol.* 2021;156(3):300-21.
[14] Brat D J, Giannini C, Scheithauer B W, et al. Primary melanocytic neoplasms of the central nervous systems. *Am. J. Surg. Pathol.* 1999;23(7):745-54.
[15] Komori T. Grading of adult diffuse gliomas according to the 2021 WHO Classification of Tumors of the Central Nervous System. *Lab. Invest.* 2022;102 (2):126-33.
[16] Santisukwongchote S, Teerapakpinyo C, Chankate P, et al. Simplified approach for pathological diagnosis of diffuse gliomas in adult patients. *Pathol. Res. Pract.* 2021; 223:153483.
[17] Wood MD, Halfpenny AM, Moore SR. Applications of molecular neuro-oncology - a review of diffuse glioma integrated diagnosis and emerging molecular entities. *Diagn. Pathol.* 2019;14(1):29.
[18] Andrews C, Prayson RA. IDH mutations in older patients with diffuse astrocytic gliomas. *Ann. Diagn. Pathol.* 2020;49:151653.
[19] Shaikh N, Brahmbhatt N, Kruser T J, et al. Pleomorphic xanthoastrocytoma: a brief review. *CNS Oncol.* 2019;8(3):Cns39.
[20] Kepes J J, Rubinstein L J, Ansbacher L, et al. Histopathological features of recurrent pleomorphic xanthoastrocytomas: further corroboration of the glial nature of this neoplasm. A study of 3 cases. *Acta Neuropathol.* 1989;78(6):585-93.

[21] Weldon-Linne C M, Victor T A, Groothuis D R, et al. Pleomorphic xanthoastrocytoma. Ultrastructural and immunohistochemical study of a case with a rapidly fatal outcome following surgery. *Cancer.* 1983;52(11):2055-63.

[22] Iwaki T, Fukui M, Kondo A, et al. Epithelial properties of pleomorphic xanthoastrocytomas determined in ultrastructural and immunohistochemical studies. *Acta Neuropathol.* 1987;74(2):142-50.

[23] Hilton DA, Hanemann CO. Schwannomas and their pathogenesis. *Brain Pathol.* 2014;24(3):205-20.

[24] Sheikh M M, De Jesus O. Schwannoma. *StatPearls.* Treasure Island (FL): StatPearls Publishing Copyright © 2022, StatPearls Publishing LLC.; 2022.

[25] Magro G. Differential diagnosis of benign spindle cell lesions. *Surg. Pathol. Clin.* 2018;11(1):91-121.

[26] Belakhoua S M, Rodriguez F J. Diagnostic pathology of tumors of peripheral nerve. *Neurosurgery.* 2021;88(3):443-56.

[27] Majumder A, Ahuja A, Chauhan DS, et al. A clinicopathological study of peripheral schwannomas. *Med. Pharm. Rep.* 2021;94(2):191-6.

[28] Chan S H, Chiang J, Ngeow J. CDKN2A germline alterations and the relevance of genotype-phenotype associations in cancer predisposition. *Hered. Cancer Clin. Pract.* 2021;19(1):21.

[29] Kamb A, Shattuck-Eidens D, Eeles R, et al. Analysis of the p16 gene (CDKN2) as a candidate for the chromosome 9p melanoma susceptibility locus. *Nat. Genet.* 1994;8(1):23-6.

[30] Romagosa C, Simonetti S, López-Vicente L, et al. p16(Ink4a) overexpression in cancer: a tumor suppressor gene associated with senescence and high-grade tumors. *Oncogene.* 2011;30(18):2087-97.

[31] Ozenne P, Eymin B, Brambilla E, et al. The ARF tumor suppressor: structure, functions and status in cancer. *Int. J. Cancer.* 2010;127(10):2239-47.

[32] Nilsson K, Landberg G. Subcellular localization, modification and protein complex formation of the cdk-inhibitor p16 in Rb-functional and Rb-inactivated tumor cells. *Int. J. Cancer.* 2006;118(5):1120-5.

[33] Katalinic A, Waldmann A, Weinstock M A, et al. Does skin cancer screening save lives?: an observational study comparing trends in melanoma mortality in regions with and without screening. *Cancer.* 2012;118(21):5395-402.

Chapter 14

Neuropathologic Findings in Familial Adenomatous Polyposis Syndrome

Hailey L. Gosnell, MD
and Richard A. Prayson*, **MD, MEd**
Department of Anatomic Pathology, Cleveland Clinic, Cleveland, Ohio, USA

Abstract

Familial adenomatous polyposis (FAP1) is an autosomal dominant genetic syndrome caused by a pathogenic, inactivating sequence variant in the tumor suppressor gene APC. While FAP1 is predominantly characterized phenotypically by the development of gastrointestinal neoplasia, formation of primary brain tumors also occurs in a small subset of these patients, a phenomenon termed brain tumor polyposis syndrome 2 (BTP2).

Medulloblastomas are the only tumor type definitively associated with BTP2. Development of these tumors is mediated by activation of the WNT signaling pathway, as a result of APC loss. Although syndromic medulloblastoma due to germline APC mutation makes up a small fraction (roughly 5%) of WNT activated medulloblastomas, both somatic and germline variants are associated with early onset (peak incidence within the first decade of life) and excellent prognosis (5-year survival > 95%).

The goal of this chapter is to describe the clinical features of FAP1, histopathologic characteristics of BTP2, and unique molecular findings associated with medulloblastomas arising in this context, as well as diagnostic and prognostic information pertaining to this rare neurologic manifestation.

---

* Corresponding Author's Email: praysor@ccf.org.

In: Central Nervous System Pathologies in Hereditary Tumor Syndromes
Editor: Richard A. Prayson
ISBN: 979-8-88697-620-5

Introduction

The association between familial colorectal polyposis and adenocarcinoma development was initially posited almost one-hundred fifty years ago and refined over the last several decades. In 1882, Dr. William Harrison Cripps, a prominent rectal surgeon, was the first to theorize that colorectal polyposis was a familial condition associated with increased risk of cancer development [1]. Fifty years later, Dr. Cuthbert Dukes, a gastrointestinal and genitourinary pathologist, developed a system for staging polyp-derived large intestinal tumors based on his clinical experience with hereditary polyposis patients [1, 2]. In 1942, C.M. Gardner established that the typical onset age of hereditary polyposis was between puberty and 30 years [3]. The clinical characteristics and natural history of hereditary polyposis, later termed familial adenomatous polyposis, was described by Dr. Richard Bussey in 1975 [4]. In 1987, a paper published by Dr. William Bodmer localized the gene associated with familial adenomatous polyposis, adenomatous polyposis (APC) gene, to chromosome 5q21-22 [5].

Familial Adenomatous Polyposis 1 (FAP1): A Clinical Overview

Familial adenomatous polyposis (FAP1) is the second most common genetic polyposis syndrome of the colon, affecting about 1 in 10,000 individuals [6]. An inactivating sequence variant in the tumor suppressor gene APC is the molecular underpinning of this disease process, displaying an autosomal dominant inheritance pattern [7]. Clinically, FAP1 is defined by the development of at least one hundred, but often, hundreds to thousands of colonic adenomas by the second decade of life, after spontaneous somatic loss of the remaining functional APC allele occurs [8]. The development of colon cancer is inevitable in these patients without prophylactic colectomy, highlighting the importance of early screening [8]. Individuals with known family history of classic FAP1 are recommended to begin screening colonoscopies at age 10-12 years and to repeat screen every one to two years [6].

Diagnosis of FAP1 is important not only for recognition and treatment of colonic manifestations, but also in the identification of less well known, but still significant extracolonic malignancies that these patients are at higher risk for developing. While FAP1 is well known for predisposition to colonic tumor development, there are a number of extracolonic malignancies that individuals affected by this syndrome are more likely to develop which include osteomas (50-90% of patients), desmoid tumors (10-15%), thyroid cancers (2-3%), hepatoblastomas (about 1%), and central nervous system (CNS) tumors (about 1%) [9]. The development of CNS tumors in the setting of FAP1, previously referred to as Turcot Syndrome Type 2, but more recently termed brain tumor polyposis syndrome (BTP2), is the topic of this chapter [10].

What Is BTP2?

Brain tumor polyposis syndrome 2 (BTP2) is a rare manifestation of FAP1, characterized by the development of primary CNS lesions, specifically medulloblastomas. While other neurologic tumor types including astrocytomas, ependymomas, craniopharyngiomas, and pineoblastomas have been reported in the setting of BTP2, the only primary brain neoplasm clearly associated with the syndrome is medulloblastoma [11-13]. In fact, the clinical criteria for the diagnosis of BTP2 are "occurrence of a brain tumor, typically WNT-activated medulloblastoma, in a patient with familial adenomatous polyposis 1," or "identification of a pathogenic germline mutation in the APC gene in a child with WNT-activated medulloblastoma lacking CTNNB1 mutation [9]."

Genetics of BTP2 Medulloblastomas and Somatic Wingless/Integrated (WNT)-Activated Medulloblastomas

BTP2 associated medulloblastomas, like other FAP1 associated lesions, arise due to somatic loss of the remaining functional APC allele [14]. The loss of APC gene functioning allows the Wingless/Integrated (WNT) signaling pathway to go unregulated, resulting in blocked phosphorylation of beta catenin [15]. Hypophosphorylated (active) beta-catenin migrates to the cell nucleus, ultimately resulting in unchecked cell differentiation and proliferation by promoting mutational inactivation of p53 transcription.

Medulloblastomas associated with BTP2 make up a very small subset of WNT-activated medulloblastomas (about 5%) [9]. The vast majority of WNT-activated medulloblastomas are mediated by somatic mutation of the GSK-3B phosphorylation domain of CTNNB1, resulting in nuclear oversaturation with active beta-catenin [16-18]. The downstream effect of active beta catenin buildup within the cell in somatic WNT-activated medulloblastomas parallels their syndromic counterparts, enabling limitless cellular differentiation and proliferation by compromising p53 transcription. While the molecular mechanisms of germline and somatic WNT-associated medulloblastomas differ, their histopathologic, clinical, and prognostic features are nearly indistinguishable.

Histopathology of BTP2 Associated Medulloblastomas and Their Somatic WNT-Activated Counterparts

Histopathologic findings characteristic of BTP2 associated medulloblastomas are largely indistinguishable from their somatic WNT-activated counterparts. Both medulloblastoma subsets are made up of small, round embryonal cells with high nuclear to cytoplasmic ratio arranged in sheets with frequent Homer Wright pseudorosettes (classic histologic type) (Figure 1) [19-20]. In addition, somatic and germline WNT mediated medulloblastomas display nuclear expression of beta catenin, a molecular feature that differentiates these entities from other medulloblastoma subtypes [21].

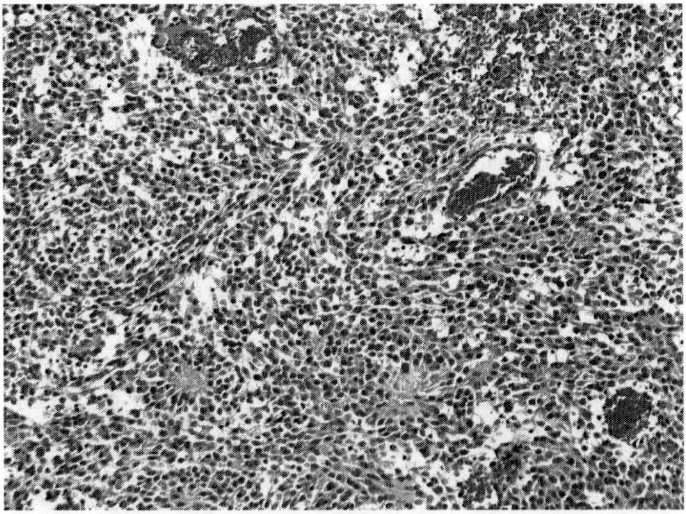

Figure 1. A classic medulloblastoma, WHO grade 4, in a familial adenomatous polyposis 1 patient. The tumor is marked by a sheet of small embryonal cells with mitoses and an occasional Homer Wright pseudorosette (hematoxylin and eosin, original magnification 200X).

Discerning BTP2 associated medulloblastomas from somatic WNT-activated medulloblastomas comes down to genetic testing. BTP2 associated medulloblastomas display a loss of function mutation in the APC gene [13]. Conversely, patients with somatic WNT-activated medulloblastomas will have a CTNNB1 mutation [22].

Histopathology of Other Brain Tumors Reported in the Context of BTP2

As previously mentioned, rare cases of craniopharyngiomas, glioblastomas, anaplastic astrocytomas, and ependymomas have been reported in the setting of BTP2. Histologically, craniopharyngiomas reported in FAP patients are consistent with the adamantinomatous variant, showing a well-differentiated, palisading basaloid epithelium, a stellate reticulum, and, often, calcifications (Figure 2) [23].

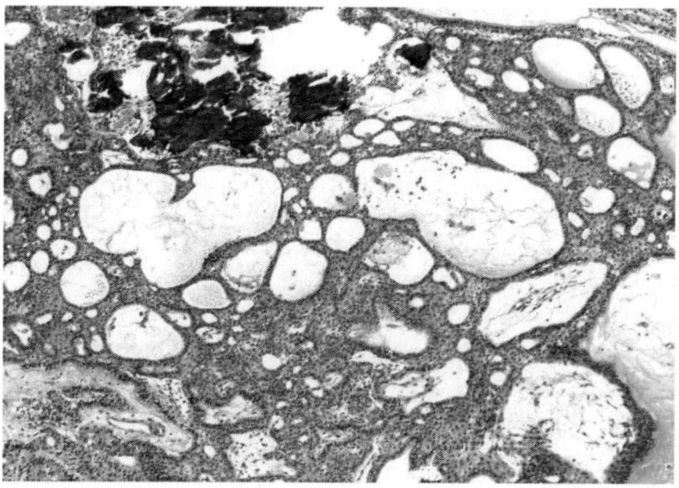

Figure 2. An adamantinomatous craniopharyngioma, WHO grade 1, with focal calcification, arising in a familial adenomatous polyposis 1 patient (hematoxylin and eosin, original magnification 100X).

Astrocytomas described in the context of BTP2 are of the anaplastic type, characterized by increased cellularity, pleomorphism, mitoses, and hyperchromasia. However, unlike glioblastomas delineated in this clinical setting, they lack vascular proliferation and necrosis [24]. Lastly, the limited number of ependymomas reported in FAP patients, like those reported in other clinical contexts, are characterized by sheets of epithelioid cells comprising pseudorosettes and/or true ependymal rosettes. Calcification and necrosis without palisading may also be present [25].

Clinical Presentation and Diagnosis of BTP2-Associated Medulloblastomas and Somatic WNT-Activated Medulloblastomas

Often, patients with a known family history of FAP1 are cognizant of their risk for adenomatous polyposis and eventual colorectal cancer. As a result, these individuals are screened and treated appropriately for colonic manifestations of this syndrome [6]. However, the rarity of medulloblastoma occurrence in the context of FAP precludes a standardized screening process for this potential manifestation [9]. Thus, patients with known FAP1 are often discovered to have BTP2 only after displaying neurologic symptoms (ex: headaches, nausea, blurred vision, confusion, seizures, loss of consciousness, etc.) progressing over a period of weeks to months. Radiologic studies most commonly reveal contrast enhancing mass lesions arising either in the midline of the medulla (occupying the fourth ventricle) [26-27], cerebellopontine angle cistern, or the cerebellar peduncle [28]. Usually, these tumors affect patients at a mean age of 15 years [29]. Patients affected by somatic WNT-associated medulloblastomas, like their germline counterparts, are often diagnosed in their second decade and only after displaying neurologic symptomology. Somatic WNT medulloblastoma localization by imaging results is also nearly identical to that of BTP2 associated tumors [28]. Genetic testing reveals a CTNN1B mutation, confirming somatic etiology. In cases of seemingly sporadic medulloblastoma without CTNN1B mutation, testing for APC pathogenic variants should always be conducted, as germline APC mutations are very common in this context [13].

Patients diagnosed with somatic and germline WNT associated medulloblastomas undergo spinal fluid cytology and cranial and spinal magnetic resonance imaging (MRI) to evaluate for metastasis [9]. Fortunately, only around 10% of patients with WNT derived medulloblastomas are found to have metastatic disease at the time of diagnosis [30].

Treatment and Prognosis of BTP2-Associated and Somatic WNT-Associated Medulloblastomas

Patients diagnosed with both germline and somatic WNT-associated medulloblastomas, like those with other forms of medulloblastoma, undergo conventional treatment, consisting of surgical resection, adjuvant chemotherapy, and radiation therapy [30, 31]. With conventional treatment, WNT-associated medulloblastomas tend to have the best prognosis of all medulloblastoma subtypes, exhibiting an overall survival of 95% in children and 100% in adults after 5 years [30].

However, conventional treatment can have many temporary and permanent sequelae. Surgical excision of the tumor can result in central nervous system infection or neurologic deficits, depending upon the extent of the procedure [32]. Patients receiving radiation can experience fatigue (80%), nausea (80%), anorexia (80%), and myelosuppression (36%) [32, 33]. In patients aged 3-7 years, radiation is associated with an intellectual deficit of 20-30 IQ points [34]. Chemotherapeutic regimens (often including Vincristine, Cisplatin, Lomustine, and/or Cyclophosphamide) are associated with CNS toxicity, gastrointestinal disturbances, nephrotoxicity, hepatotoxicity, ototoxicity, and compromised fertility [32]. Thus, alternative treatment modalities with less severe short- and long-term side effects would be beneficial in this setting.

The molecular subtyping of medulloblastomas has opened the door for targeted therapies with promising implications for patient quality of life and survival. Clinical trials for therapeutic agents targeting the WNT pathway including beta-catenin-T cell factor antagonists, mechanism-based inhibitors targeting essential enzymes in the WNT cascade, biologics, and drugs targeting WNT co-activators are currently underway [35, 37]. Currently, no targeted therapies modulating the WNT cascade have been approved by the Food and Drug Administration.

Conclusion

The near certain likelihood of developing adenomatous polyps and eventual colorectal cancer for patients affected by FAP1 is a well-known sequela of this genetic syndrome. However, rarely, patients with FAP1 also develop BTP2. Medulloblastomas are the main brain tumor subtype associated with BTP2.

These tumors arise as a result of WNT activation secondary to the loss of function APC gene mutation that drives other syndromic features of FAP1. These medulloblastomas usually occur during the second decade of life. No specific screening protocol is in place to detect these tumors in patients with FAP1. Thus, FAP1 patients are diagnosed only after displaying progressive neurologic symptoms over the course of weeks to months.

Imaging reveals a cerebellar (cerebellopontine angle or cerebellar peduncle) or medullary (midline) contrast enhancing mass lesion. BTP2 associated medulloblastomas display classic type histopathologic features (sheets of small, round cells with high nuclear to cytoplasmic ratios and interspersed Homer Wright pseudorosettes). Patients diagnosed with BTP2 associated medulloblastomas have an excellent prognosis with conventional therapy (95% overall survival rate in children and 100% in adults) in comparison to non-WNT associated medulloblastoma subtypes (70% in children and 58-84% in adults) [38-39]. However numerous debilitating side effects and long-term complications arise from conventional therapy, prompting the need for targeted therapies in this setting.

Though BTP2 associated medulloblastomas only make up a small subset of WNT driven medulloblastomas, their demographic, histopathologic, radiologic, and prognostic features are nearly identical to their somatic counterparts.

References

[1] Gardner EJ. A genetic and clinical study of intestinal polyposis, a predisposing factor for carcinoma of the colon and rectum. *Am J Hum Genet.* 1951;3(2):167-76.

[2] Dukes CE, Bussey HJ. The spread of rectal cancer and its effect on prognosis. *Br J Cancer.* 1958;12(3):309-20.

[3] Gardner CM. Polyposis of the colon. *Arch Surg.* 1948;56(1):75-8.

[4] Bussey HJ, Veale AM, Morson BC. Genetics of gastrointestinal polyposis. *Gastroenterology.* 1978;74(6):1325-30.

[5] Bodmer, WF, Bailey, CJ, Bodmer, J, et al. Localization of the gene for familial adenomatous polyposis on chromosome 5. *Nature.* 1987;328(6131):614-6.

[6] Jasperson, KW, Tuohy, TM, Neklason, DW, et al. Hereditary and familial colon cancer. *Gastroenterology.* 2010;138(6):2044-2058.

[7] Half E, Bercovich D, Rozen P. Familial adenomatous polyposis. *Orphanet J Rare Dis.* 2009;4:22.

[8] Bosman FT, Carneiro F, Hruban RH, et al. *World Health Organization Histological Classification of Tumours of the Digestive System.* 4th ed. Lyon: International Agency for Research on Cancer; 2010.

[9] Louis DN, Ohgaki H, Wiestler OD, et al. *World Health Organization Histological Classification of Tumours of the Central Nervous System*. 4th ed. Lyon: International Agency for Research on Cancer; 2007.

[10] Perry A, Brat DJ. *Practical Surgical Neuropathology: A Diagnostic Approach*. Philadelphia, PA: Churchill Livingstone/Elsevier; 2010.

[11] Van Meir EG. "Turcot's Syndrome": phenotype of brain tumors, survival, and mode of inheritance. *Int J Cancer*. 1998; 75:162-164.

[12] Kim B, Tabori U, Hawkins C. An update on the CNS manifestations of brain tumor polyposis syndromes. *Acta Neuropathol*. 2020 Apr;139(4):703-15.

[13] Waszak Sebastian M, Paul A Northcott, Ivo Buchhalter, et al. Spectrum and prevalence of genetic predisposition in medulloblastoma: a retrospective genetic study and prospective validation in a clinical trial cohort. *Lancet Oncol*. 2018 Jun;19(6):785-798.

[14] Hamilton SR, Liu B, Parsons RE, et al. The molecular basis of Turcot's syndrome. *N Engl J Med*. 1995;332(13):839-847.

[15] Damalas A, Ben-Ze'ev A, Simcha I, et al. Excess beta-catenin promotes accumulation of transcriptionally active p53. *EMBO J*. 1999;18(11):3054-3063.

[16] Taylor, MD, Northcott, PA, Korshunov, A, et al. Molecular subgroups of medulloblastoma: the current consensus. *Acta Neuropathol*. 2012;123(4):465-472.

[17] Hamilton SR, Liu B, Parsons RE, et al. The molecular basis of Turcot's syndrome. *N Engl J Med*. 1995;332:839–847.

[18] Zurawel RH, Chiappa SA, Allen C, et al. Sporadic medulloblastomas contain oncogenic beta-catenin mutations. *Cancer Res*. 1998;58(5):896-9.

[19] Orr BA. Pathology, diagnostics, and classification of medulloblastoma. *Brain Pathol*. 2020;30(3):664-678.

[20] Surun Aurore, Pascale Varlet, Laurence Brugières, et al. Medulloblastoma associated with an APC germline pathogenic variant share the good prognosis of CTNNB1-mutated medulloblastomas. *Neuro Oncol*. 2020;22(1):128-138.

[21] Ellison DW, Dalton J, Kocak M,et al. Medulloblastoma: clinicopathological correlates of SHH, WNT, and non-SHH/WNT molecular subgroups. *Acta Neuropathol*. 2011;121(3):381-96.

[22] Rogers HA, Miller S, Lowe J, et al. An investigation of WNT pathway activation and association with survival in central nervous system primitive neuroectodermal tumours (CNS PNET). *Br J Cancer*. 2009;100(8): 1292–1302.

[23] Dahl NA, Pratt D, Camelo-Piragua S, et al. Pediatric craniopharyngioma in association with familial adenomatous polyposis. *Fam Cancer*. 2019;18(3):327-330.

[24] Attard TM, Giglio P, Koppula S, et al. Brain tumors in individuals with familial adenomatous polyposis: a cancer registry experience and pooled case report analysis. *Cancer*. 2007;109(4):761-6.

[25] Tarapore PE, Modera P, Naujokas A, et al. Pathology of spinal ependymomas: an institutional experience over 25 years in 134 patients. *Neurosurgery*. 2013;73(2): 247-55.

[26] Teo Wan-Yee, Jianhe Shen, Jack Meng Fen Su, et al. Implications of tumor location on subtypes of medulloblastoma. *Pediatr Blood Cancer*. 2013;60(9):1408-10.

[27] Gibson Paul, Yiai Tong, Giles Robinson, et al. Subtypes of medulloblastoma have distinct developmental origins. *Nature.* 2010;468:1095–1099.

[28] Perreault S, Ramaswamy V, Achrol AS, et al. MRI surrogates for molecular subgroups of medulloblastoma. *AJNR Am J Neuroradiol.* 2014;35(7):1263–9.

[29] Van Meir EG, "Turcot's syndrome": phenotype of brain tumors, survival, and mode of inheritance. *Int J Cancer.* 1998; 75:162-164.

[30] Millard NE, De Braganca KC. Medulloblastoma. *J Child Neurol.* 2016;31(12):1341-53.

[31] Khatua S, Song A, Citla Sridhar D, et al. Childhood medulloblastoma: current therapies, emerging molecular landscape and newer therapeutic insights. *Curr Neuropharmacol.* 2018;16(7):1045-1058.

[32] De Braganca KC, Packer RJ. Treatment options for medulloblastoma and CNS primitive neuroectodermal tumor (PNET). *Curr Treat Options Neurol.* 2013; 15(5):593-606.

[33] Jakacki RI, Burger PC, Zhou T, et al. Outcome of children with metastatic medulloblastoma treated with carboplatin during craniospinal radiotherapy: a Children's Oncology Group Phase I/II study. *J Clin Oncol.* 2012;30(21):2648-53.

[34] Packer RJ, Vezina G. Management of and prognosis with medulloblastoma: therapy at a crossroads. *Arch. Neurol.* 2008;65:1419–1424.

[35] Maier H, Dalianis T, Kostopoulou ON. New approaches in targeted therapy for medulloblastoma in children. *Anticancer Res.* 2021;41(4):1715-1726.

[36] Anastas JN, Moon RT. WNT signaling pathways as therapeutic targets in cancer. *Nat Rev Cancer.* 2013;13(1):11–26.

[37] Kahn M. Can we safely target the WNT pathway? *Nat Rev Drug Discov.* 2014; 13(7):513–32.

[38] Johnston DL, Keene D, Strother D, et al. Survival following tumor recurrence in children with medulloblastoma. *J Pediatr Hematol Oncol.* 2018;40(3):e159-e163.

[39] Prados MD, Warnick RE, Wara WM, et al. Medulloblastoma in adults. *Int J Radiat Oncol Biol Phys.* 1995;32:1145–52.

Chapter 15

BAP1 Tumor Predisposition Syndrome: Central Nervous System Pathology

Maeve Pascoe[1], BS
and Richard A. Prayson[2,*], MD, MEd
[1] Cleveland Clinic Lerner College of Medicine, Cleveland, Ohio, USA
[2] Department of Anatomic Pathology, Cleveland Clinic, Cleveland, Ohio, USA

Abstract

BAP1 tumor predisposition syndrome (*BAP1*-TPDS) is a syndrome caused by autosomal dominant germline variants of *BAP1*, which lead to BAP1 protein loss of tumor suppressing function. The syndrome is associated with a predisposition for the development of a variety of tumors including uveal and cutaneous melanomas, mesotheliomas, and meningiomas, among others. Meningiomas are the primary central nervous system tumors associated with *BAP1*-TPDS and are typically high grade and have rhabdoid morphology.

This chapter will review *BAP1*-TPDS and its associated tumors, with a focus on the neuropathological features of its associated meningiomas.

Introduction

While families with multiple members affected by malignant mesothelioma were identified as early as the 1980s [1], *BAP1* tumor predisposition syndrome was first identified as a syndrome by several investigators in 2011 studying families with multiple tumor types, including malignant mesothelioma,

* Corresponding Author's Email: praysor@ccf.org.

In: Central Nervous System Pathologies in Hereditary Tumor Syndromes
Editor: Richard A. Prayson
ISBN: 979-8-88697-620-5

melanomas, and meningiomas, among others [2-5]. Although only found in 1/50,000 people without cancer, *BAP1* pathologic germline variants are found in 1/1900 people with cancer [6]. In fact, the lifetime risk of developing cancer in people with a *BAP1* pathologic variant is nearly 100% in some studies, and most affected families report multiple tumor types among those affected [7, 8].

This chapter will review *BAP1* tumor predisposition syndrome (*BAP1*-TPDS), covering both its non-neurological and neurological findings with a focus on the neuropathological features of its associated central nervous tumors.

Molecular Genetics

This syndrome is caused by autosomal dominant (and rarely, de novo) germline mutations in the *BAP1* tumor suppressor gene, composed of 17 exons located on chromosome 3p21.1 [9]. There are 140 known pathologic variants (null and missense) of *BAP1*, with the most prevalent being *BAP1 p.L573Wfs*2;* null variants which typically predispose to earlier tumor formation [8]. The BAP1 protein, as its name suggests, is a BRCA1-associated protein (BAP), which plays a role in DNA repair via homologous recombination; however, it has also been found to serve as a deubiquitinase acting on ASXL proteins as part of the polycomb group epigenetic regulatory complex and on IP3R3 to regulate apoptosis [10-13]. As such, mutations in *BAP1* result in loss of BAP1 protein functions, including transcriptional regulation, cell cycle regulation and lineage differentiation, and immunomodulation [14].

Clinical Manifestations Outside of the Central Nervous System

As previously mentioned, loss of function of *BAP1* predisposes to both neurological and non-neurological tumors. Among the non-neurological tumors, uveal melanoma is the most common cancer and cancer with earliest reported age of onset (16 years) in patients with *BAP1*-TPDS [8, 15]. Additionally, loss of *BAP1* function can lead to the development of pulmonary, pleural, and peritoneal cancers, including malignant mesothelioma, the second most common cancer in patients with *BAP1*-TPDS, and pulmonary adenocarcinomas [2, 4, 16]. Dermatological manifestations include cutaneous melanocytic tumors, melanocytic BAP1-mutated atypical intradermal tumors (MBAITs), and basal cell carcinomas [3, 5, 7, 17]. Additional tumors that have been seen are breast cancer, hepatocellular carcinoma, cholangiocarcinoma, and clear cell/sarcomatous renal carcinoma [4, 18-21].

While BAP1-deficient tumors themselves can be diagnosed with immunohistochemistry, clinical diagnosis of *BAP1*-TPDS relies on the presence of a BAP1 pathogenic variant identified with genetic testing in the context of the presence of characteristic tumors. Criteria for genetic testing for *BAP1*-TPDS include either (a) a history of at least two *BAP1*-TPDS-associated tumors, (b) one *BAP1*-TPDS tumor plus one first/second degree relative with a *BAP1*-TPDS tumor, and/or (c) early age of tumor onset [7, 8, 22].

Neurologic Clinical and Imaging Features

The primary central nervous system pathology associated with *BAP1*-TPDS is meningioma, and neurologic clinical features seen in patients with *BAP1*-TPDS are associated with meningioma tumor burden. Meningiomas have an annual incidence in adults of 8.83 per 100,000 and are seen in 8.5% of patients with *BAP1*-TPDS, with BAP1-variant meningiomas accounting for <1% of all meningiomas [23]. Onset in the general population typically occurs over age 65 years and in females more commonly than males [24].

Patients with meningiomas may not have any obvious clinical symptoms, but the symptoms most commonly reported are headaches, seizures, and focal neurological deficits based on tumor location and mass effect (e.g., weakness, sensory loss, aphasia, visual loss) [24]. Additional symptoms may include memory problems, mood disturbances, personality changes, and nausea/vomiting or loss of consciousness due to increased intracranial pressure.

If a brain lesion is suspected based on history and physical exam, computed tomography (CT) and magnetic resonance imaging (MRI) with contrast are useful imaging modalities for visualizing and identifying the lesion in question. Meningiomas have characteristic features that can be easily identified on CT and MRI, and MRI images are typically used for diagnosis [25]. On a CT scan, meningiomas appear as well-defined, extra-axial, dural-adjacent masses that have smooth contours. They may also be multilobulated or have areas of calcification and are often contrast-enhancing. On MRI scans, meningiomas will be hypo- or isointense to gray matter on T1 images and iso-

or hyperintense on proton density and T2 images, with strong contrast enhancement and a "tail sign" of marginal dural thickening with peripheral tapering.

Neuropathological Features

BAP1-variant meningiomas are typically high-grade (usually World Health Organization (WHO) grade 3 but occasionally grade 2 and rarely grade 1); they most commonly have rhabdoid cytomorphology [26-28]. Less commonly, they may have papillary cytomorphology, characteristic of some WHO grade 3 meningiomas, and occasionally may have epithelioid cellular components [26, 27, 29]. In general, rhabdoid meningiomas present on histology with eosinophilic meningothelial cells with peripheral and enlarged nuclei (Figures 1 and 2), while papillary meningiomas present with papillary or pseudopapillary cellular patterns of fibrovascular cores surrounded by meningothelial cells [28].

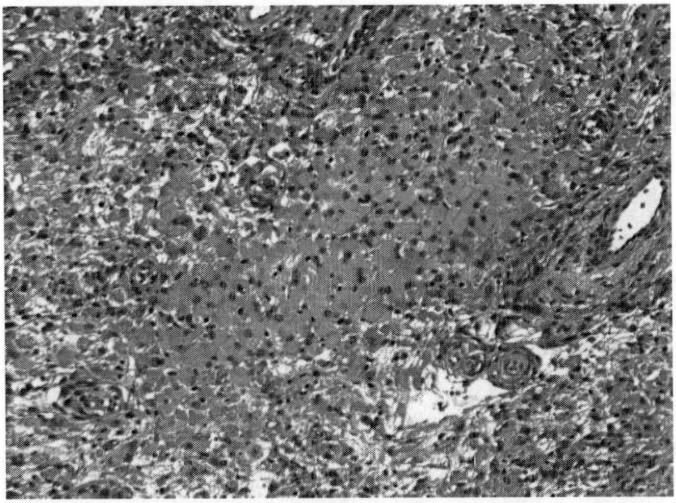

Figure 1. A rhabdoid meningioma (WHO grade 3) marked by a proliferation of cells with an eosinophilic cytoplasmic globular-like appearance and eccentrically placed nuclei (hematoxylin and eosin, original magnification 200X).

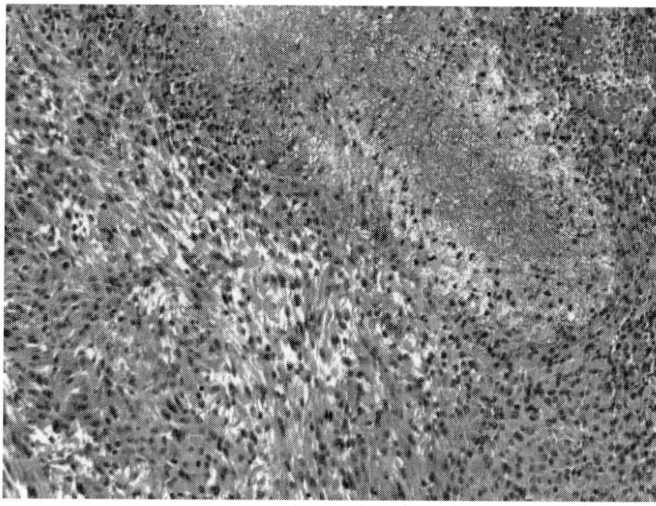

Figure 2. The same tumor as in Figure 1 with an area of geographic necrosis (hematoxylin and eosin, original magnification 200X).

Immunohistochemistry can also be used to identify meningiomas, particularly those associated with *BAP1*-TPDS. Generally, somatostatin receptor 2A (SSTR2A), epithelial membrane antigen (EMA), and progesterone receptor (PR) expression is seen in meningiomas [28, 30]. Loss of nuclear BAP1 immunoreactivity can be used to identify BAP1-associated tumor cells, with good concordance between BAP1 loss on immunohistochemistry and BAP1 pathological variants identified with genotyping [31-34].

Histologic and immunohistochemical features of meningiomas can be used to narrow the differential diagnosis and distinguish them from other central nervous system tumors. Meningioma mimics include solitary fibrous tumors (will have STAT6 immunoreactivity), sarcomas (generally lack SSTR2a and progesterone receptor immunoreactivity), pachymeningitis due to IgG4 disease (will have >10% IgG4:IgG), papillary carcinomas (will express other immunomarkers such as PAX8 or thyroid transcription factor-1), rhabdomyosarcoma (will stain with antibodies to myoD1, myogenin, and desmin), or metastatic melanoma (will express neural crest markers such as S-100 protein, SOX10 and HMB45) [28].

Treatment and Prognosis

For WHO grade 2 and 3 meningiomas, guidelines for treatment include gross total surgical resection (if possible), along with adjuvant radiation therapy, followed by surveillance for recurrent disease [25, 35]. Though not currently standard of care, there is growing evidence for the utility of chemotherapies and immunotherapies (e.g., EZH2 and PARP inhibitors, checkpoint inhibitors) in recurrent and aggressive meningiomas, such as those associated with *BAP1*-TPDS [27, 36]. Recurrence is less likely with complete resection, but certain clinical features may confer greater risk for recurrence, including older age and incomplete resection [37]. Additionally, patients with BAP1-deficient meningiomas tend to have a significantly reduced time to recurrence [26].

Regarding prognosis, *BAP1* variants may have different prognostic significance within different cancer types but does not appear to have prognostic significance across all cancers [38]. While patients with mesothelioma have less aggressive tumors and a greatly increased 5-year survival rate in the context of BAP1 mutations, BAP1-variant meningiomas are generally more aggressive with worse progression-free and overall survival [39, 40]. In general, WHO grade 2 and 3 meningiomas, like those seen in *BAP1*-TPDS, confer a median progression-free survival (PFS) around 3 years and overall survival (OS) between 5-10 years, with recent studies showing ~35-53% PFS and ~66-71% OS at 5 years in grade 2 and 3 tumors [41, 42]. Use of adjuvant radiotherapy is associated with improved progression free survival, while indicators of greater cell proliferation (Ki-67 index >10%) are associated with worse progression free survival [42, 43].

Conclusion

BAP1 tumor predisposition syndrome is an autosomal dominant condition associated with germline mutations of the BAP1 tumor suppressor gene located on chromosome 3p. The condition is associated with a predisposition for the development of meningiomas in the central nervous system. Meningiomas which arise in this setting are more likely to be more aggressive behaving tumors (WHO grade 2 or 3 lesions).

References

[1] Risberg B., Nickels J., Wågermark J. Familial clustering of malignant mesothelioma. *Cancer*. May 1 1980;45(9):2422-7.

[2] Testa J. R., Cheung M., Pei J., et al., Germline BAP1 mutations predispose to malignant mesothelioma. *Nat Genet*. Aug 28 2011;43(10):1022-5.

[3] Wiesner T., Obenauf A. C., Murali R., et al., Germline mutations in BAP1 predispose to melanocytic tumors. *Nat Genet*. Aug 28 2011;43(10):1018-21.

[4] Abdel-Rahman M. H., Pilarski R., Cebulla C. M., et al., Germline BAP1 mutation predisposes to uveal melanoma, lung adenocarcinoma, meningioma, and other cancers. *J Med Genet*. Dec 2011;48(12):856-9.

[5] Carbone M., Ferris L. K., Baumann F., et al., BAP1 cancer syndrome: malignant mesothelioma, uveal and cutaneous melanoma, and MBAITs. *J Transl Med*. Aug 30 2012;10:179.

[6] Massengill J. B., Sample K. M., Pilarski R., et al., Analysis of the exome aggregation consortium (ExAC) database suggests that the BAP1-tumor predisposition syndrome is underreported in cancer patients. *Genes Chromosomes Cancer*. Sep 2018;57(9):478-481.

[7] Rai K., Pilarski R., Cebulla C. M., Abdel-Rahman M. H. Comprehensive review of BAP1 tumor predisposition syndrome with report of two new cases. *Clin Genet*. Mar 2016;89(3):285-94.

[8] Walpole S., Pritchard A. L., Cebulla C. M., et al., Comprehensive study of the clinical phenotype of germline BAP1 variant-carrying families worldwide. *J Natl Cancer Inst*. Dec 1 2018;110(12):1328-1341.

[9] Jensen D. E., Proctor M., Marquis S. T., et al., BAP1: a novel ubiquitin hydrolase which binds to the BRCA1 RING finger and enhances BRCA1-mediated cell growth suppression. *Oncogene*. Mar 5 1998;16(9):1097-112.

[10] LaFave L. M., Béguelin W., Koche R., et al., Loss of BAP1 function leads to EZH2-dependent transformation. *Nat Med*. Nov 2015;21(11):1344-9.

[11] Ismail I. H., Davidson R., Gagné J. P., et al., Germline mutations in BAP1 impair its function in DNA double-strand break repair. *Cancer Res*. Aug 15 2014;74(16):4282-94.

[12] Daou S., Hammond-Martel I., Mashtalir N., et al., The BAP1/ASXL2 histone H2A deubiquitinase complex regulates cell proliferation and is disrupted in cancer. *J Biol Chem*. Nov 27 2015;290(48):28643-63.

[13] Bononi A., Giorgi C., Patergnani S., et al., BAP1 regulates IP3R3-mediated Ca(2+) flux to mitochondria suppressing cell transformation. *Nature*. Jun 22 2017;546 (7659):549-553.

[14] Carbone M., Harbour J. W., Brugarolas J., et al., Biological mechanisms and clinical significance of BAP1 mutations in human cancer. *Cancer Discov*. Aug 2020;10 (8):1103-1120.

[15] Gupta M. P., Lane A. M., DeAngelis M. M., et al., Clinical characteristics of uveal melanoma in patients with germline BAP1 mutations. *JAMA Ophthalmol*. Aug 2015;133(8):881-7.

[16] Cheung M., Testa J. R. BAP1, a tumor suppressor gene driving malignant mesothelioma. *Transl Lung Cancer Res*. Jun 2017;6(3):270-278.

[17] Wadt K. A., Aoude L. G., Johansson P., et al., A recurrent germline BAP1 mutation and extension of the BAP1 tumor predisposition spectrum to include basal cell carcinoma. *Clin Genet*. Sep 2015;88(3):267-72.

[18] Jager M. J., Shields C. L., Cebulla C. M., et al., Uveal melanoma. *Nat Rev Dis Primers*. Apr 9 2020;6(1):24.

[19] Popova T., Hebert L., Jacquemin V., et al., Germline BAP1 mutations predispose to renal cell carcinomas. *Am J Hum Genet*. Jun 6 2013;92(6):974-80.

[20] Bell H. N., Kumar-Sinha C., Mannan R., et al., Pathogenic ATM and BAP1 germline mutations in a case of early-onset, familial sarcomatoid renal cancer. *Cold Spring Harb Mol Case Stud*. Apr 2022;8(3).

[21] Blatnik A., Ribnikar D., Šetrajčič Dragoš V., et al., BAP1-defficient breast cancer in a patient with BAP1 cancer syndrome. *Breast Cancer*. Sep 2022;29(5):921-927.

[22] Chau C., van Doorn R., van Poppelen N. M., et al., Families with BAP1-tumor predisposition syndrome in the Netherlands: path to identification and a proposal for genetic screening guidelines. *Cancers (Basel)*. Aug 4 2019;11(8).

[23] Ostrom Q. T., Cioffi G., Gittleman H., et al., CBTRUS statistical report: primary brain and other central nervous system tumors diagnosed in the United States in 2012-2016. *Neuro Oncol*. Nov 1 2019;21(Suppl 5):v1-v100.

[24] Zouaoui S., Darlix A., Rigau V., et al., Descriptive epidemiology of 13,038 newly diagnosed and histologically confirmed meningiomas in France: 2006-2010. *Neurochirurgie*. Mar 2018;64(1):15-21.

[25] Maggio I., Franceschi E., Tosoni A., et al., Meningioma: not always a benign tumor. A review of advances in the treatment of meningiomas. *CNS Oncol*. Jun 1 2021;10(2):Cns72.

[26] Shankar G. M., Abedalthagafi M., Vaubel R. A., et al., Germline and somatic BAP1 mutations in high-grade rhabdoid meningiomas. *Neuro Oncol*. Apr 1 2017;19(4): 535-545.

[27] Shankar G. M., Santagata S. BAP1 mutations in high-grade meningioma: implications for patient care. *Neuro Oncol*. Oct 19 2017;19(11):1447-1456.

[28] Toland A., Huntoon K., Dahiya S. M. Meningioma: a pathology perspective. *Neurosurgery*. Jun 15 2021;89(1):11-21.

[29] Louis D. N., Perry A., Reifenberger G., et al., The 2016 World Health Organization Classification of Tumors of the Central Nervous System: a summary. *Acta Neuropathol*. Jun 2016;131(6):803-20.

[30] Menke J. R., Raleigh D. R., Gown A. M., et al., Somatostatin receptor 2a is a more sensitive diagnostic marker of meningioma than epithelial membrane antigen. *Acta Neuropathol*. Sep 2015;130(3):441-3.

[31] Bott M., Brevet M., Taylor B. S., et al., The nuclear deubiquitinase BAP1 is commonly inactivated by somatic mutations and 3p21.1 losses in malignant pleural mesothelioma. *Nat Genet*. Jun 5 2011;43(7):668-72.

[32] Koopmans A. E., Verdijk R. M., Brouwer R. W., et al., Clinical significance of immunohistochemistry for detection of BAP1 mutations in uveal melanoma. *Mod Pathol*. Oct 2014;27(10):1321-30.

[33] Nasu M., Emi M., Pastorino S., et al., High incidence of somatic BAP1 alterations in sporadic malignant mesothelioma. *J Thorac Oncol.* Apr 2015;10(4):565-76.

[34] van de Nes J. A., Nelles J., Kreis S., et al., Comparing the prognostic value of BAP1 mutation pattern, chromosome 3 status, and BAP1 immunohistochemistry in uveal melanoma. *Am J Surg Pathol.* Jun 2016;40(6):796-805.

[35] Goldbrunner R., Stavrinou P., Jenkinson M. D., et al., EANO guideline on the diagnosis and management of meningiomas. *Neuro Oncol.* Nov 2 2021;23(11): 1821-1834.

[36] Graillon T., Tabouret E., Chinot O. Chemotherapy and targeted therapies for meningiomas: what is the evidence? *Curr Opin Neurol.* Dec 1 2021;34(6):857-867.

[37] Aghi M. K., Carter B. S., Cosgrove G. R., et al., Long-term recurrence rates of atypical meningiomas after gross total resection with or without postoperative adjuvant radiation. *Neurosurgery.* Jan 2009;64(1):56-60; discussion 60.

[38] Wang Z., Wang X. Y., Li J., Zhu W. W. Prognostic and clinicopathological significance of BAP1 protein expression in different types of cancer-a meta-analysis. *Genet Test Mol Biomarkers.* Feb 2018;22(2):115-126.

[39] Baumann F., Flores E., Napolitano A., et al., Mesothelioma patients with germline BAP1 mutations have 7-fold improved long-term survival. *Carcinogenesis.* Jan 2015;36(1):76-81.

[40] Ruzevick J., Gibson A., Tatman P., et al., WHO grade III meningioma: De novo tumors show improved progression free survival as compared to secondary progressive tumors. *J Clin Neurosci.* Sep 2021;91:105-109.

[41] Recker M. J., Kuo C. C., Prasad D., et al., Incidence trends and survival analysis of atypical meningiomas: a population-based study from 2004 to 2018. *J Neurooncol.* Jul 11 2022.

[42] Kent C. L., Mowery Y. M., Babatunde O., et al., Long-term outcomes for patients with atypical or malignant meningiomas treated with or without radiation therapy: a 25-year retrospective analysis of a single-institution experience. *Adv Radiat Oncol.* May-Jun 2022;7(3):100878.

[43] Liu N., Song S. Y., Jiang J. B., et al., The prognostic role of Ki-67/MIB-1 in meningioma: A systematic review with meta-analysis. *Medicine (Baltimore).* Feb 2020;99(9):e18644.

Chapter 16

ELP1-Medulloblastoma Syndrome

Mario-Cyriac Tcheukado[1], BS
Derrick Obiri-Yeboah[1], BS
and Richard A. Prayson[2,1], MD, MEd
[1] Cleveland Clinic Lerner College of Medicine, Cleveland, Ohio, USA
[2] Department of Anatomic Pathology, Cleveland Clinic, Cleveland, Ohio, USA

Abstract

ELP1-medulloblastoma syndrome is an autosomal dominant disorder caused by mutations in the ELP1 gene. ELP1 is the most common medulloblastoma predisposition gene with a prevalence of 30% among pediatric patients with the sonic hedgehog-activating subtype. The inactivation of ELP1 characterizes the pathogenesis of this syndrome due to somatic loss of chromosome 9q. Additionally, most of these medulloblastomas also exhibit alteration in PTCH1, leading to biallelic inactivation along with amplification of PPM1D and MDM4 which are components that regulate p53 signaling. The median age of diagnosis of ELP1-associated medulloblastomas is 6.3 years with favorable clinical outcomes seen in preliminary data.

This chapter will review the clinicopathologic features of this disorder, with a primary focus on central nervous system-associated pathology.

Introduction

Posterior fossa tumors seen in pre-adolescents were first named "medulloblastoma" by Harvey Cushing and Percival Bailey in 1925 [1].

In: Central Nervous System Pathologies in Hereditary Tumor Syndromes
Editor: Richard A. Prayson
ISBN: 979-8-88697-620-5

Cushing characterized these tumors as arising from the cerebellum or posterior cranial fossa and metastasizing to distant locations, affecting younger male patients, and presenting with a short duration of symptoms prior to diagnosis [1]. Medulloblastoma (MB) is the most common brain tumor in children, comprising up to 20% of all pediatric brain tumors and 64% of all embryonal brain tumors [2]. They are considered to be one of the most threatening malignant brain tumors with a higher mortality [3]. MBs can be classified into four molecular subgroups: WNT, SHH, group 3, and group 4, all of which have unique clinical features and prognoses [4]. This chapter will focus specifically on the SHH subtype (SHH-MB) which accounts for approximately 30% of all MB cases [5]. In SHH-MB, germline heterozygous loss-of-function variants across ELP1 are the most common MB predisposition gene abnormalities which are detected in 14% of pediatric SHH-MB patients [4]. This chapter will review the clinical and pathologic features of ELP1-medulloblastoma syndrome, focusing on the neuropathologic findings.

Genetics of ELP1-Medulloblastoma Syndrome

The prevalence of MB molecular subtypes varies in their prevalence with 40% of patients with SHH-MB harboring germline variations in different genes [6]. There is a lower prevalence of around 6-8% in APC germline variations noted in the WNT-MB group with rare BRCA2 or PALB2 variations (1% prevalence) found within group 3 or 4 MB [6]. However, despite differences in molecular subgroups of MB, the therapeutic approach remains generally similar.

Nearly 40% of patients with MB harbor a sonic hedgehog germline alteration [4]. Specifically, Waszak et al. identified germline loss-of-function (LoF) mutations in elongator complex protein 1 (ELP1) to be the most common MB predisposition gene (14% of pediatric patients with SHH-MB) and is strongly associated with MBs in pediatric age patients [7]. ELP1-medulloblastoma syndrome is caused by a germline sequence variant in the ELP1 gene, located on chromosome 9 at position 9q31.3, resulting in loss of heterozygosity and biallelic inactivation coupled with monoallelic loss of PTCH1 [7]. Since ELP1 is the largest component of the elongator complex, inactivation leads to translational dysregulation and disruption in protein homeostasis. It has further been postulated that there may be additional mutations or focal deletions in PTCH1 seen in ELP-MB leading to amplification of PPMD1 and MDM4 (regulators of p53 signaling) [7].

General Clinical Features

Germline heterozygous LoF mutations in ELP1 represent the most common predisposition gene to MBs which were detected in 14% of pediatric patients with SHH-MB [7]. Patients are diagnosed at a median age of 6.3 years with ELP1-associated MBs being the predominant histological diagnosis. While some patients may be the first in their families to develop MB, a considerable number of them often have a family history of MB [7].

Affected patients with MB often present with specific signs and symptoms due to increased intracranial pressure and cerebellar dysfunction, both of which evolve over a period of weeks to months [8]. The most common symptoms of MB are nausea, vomiting, altered mental status, and nocturnal or morning headaches [8]. In addition to increased intracranial pressure and cerebellar dysfunction, the location of the tumor can also determine the specific symptoms. For example, tumors located near the midline may cause gait ataxia or truncal instability, whereas those more lateral may present with difficulty moving a limb [9]. Dizziness and double vision are common in tumors located in the cerebellum, brainstem, or cranial nerve tumors [9].

Neurologic Clinical Features

ELP1-medulloblastoma syndrome is caused by a germline sequence variant in the ELP1 gene, located on chromosome 9 at position 9q31.3, resulting in loss of heterozygosity and biallelic inactivation coupled with monoallelic loss of PTCH1 [7]. Patients typically present with signs of increased intracranial pressure related to obstructive hydrocephalus, a finding most likely due to tumor growth and compression of the fourth ventricle [8]. Other signs of intracranial pressure include an increased head circumference and early morning headaches with vomiting, irritability, and fatigue [10]. MBs are common in the cerebellar midline and may be associated with axial instability, which manifests as an unsteady gait [11]. Rarely, MBs may involve the lateral cerebellum which may lead to appendicular ataxia and dysmetria. Altered eye movements and disequilibrium may indicate flocculonodular lobe inclusion [11].

Diagnosis of a MB includes a well-detailed history, physical exam, and imaging. The neurological exam findings depend on the location of the tumor within the posterior fossa. Patients with midline tumors typically present with gait or lower limb functional abnormalities, which manifest as a broad-based gait or difficulty with heel-to-tie talking [12]. Other common signs are head titubation (bobbing) or rapid, repetitive, and uncontrolled eye movements (nystagmus) [13]. On the other hand, patients with lateral tumors may present with difficulty coordinating limb movement (dysmetria) and this will show as difficulty completing the finger-to-nose test [13]. Other lateral tumor symptoms include intention tremors and faculty performing the heal-to-shin test [12].

Imaging Findings

The appearance of medulloblastomas on magnetic resonance imaging (MRI) can be variable. Typically, MBs appear as round, slightly lobulated, and T1-iso-/hypointense masses [14]. Furthermore, the T2 signal can be heterogeneous with the solid portion often being T2-hypo- to isointense compared to the gray matter [15]. MRI with contrast enhancement is present but may vary in degree from diffuse and homogenous to focal and patchy [16]. However, a lack of enhancement has been reported in 7.5% of tumors [17]. Cysts are very common in MBs and are found in approximately 50% of cases that appear small and numerous. Solitary and isolated cysts are less frequent, seen in about 30-35% and 5-15% of cases respectively. Enhanced nodules in the ventricles or over the surface of the brain or spinal cord may be indicative of leptomeningeal dissemination [17]. Metastases of MBs can occur and can be discovered via MRI imaging with intracranial ones being commonly found in the vermis, basal cisterns, subependymal region of the lateral ventricles, floor of the third ventricle, and subfrontal regions [17]. Finally, dissemination of the tumor to the cerebrospinal fluid is common and can best be seen on T1-weighted sequences with paramagnetic contrast [18].

The typical features of MB on contrast-enhanced computer tomography (CT) is a midline, well-defined, and homogenous mass [17]. MBs are commonly hyperdense or isodense compared to the surrounding tissue and this is due to their high cellularity marked by cells with dense, hyperchromatic nuclei and cytoplasm [17]. Edema have been reported in 90-90% of patients [17]. Finally, calcifications have been found in 20% of cases, and cysts or necrosis in 50%. Hemorrhages are rarely seen in either imaging modality (MRI or CT) [19, 20].

Neuropathological Findings

Biopsies are rarely performed in patients suspected of having a MB upon imaging because total resection is integral in the treatment. Therefore, diagnosis of MB requires histopathologic confirmation after surgical resection. At surgery, MBs are said to be soft and brittle often with necrosis [21]. With histological analysis, MBs are highly cellular with round or oval nuclei and low cytoplasm [21]. Their histopathological appearance can range from tumors with extensive nodularity to those with large cell/anaplastic features (Figures 1 and 2) [21].

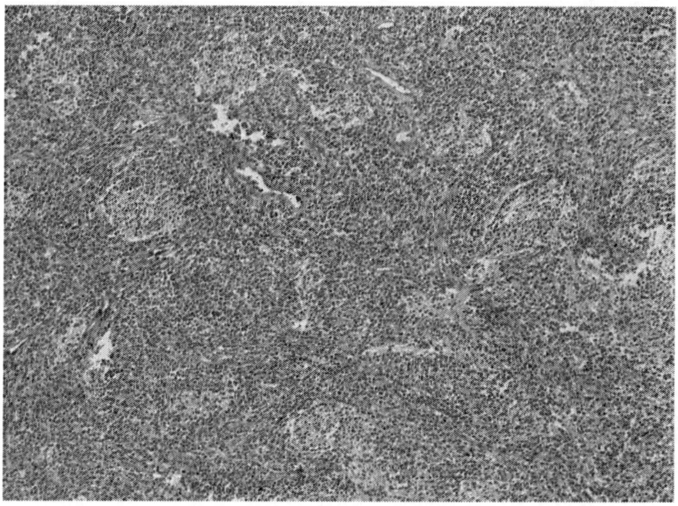

Figure 1. A desmoplastic/nodular cerebellar medulloblastoma, WHO grade 4, presenting in a 4-year-old male with ELP-1 Medulloblastoma syndrome (hematoxylin and eosin, original magnification 100X).

MBs are also characterized by mitotic activity and the presence of Homer Wright rosettes [22]. Immunochemical studies have also shown the common expression of synaptophysin, a neuronal marker, in MBs as well as neuron-specific enolase and nestin [23]. Other studies have shown that cerebellar granular cell markers are present in MBs, such as PAX6, EN1, and EN2, supporting the hypothesis that this type of tumor may originate in the external granular layer of the cerebellum in some cases [24]. Zinc protein has also been detected in MB cases suggesting their development from the cerebellum [25].

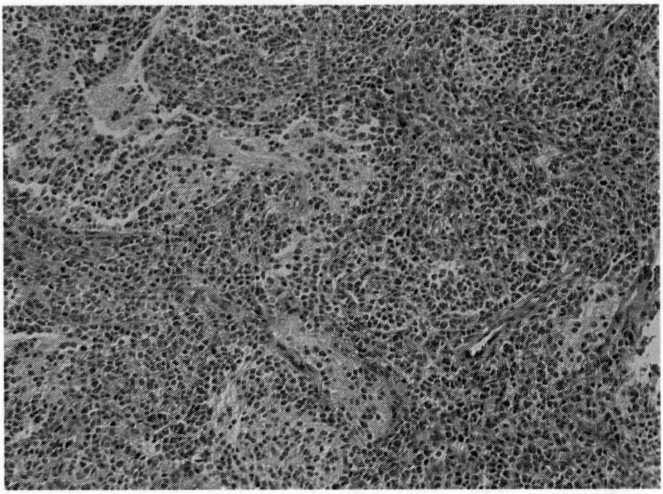

Figure 2. The same tumor as in Figure 1. The tumor is characterized by nodular, reticulin free zones with intervening more densely cellar areas (hematoxylin and eosin, original magnification 200X).

Approximately a third of MBs metastasize throughout the central nervous system via the cerebrospinal fluid tracts [21, 26]. In cases of metastasis, neoplastic cells can be seen within the cerebrospinal fluid. This has also been associated with elevated protein and mild pleocytosis [26].

As demonstrated by Change et al. 1969, the combination of imaging and cerebrospinal fluid cytology can determine the clinical staging of MBs as detailed below [27, 28]:

- M0: No evidence of subarachnoid or hematogenous metastasis.
- M1: Microscopic tumor cells in the cerebrospinal fluid.
- M2: Gross nodular seeding in the cerebellar/cerebral subarachnoid space or in the 3rd or lateral ventricles.
- M3: Gross nodular seeding of the spinal subarachnoid space.
- M4: Metastasis outside the cerebrospinal axis.

Treatment and Prognosis

Although medulloblastoma are considered high grade neoplasms (World Health Organization grade 4 tumors), ELP1-associated medulloblastoma is associated with a favorable clinical outcome with a 5-year overall survival rate seen in 92% of cases [7]. Treatment consists of a combination of surgery, radiation therapy, and chemotherapy [29]. Studies have also shown excellent local control of childhood medulloblastoma with the use of intensity-modulated radiotherapy (IMRT) boost [30]. Treatment with radiotherapy is associated with a 5-year disease-free survival rate in 50-60% of average-risk patients and 40% in high-risk patients [29, 31, 32]. Relapses in MBs have been noted in approximately 30% of patients and are usually associated with metastases and therefore almost always fatal [33, 34].

Conclusion

ELP-1 medulloblastoma syndrome is an autosomal dominant disorder which can arise in association with germline mutations in the ELP1 gene situated on chromosome 9q often coupled with monoallelic loss of PTCH1. Patients are prone to develop medulloblastomas (WHO grade 4). A significant subset of patients harbor a sonic hedgehog germline alteration.

References

[1] Bailey P, Cushing H. Medulloblastoma cerebelli: a common type of midcerebellar glioma of childhood. *Arch Neurol Psych.* 1925; 14: 192–224.

[2] CBTRUS Statistical Report: Primary Brain and Other Central Nervous System Tumors Diagnosed in the United States in 2009–2013 | Neuro-Oncology | Oxford Academic Available online: https://academic.oup.com/neuro-oncology/article/18/suppl_5/v1/2590014 (accessed on Sep 26, 2022).

[3] Mollashahi B, Aghamaleki FS, Movafagh A. The roles of miRNAs in medulloblastoma: a systematic review. *J Cancer Prev.* 2019; 24: 79–90.

[4] Farouk Sait S, Walsh MF, Karajannis MA. Genetic syndromes predisposing to pediatric brain tumors. *Neurooncol Pract.* 2021; 8: 375–390.

[5] Li Y, Song Q, Day BW. Phase I and phase II sonidegib and vismodegib clinical trials for the treatment of paediatric and adult MB patients: a systemic review and meta-analysis. *Acta Neuropathol Commun.* 2019; 7: 123.

[6] Spectrum and prevalence of genetic predisposition in medulloblastoma: a retrospective genetic study and prospective validation in a clinical trial cohort - The Lancet Oncology Available online: https://www.thelancet.com/journals/lanonc/article/PIIS1470-2045(18)30242-0/fulltext (accessed on Sep 26, 2022).

[7] Waszak SM, Robinson GW, Gudenas BL, et al. Germline Elongator mutations in Sonic Hedgehog medulloblastoma. *Nature.* 2020; 580: 396–401.

[8] Millard NE, De Braganca KC. Medulloblastoma. *J Child Neurol.* 2016; 31: 1341–1353.

[9] Wilne S, Collier J, Kennedy C, et al. Presentation of childhood CNS tumours: a systematic review and meta-analysis. *Lancet Oncol.* 2007; 8: 685–695.

[10] Halperin EC, Friedman HS. Is there a correlation between duration of presenting symptoms and stage of medulloblastoma at the time of diagnosis? *Cancer.* 1996; 78: 874–880.

[11] *Duration of symptoms prior to diagnosis is related inversely to presenting disease stage in children with medulloblastoma - Halperin* - 2001 - Cancer - Wiley Online Library Available online: https://acsjournals.onlinelibrary.wiley.com/doi/10.1002/1097-0142(20010415)91:8%3C1444::AID-CNCR1151%3E3.0.CO;2-U (accessed on Sep 18, 2022).

[12] *Symptoms and time to diagnosis in children with brain tumours* Available online: https://ugeskriftet.dk/dmj/symptoms-and-time-diagnosis-children-brain-tumours (accessed on Sep 25, 2022).

[13] Quinlan A, Rizzolo D. Understanding medulloblastoma. *JAAPA.* 2017; 30: 30–36.

[14] Poretti A, Meoded A, Huisman TAGM. Neuroimaging of pediatric posterior fossa tumors including review of the literature. *J Magnetic Res Imag.* 2012; 35: 32–47.

[15] Koeller KK, Rushing EJ. Medulloblastoma: a comprehensive review with radiologic-pathologic correlation. *AFIP Arch.* 2003; 1613-1637.

[16] Kumar R, Achari G, Banerjee D, et al Uncommon presentation of medulloblastoma. *Child's Nerv Syst.* 2001; 17: 538–542.

[17] Nelson M, Diebler C, Forbes WS. Paediatric medulloblastoma: atypical CT features at presentation in the SIOP II trial. *Neuroradiology.* 1991; 33: 140–142.

[18] Shaw DW, Weinberger E, Brewer DK, et al. Spinal subdural enhancement after suboccipital craniectomy. *Am J Neuroradiol.* 1996; 17: 1373–1377.

[19] Types, causes, and outcome of intracranial hemorrhage in children with cancer in: *Journal of Neurosurgery: Pediatrics,* Volume 102 Issue 1 (2005). Available online: https://thejns.org/pediatrics/view/journals/j-neurosurg-pediatr/102/1/article-p31.xml (accessed on Sep 25, 2022).

[20] Eran A, Ozturk A, Aygun N, et al. Medulloblastoma: atypical CT and MRI findings in children. *Pediatr Radiol.* 2010; 40: 1254–1262.

[21] Eberhart CG, Kepner JL, Goldthwaite PT, et al. Histopathologic grading of medulloblastomas. *Cancer.* 2002; 94: 552–560.

[22] Louis DN, Perry A, Reifenberger G, et al. The 2016 World Health Organization Classification of Tumors of the Central Nervous System: a summary. *Acta Neuropathol.* 2016; 131: 803–820.

[23] McLendon, Friedman, Fuchs, et al. Diagnostic markers in paediatric medulloblastoma: a Paediatric Oncology Group Study. *Histopathology.* 1999; 34: 154–162.

[24] Kozmik Z, Sure U, Rüedi D, et al. Deregulated expression of PAX5 in medulloblastoma. *Proc Natl Acad of Sci.* 1995; 92: 5709–5713.

[25] Yokota N, Aruga J, Takai S, et al. Predominant expression of human zic in cerebellar granule cell lineage and medulloblastoma. *Cancer Res.* 1996; 56: 377–383.

[26] Evaluation of intracranial cerebrospinal fluid cytology in staging pediatric medulloblastomas, supratentorial primitive neuroectodermal tumors, and

ependymomas. *J Neurosurg Pediatr*. Volume 6 Issue 2 (2010) Journals Available online: https://thejns.org/pediatrics/view/journals/j-neurosurg-pediatr/6/2/article-p131.xml (accessed on Sep 25, 2022).

[27] Chang CH, Housepian EM, Herbert C. An operative staging system and a megavoltage radiotherapeutic technic for cerebellar medulloblastomas. *Radiology*. 1969; 93: 1351–1359.

[28] Sure U, Berghorn WJ, Bertalanffy H, et al. Staging, scoring and grading of medulloblastoma. *Acta Neurochir*. 1995; 132: 59–65.

[29] MacDonald TJ, Rood BR, Santi MR, et al. Advances in the diagnosis, molecular genetics, and treatment of pediatric embryonal CNS tumors. *Oncologist*. 2003; 8: 174–186.

[30] *Local control after craniospinal irradiation, intensity-modulated radiotherapy boost, and chemotherapy in childhood medulloblastoma* - Paulino - 2011 - Cancer - Wiley Online Library Available online: https://acsjournals.onlinelibrary.wiley.com/doi/10.1002/cncr.25601 (accessed on Sep 26, 2022).

[31] Packer RJ, Vezina G. Management of and prognosis with medulloblastoma: therapy at a crossroads. *Arch Neurol*. 2008; 65: 1419–1424.

[32] Packer RJ, Cogen P, Vezina G, et al. Medulloblastoma: clinical and biologic aspects. *Neuro-Oncology*. 1999; 1: 232–250.

[33] Combined MYC and p53 defects emerge at medulloblastoma relapse and define rapidly progressive, therapeutically targetable disease: *Cancer Cell*. Available online: https://www.cell.com/cancer-cell/fulltext/S1535-6108(14)00453 (accessed on Sep 26, 2022).

[34] Ramaswamy V, Remke M, Bouffet E, et al. Recurrence patterns across medulloblastoma subgroups: an integrated clinical and molecular analysis. *The Lancet Oncology*. 2013; 14: 1200–1207.

Chapter 17

Nevoid Basal Cell Carcinoma Syndrome: Neuropathologic Features

Derrick Obiri-Yeboah[1], BS
Mario-Cyriac Tcheukado[1], BS
and Richard A. Prayson[2,*], MD, MEd
[1] Cleveland Clinic Lerner College of Medicine, Cleveland, Ohio, USA
[2] Department of Anatomic Pathology, Cleveland Clinic, Cleveland, Ohio, USA

Abstract

Nevoid basal cell carcinoma syndrome, also known as Gorlin syndrome, is a rare neurocutaneous disorder that is marked by developmental anomalies such as dyskeratotic palmar and plantar pitting, rib anomalies, basal cell carcinomas and odontogenic keratocysts of the jaw. Classically, Gorlin syndrome is inherited in an autosomal dominant fashion and characterized by increased tumorigenesis from an early age, prone to developing basal cell carcinomas and medulloblastoma. The syndrome occurs usually because of a frameshift, missense, or nonsense mutation in PTCH1, a human homologue of Drosophila.

As a member of the highly conserved hedgehog signaling pathway that modulates cell growth and development, PTCH1 dysfunction gives rise to not only developmental anomalies but also the diverse tumors observed in nevoid basal cell carcinoma syndrome.

This chapter will review the clinicopathologic features of this disorder, with a primary focus on the central nervous system associated pathology.

* Corresponding Author's Email: praysor@ccf.org.

In: Central Nervous System Pathologies in Hereditary Tumor Syndromes
Editor: Richard A. Prayson
ISBN: 979-8-88697-620-5

Introduction

Nevoid basal cell carcinoma syndrome (NBCCS) also referred to as Gorlin-Goltz syndrome is believed to have first being described in the literature in 1894. However, the syndrome was not categorized as a distinct entity until the mid – twentieth century at which point the relationship between the syndrome and development of multiple basal cell carcinomas (BCCs), keratocystic odontogenic tumors (KOTs), palmar and plantar pitting, etc. were made [1-3]. Over the years, further investigation has led to the establishment of the genetic basis of NBCCS and potential drug therapies aimed at exploiting the current understanding. This chapter will review the clinical and pathologic features of NBCCS, focusing on the neuropathological findings that have been described in this syndrome.

Genetics of Nevoid Basal Cell Carcinoma Syndrome

NBCCS is known to be caused by heterozygous germline mutations in the human homolog *PTCH1* (Chr9q22.32) of the *Drosophila* gene, *patched 1* [4, 5]. This syndrome is inherited in an autosomal dominant pattern and has been shown to demonstrate variable expressivity with an equivalent prevalence in males and females [6-8]. In most cases of NBCCS, germline mutations of the PTCH1 gene result in premature termination of the patched protein [4]; however, since the PTCH1 gene was linked to the syndrome, numerous mutations in the gene including missense, nonsense and various splicing variants have been reported [4, 8]. While there abounds numerous literature evidence linking the various gene mutations involved in the etiology of NBCCS, there have been some patients in whom PTCH1 mutations could not be determined, most likely a result of large deletions or mutations outside the regions that were analyzed [4].

In addition to the PTCH1 gene, other rare causative genes have been identified in NBCCS including SUFU and PTCH2, encoding for suppressor of fused homolog proteins and patched 2 respectively [9-11]. As noted above, NBCCS is often associated with variable expressivity. Specifically, it has been demonstrated that the genotype-phenotype correlation is not consistently present, such that family members with the same PTCH1 germline mutation demonstrate variable phenotype, which suggests the existence of a complex syndrome variability most likely a result of interaction between patient's genetic background and their environmental factors or possibly additional simultaneous mutations that influence phenotype variation [12-15].

The malignancies and developmental deficits associated with NBCCS are believed to arise via a two-hit mechanism [1, 16]. Under physiological conditions, PTCH1 is a membrane bound protein that maintains a smoothened (SMO) or inactive/unphosphorylated state, which makes it susceptible to degradation and endocytosis as well as being incapable of GLI protein repression or activation, which is required for pathway dependent genes [1, 17, 18]. In the presence of a hedgehog ligand (such as Indian hedgehog, desert hedgehog, sonic hedgehog (SHH)) and PTCH1 binding, SMO becomes hyperphosphorylated, resulting in GLI relocalization to the nucleus [18]. This causes transcriptional modulation and other various downstream effects, such as proliferation, migration and progenitor cell differentiation under normal circumstances, all of which occur in almost all stages of vertebrate development [1, 18]. However, under pathologic conditions, there is a constitutive hedgehog signaling pathway activation due to mutation of regulatory proteins which causes tumor cell proliferation [1]. These mutations, as highlighted above, occur mostly in the PTCH1, PTCH2 and SUFU genes and result in the aberrant functioning of the pathway described above [1, 4].

General Clinical and Neurologic Features

NBCCS, as previously mentioned, is inherited mostly in an autosomal dominant fashion and the syndrome is characterized by development of basal cell carcinomas (BCCs) at a young age [1]. The prevalence of NBCCS is currently estimated at 1 in 57,000 – 1 in 164,000 with equal incidence in both men and women [1, 19, 20]. In individuals affected by this syndrome, the occurrence of BCCs can be as many as 500 often presenting very aggressive clinically and having a predilection for lighter pigmented individuals as well as those with increased ultraviolet light exposure [1]. When the BCCs occur in NBCCS patients, they do follow a similar distribution pattern as that observed in non – syndromic basal cell carcinoma patients developing more commonly on the sun exposed areas like the face, trunk and limbs [1, 19].

In addition to the cutaneous BCCs that occur at a young age, other clinical features such as keratocystic odontogenic tumors (KOTs), dyskeratotic palmar and plantar pitting, spine and rib anomalies as well as early falx cerebri calcification also characterize NBCCS [1]. These are common and occur in an estimated 70-80% of patients [1, 19]. Furthermore, certain facial features such as hypertelorism, frontal bossing, macrocephaly, and cleft lip and palate have been noted in a significant subset of NBCCS patients [19]. While less commonly occurring than the conditions described above, NBCCS patients have also been shown to be more susceptible to childhood desmoplastic medulloblastoma (Figures 1 and 2) and other neoplasms such as rhabdomyosarcomas, mesenteric keratocysts, meningiomas and cardiac and ovarian fibromas, etc. [19, 21]. Much rarer clinical abnormalities, such as corpus callosum agenesis, continue to be described as understanding of the syndrome grows [1].

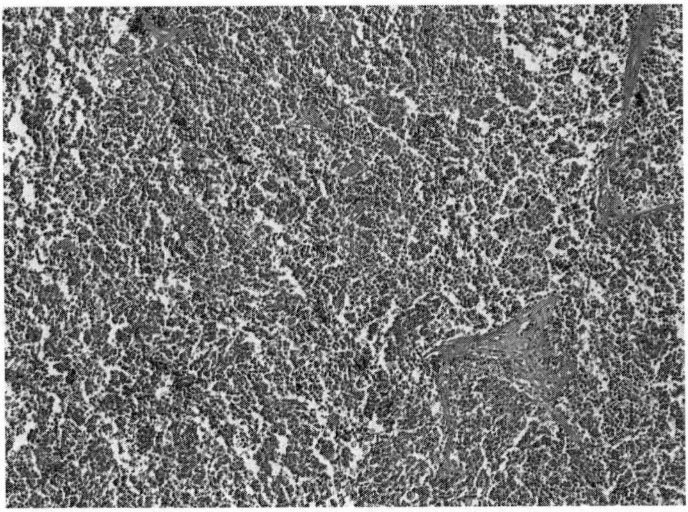

Figure 1. Cerebellar medulloblastoma in a nevoid basal cell carcinoma syndrome marked by sheet-like proliferation of embryonal cells (hematoxylin and eosin, original magnification 100X).

About 50% of reported NBCCS cases occur as a result of sporadic development, even though the syndrome was initially understood to only be an inherited condition [22]. Likewise, while NBCCS is understood to be characterized by high disease penetrance, individuals often display varying disease expressivity even among the same family members which poses an increased diagnostic challenge [1, 23]. Nonetheless, diagnostic criteria for NBCCS were proposed about two decades ago, drawing from numerous large clinical case series that included several discrepancies, most likely reflecting the variable expressivity of the syndrome [1, 24]. Over the years, these criteria have been refined and added onto to streamline diagnosis even though a final consensus remains to be reached.

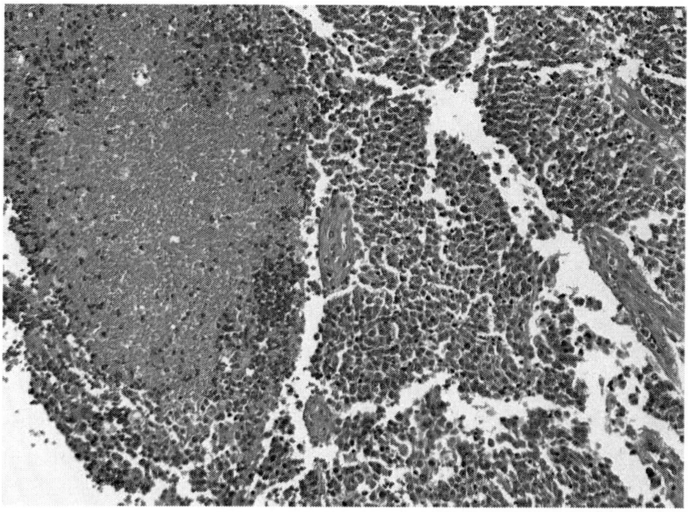

Figure 2. Same tumor as in Figure 1 showing an area of geographic necrosis (hematoxylin and eosin, original magnification 200X).

Table 1. Diagnostic criteria for nevoid basal cell carcinoma syndrome (adapted from 1)

Major criteria	Minor criteria
1. Basal cell carcinoma before 20 years of age or excessive numbers of basal cell carcinomas out of proportion to prior sun exposure and skin type	1. Rib abnormalities
2. Keratocystic odontogenic tumor before 20 years of age	2. Other specific skeletal malformations and radiologic changes (i.e., vertebral anomalies, kyphoscoliosis, short fourth metacarpals, postaxial polydactyly)
3. Palmar or plantar pitting	3. Macrocephaly
4. Lamellar calcification of the falx cerebri	4. Cleft lip or palate
5. Medulloblastoma, typically desmoplastic	5. Ovarian or cardiac fibroma
6. First degree relative with nevoid basal cell carcinoma syndrome	6. Lymphomesenteric cysts
	7. Ocular abnormalities (i.e., strabismus, hypertelorism, congenital cataracts, glaucoma, coloboma)

In summary, as can be seen in Table 1, the diagnosis of NBCCS requires presence of either two major criteria or one major criteria in addition to two minor criteria [1, 24]. All suspected patients are required to complete dermatologic exam in addition to radiologic tests such as baseline brain magnetic resonance imaging (MRI), cardiac and pelvic (if female) ultrasound, and panoramic dental and spine radiographs [1, 24].

Imaging Findings

Numerous literature studies have detailed the imaging findings common with NBCCS. Of note is a study by Kimonis et al. 2004, wherein radiological features of 82 NBCCS patients were described [25]. In their study, they highlighted peculiar findings in patients with NBCCS relative to unaffected siblings who served as controls [25]. The most consistent imaging finding described in the literature on patients with NBCCS is falx cerebri calcification [25]. In their study, Kimonis et al., demonstrated falx cerebri calcification on skull films, a finding that appeared to increase in frequency with age of patients with patients over 40 years having the most cases of falx calcification [25]. Additional skull film findings described in NBCCS include tentorium cerebellum calcification, petroclinoid ligament calcification, pituitary calcification as well as hyperaeration of the frontal sinuses [25].

On computed tomography (CT) and MRI studies, NBCCS patients have been observed to have asymmetric ventricles, often times due to previous surgery for medulloblastoma and as a result of communicating hydrocephalus [25]. Cerebral atrophy, cavum septum pellucidum, corpus callosum dysgenesis/agenesis are all other notable MRI findings reported in patients with NBCCS. The presence of other intracranial masses consistent with the appearance of meningiomas has also been reported [25].

Lateral skull and neck films in NBCCS patients have been shown to demonstrate nuchal ligament calcification as well as an increased rate of bifid spinous process in this patient population [25]. Notably, thoracolumbar spine films in these patients have shown increased incidence of scoliosis, predominantly at sites of other anomalies such as hemivertebrae, spina bifida occulta, elongation of the vertebral bodies or vertebral body fusions [25]. Interestingly, no difference in incidence of spondylolisthesis and spondylosis have been reported in NBCCS patients.

Neuropathologic Findings

The most common central nervous system pathology in NBCCS is medulloblastoma [1]. An estimated 5% of NBCCS patients are believed to develop medulloblastoma, which all present with specific features [26]. Contrary to sporadic medulloblastomas which have an approximate mean age of onset of 6 years, NBCCS patients who develop medulloblastomas have an approximate first age of onset of 2 years [26]. The association between NBCCS and medulloblastoma was first described in 1963 by Herzberg and Wiskemann following which several other authors have validated this association [26]. Of note, most of these studies are in agreement that the histopathologic characteristics of medulloblastomas associated with NBCCS patients are the same as that observed in sporadic medulloblastomas; the disease course is sometimes different in NBCCS patients primarily due to these patients' earlier tumor development [26]. Like sporadically occurring medulloblastomas, NBCCS associated medulloblastomas are characterized histologically by sheet-like proliferation of embryonal cells, often with foci of necrosis and prominent mitotic activity (Figures 1 and 2). Additional histological findings present in sporadic medulloblastomas that can also be found in NBCCS associated medulloblastomas include synaptophysin, nestin and neuron specific enolase expression [27]. The presence of cerebellar granule markers such as PAX6 and EN2 have also been demonstrated in these tumors [28].

A notable difference is the finding that most medulloblastomas observed in NBCCS are of the desmoplastic subtype [26, 29]. This specific association between desmoplastic medulloblastoma subtype and NBCCS was first noted by Schofield and colleagues when they showed in their study that all the NBCCS patients with medulloblastomas had the desmoplastic subtype [30].

Treatment and Prognosis

Standard treatment of medulloblastoma seen in NBCCS patients includes surgery in combination with chemotherapy and irradiation [26]. Unfortunately, because patients with NBCCS are already predisposed to developing multiple BCCS as well as other radiation – induced tumors like meningiomas, fibrosarcoma, and ependymomas in irradiated areas, critical consideration must be given to use of adjuvant radiation in these patients [26].

Thus, because most NBCCS patients who develop medulloblastomas often have this as the first presenting disease symptom at a mean age of 2 years, use of radiation is not recommended in children younger than 5 years [26]. In these patients, use of chemotherapy alone has been proven to have good outcomes [26]. Interestingly, NBCCS patients affected with medulloblastomas are believed to have a better prognosis than sporadic medulloblastomas [26, 31, 32]. The precise mechanism behind this remains to be explored but several case studies have shown increased treatment response in NBCCS patient diagnosed with medulloblastomas.

Furthermore, patients with NBCCS requires frequent dermatologic monitoring and sun protection. Radiologic screening for presence of KOTs and medulloblastomas is additionally recommended for patients younger than 8 years and is often performed annually [1]. In patients with BCCs, treatment is dependent on histologic subtype, location and size of the tumor. Excision is recommended if possible but because of the large tumor burden often present in these patients, the number of excisions can be extensive, often times causing disfigurement in patients [1]. In this case, other treatment modalities can including 5-fluorouracil (5-FU) and imiquimod can be considered, especially for localized disease [1].

Early diagnosis of NBCCS is critical as it allows for detection and management of potentially lethal skin and brain malignancies. This is important in informing preventive multidisciplinary approach, which can positively impact patient prognosis [33].

Conclusion

Nevoid basal cell carcinoma syndrome or Gorlin syndrome is an autosomal dominant condition associated with frameshift, missense or nonsense mutations in the PTCH1 gene on chromosome 9q. The most common central nervous system pathology associated with the condition is the development of medulloblastomas (WHO grade 4), particularly the desmoplastic variant. Tumors in this setting tend to arise at an earlier age than tumors which arise outside this setting.

References

[1] Bresler SC, Padwa BL, Granter SR. Nevoid basal cell carcinoma syndrome (Gorlin syndrome). *Head Neck Pathol.* 2016; 10: 119–124.

[2] Howell JB, Caro MR. The basal-cell nevus: its relationship to multiple cutaneous cancers and associated anomalies of development. *AMA Arch Derm.* 1959; 79: 67–77; discussion 77-80.

[3] Gorlin RJ, Goltz RW. Multiple nevoid basal-cell epithelioma, jaw cysts and bifid rib. A syndrome. *N Engl J Med.* 1960; 262: 908–912.

[4] Bellei B, Caputo S, Carbone A, Silipo, V, Papaccio, F, Picardo, M, & Eibenschutz, L. The role of dermal fibroblasts in nevoid basal cell carcinoma syndrome patients: an overview. *Int J Mol Sci.* 2020; 21: 720.

[5] Hahn H, Wicking C, Zaphiropoulous PG, et al. Mutations of the human homolog of Drosophila patched in the nevoid basal cell carcinoma syndrome. *Cell.* 1996; 85: 841–851.

[6] Boutet N, Bignon Y-J, Drouin-Garraud V, et al. Spectrum of PTCH1 mutations in French patients with Gorlin syndrome. *J Invest Dermatol.* 2003; 121: 478–481.

[7] Wicking C, Shanley S, Smyth I, et al. Most germ-line mutations in the nevoid basal cell carcinoma syndrome lead to a premature termination of the PATCHED protein, and no genotype-phenotype correlations are evident. *Am J Hum Genet.* 1997; 60: 21–26.

[8] Savino M, d'Apolito M, Formica V, et al. Spectrum of PTCH mutations in Italian nevoid basal cell-carcinoma syndrome patients: identification of thirteen novel alleles. *Hum Mutat.* 2004; 24: 441.

[9] Fujii K, Ohashi H, Suzuki M, et al. Frameshift mutation in the PTCH2 gene can cause nevoid basal cell carcinoma syndrome. *Fam Cancer.* 2013; 12: 611–614.

[10] Fan Z, Li J, Du J, et al. A missense mutation in PTCH2 underlies dominantly inherited NBCCS in a Chinese family. *J Med Genet.* 2008; 45: 303–308.

[11] Pastorino L, Ghiorzo P, Nasti S, et al. Identification of a SUFU germline mutation in a family with Gorlin syndrome. *Am J Med Genet A.* 2009; 149A: 1539–1543.

[12] Ogden T, Higgins S, Elbaum D, et al. The relevance of a suppressor of fused (SUFU) mutation in the diagnosis and treatment of Gorlin syndrome. *JAAD Case Rep.* 2018; 4: 196–199.

[13] Evans DG, Ladusans EJ, Rimmer S, et al. Complications of the nevoid basal cell carcinoma syndrome: results of a population based study. *J Med Genet.* 1993; 30: 460–464.

[14] Shimkets R, Gailani MR, Siu VM, et al. Molecular analysis of chromosome 9q deletions in two Gorlin syndrome patients. *Am J Hum Genet.* 1996; 59: 417–422.

[15] Onodera S, Saito A, Hasegawa D, et al. Multi-layered mutation in hedgehog-related genes in Gorlin syndrome may affect the phenotype. *PLoS One.* 2017; 12: e0184702.

[16] Levanat S, Gorlin RJ, Fallet S, et al. A two-hit model for developmental defects in Gorlin syndrome. *Nat Genet.* 1996; 12: 85–87.

[17] Atwood SX, Chang ALS, Oro AE. Hedgehog pathway inhibition and the race against tumor evolution. *J Cell Biol.* 2012; 199: 193–197.

[18] Varjosalo M, Taipale J. Hedgehog: functions and mechanisms. *Genes Dev.* 2008; 22: 2454–2472.

[19] Kimonis VE, Goldstein AM, Pastakia B, et al. Clinical manifestations in 105 persons with nevoid basal cell carcinoma syndrome. *Am J Med Genet.* 1997; 69: 299–308.

[20] Anderson DE, Taylor WB, Falls HF, et al. The nevoid basal cell carcinoma syndrome. *Am J Hum Genet.* 1967; 19: 12–22.

[21] Johnson RL, Rothman AL, Xie J, et al. Human homolog of patched, a candidate gene for the basal cell nevus syndrome. *Science.* 1996; 272: 1668–1671.

[22] Klein RD, Dykas DJ, Bale AE. Clinical testing for the nevoid basal cell carcinoma syndrome in a DNA diagnostic laboratory. *Genet Med.* 2005; 7: 611–619.

[23] Shanley S, Ratcliffe J, Hockey A, et al. Nevoid basal cell carcinoma syndrome: review of 118 affected individuals. *Am J Med Genet.* 1994; 50: 282–290.

[24] Bree AF, Shah MR, BCNS Colloquium Group. Consensus statement from the first international colloquium on basal cell nevus syndrome (BCNS). *Am J Med Genet A.* 2011; 155A: 2091–2097.

[25] Kimonis VE, Mehta SG, Digiovanna JJ, et al. Radiological features in 82 patients with nevoid basal cell carcinoma (NBCC or Gorlin) syndrome. *Genet Med.* 2004; 6: 495–502.

[26] Amlashi SFA, Riffaud L, Brassier G, et al. Nevoid basal cell carcinoma syndrome: Relation with desmoplastic medulloblastoma in infancy. *Cancer.* 2003; 98: 618–624.

[27] McLendon RE, Friedman HS, Fuchs HE, et al. Diagnostic markers in paediatric medulloblastoma: a Paediatric Oncology Group Study. *Histopathology.* 1999; 34: 154–162.

[28] Kozmik Z, Sure U, Rüedi D, et al. Deregulated expression of PAX5 in medulloblastoma. *Proc Natl Acad Sci USA.* 1995; 92: 5709–5713.

[29] Korczak JF, Brahim JS, DiGiovanna JJ, et al. Nevoid basal cell carcinoma syndrome with medulloblastoma in an African-American boy: a rare case illustrating gene-environment interaction. *Am J Med Genet.* 1997; 69: 309–314.

[30] Schofield D, West DC, Anthony DC, et al. Correlation of loss of heterozygosity at chromosome 9q with histological subtype in medulloblastomas. *Am J Pathol.* 1995; 146: 472–480.

[31] Neblett CR, Waltz TA, Anderson DE. Neurological involvement in the nevoid basal cell carcinoma syndrome. *J Neurosurg.* 1971; 35: 577–584.

[32] Lacombe D, Chateil JF, Fontan D, et al. Medulloblastoma in the nevoid basal-cell carcinoma syndrome: case reports and review of the literature. *Genet Couns.* 1990; 1: 273–277.

[33] Kiran NK, Tilak Raj TN, Mukunda KS, et al. Nevoid basal cell carcinoma syndrome (Gorlin-Goltz syndrome). *Contemp Clin Dent.* 2012; 3: 514–518.

Chapter 18

Constitutional Mismatch Repair Deficiency Syndrome: Central Nervous System Pathology

Lauren E. Heusinkveld[1], BS
and Richard A. Prayson[2,*], MD, MEd
[1] Cleveland Clinic Lerner College of Medicine, Cleveland, Ohio, USA
[2] Department of Anatomic Pathology, Cleveland Clinic, Cleveland, Ohio, USA

Abstract

Constitutional mismatch repair deficiency syndrome (CMMRD) is a rare genetic cancer syndrome characterized by early-onset central nervous system (CNS), gastrointestinal, and hematologic malignancies. CMMRD is caused by autosomal recessive mutations in DNA mismatch repair genes. Loss of mismatch repair function results in microsatellite instability and accumulation of mutations, predisposing patients to the development of multiple ultramutated cancers in childhood and young adulthood.

Children with CMMRD typically present with café-au-lait cutaneous macules, pilomatrixomas, and skin pigmentation changes. CNS and gastrointestinal cancers typically develop within the first decade of life, and one third of patients are diagnosed with a hematologic malignancy. The most common CNS pathology is high-grade glioma, typically manifesting as glioblastoma. Other rare CNS tumors have also been described in CMMRD patients.

Prognosis is poor; the most common cause of death is CNS malignancy. Management consists of surveillance for cancers and treatment of malignancy with surgery, radiation, and chemotherapy.

---

* Corresponding Author's Email: praysor@ccf.org.

In: Central Nervous System Pathologies in Hereditary Tumor Syndromes
Editor: Richard A. Prayson
ISBN: 979-8-88697-620-5

Introduction

Constitutional mismatch repair deficiency syndrome (CMMRD; OMIM #276300) is a genetic cancer syndrome characterized by early-onset CNS and extra-CNS tumors. CMMRD is one of several syndromes associated with both CNS and gastrointestinal cancers. In 1949, Crail reported the first case of concurrent medulloblastoma, colonic polyposis and adenocarcinoma, and papillary thyroid carcinoma in a 24-year-old male patient presenting with symptoms of hydrocephalus and cerebellar dysfunction [1]. A 1959 report of two teenaged siblings with colorectal adenocarcinoma and primary CNS tumors by Turcot et al., gave rise to the eponym "Turcot syndrome" [2].

Hamilton et al., defined two molecularly and clinically distinct variants of Turcot syndrome: brain tumor polyposis syndrome type 1 (BTPS1), caused by DNA mismatch repair gene mutations, and BTPS2, caused by *APC* mutations [3]. Currently two subtypes of BTPS1 are recognized: CMMRD and hereditary nonpolyposis colorectal cancer (HNPCC; also known as Lynch) syndrome. Although both are caused by mismatch repair gene mutations, their clinical features and patterns of inheritance are distinct [4–6].

CMMRD is also known as biallelic mismatch repair deficiency syndrome and mismatch repair cancer syndrome. Although only about 300 cases have been reported in the literature, the true incidence is unknown. It is important to acknowledge that most of the published CMMRD literature consists of case reports and case series. The full spectrum of features associated with CMMRD is most likely incompletely defined at present.

This chapter will review the clinical and pathologic features of CMMRD, with a focus on the neurologic findings associated with the disorder.

Genetics of Constitutional Mismatch Repair Deficiency Syndrome

CMMRD is caused by a homozygous or compound heterozygous inactivating germline mutation in one of the four DNA mismatch repair genes: *MSH2*, *MSH6*, *MLH1*, *PMS2*. *MSH6* and *PMS2* are most commonly mutated in CMMRD [7]. CMMRD is marked by an autosomal recessive pattern of inheritance. Homozygous mutations are associated with consanguinity [7]. Loss of any of the mismatch repair genes results in microsatellite instability and accumulation of mutations, predisposing patients to the development of multiple cancers in childhood and young adulthood. As a result, tumors in CMMRD demonstrate a very high mutational burden, in excess of 100 mutations/Mb [8].

Extra-Neurologic Clinical Features

Children with CMMRD typically present with café-au-lait cutaneous macules, similar to those associated with neurofibromatosis type 1 [9]. Pilomatricomas and abnormally hyper- or hypopigmented patches of skin are also common [10]. One third of patients develop hematologic malignancies, most commonly non-Hodgkin's T cell lymphoma. Non-Hodgkin's B cell lymphoma, acute lymphoblastic leukemia, and acute myeloid leukemia have also been reported [7]. By the second decade of life, all patients develop gastrointestinal polyposis which often progresses to cancer. Colorectal carcinoma is the most common gastrointestinal malignancy encountered in CMMRD, although tumors may also arise in the small bowel [7]. The European Care for CMMRD Consortium suggested guidelines for genetic testing in patients with suspected CMMRD based on cancer or pre-cancer lesions, other clinical features, and family history [7].

Although gastrointestinal, hematologic, and CNS cancers are most characteristic of CMMRD, a variety of other cancers have been reported, including urothelial carcinoma [7], rhabdomyosarcoma [11, 12], ovarian and endometrial cancer [7], transitional renal cell carcinoma [13], and parotid mucoepidermoid carcinoma [7]. CMMRD may increase the risk for the development of systemic lupus erythematosus in female patients [14].

Neurologic Clinical Features

Central nervous system (CNS) tumors in CMMRD most commonly manifest as high-grade glioma, especially glioblastoma [7, 9, 13]. Other high-grade gliomas encountered in CMMRD include oligodendroglioma, anaplastic astrocytoma, and gliosarcoma [7]. Patients are also predisposed to CNS embryonal tumors, in particular medulloblastoma. Single cases each of infiltrating pleomorphic xanthoastrocytoma [13], cerebral angiosarcoma [7], meningioma [9], anaplastic ganglioglioma [7, 9], and papillary glioneural tumor [7] have been reported. Although highly penetrant in CMMRD, developmental venous anomalies have not been reported to cause clinically significant bleeding [9, 15, 16].

The clinical presentation of CNS disease in patients with CMMRD is as expected for sporadic tumors, with the exception that tumors arise at a much younger age than is typical. In one cohort, the median age at diagnosis of first brain tumor was 9.2 years [9]. High-grade gliomas often present with seizures and symptoms of increased intracranial pressure such as vomiting and headaches [17, 18]. A 13-month-old with medulloblastoma initially presented with ataxia, strabismus, and vomiting [19].

Imaging Findings

Cancers arising due to CMMRD appear identical to sporadic cancers on imaging. Gliomas manifest as hemispheric or irregularly shaped supratentorial masses located in the white matter or deep nuclei. Evidence of mass effect is common. Anaplastic astrocytomas may demonstrate scattered contrast enhancement. Glioblastomas usually show focal necrosis with ring enhancement and may cross the corpus callosum ("butterfly glioma"). Oligodendrogliomas are usually located in the frontal lobe and less commonly in the parietal and temporal lobes. High-grade oligodendrogliomas (WHO grade 3) are usually enhancing. Medulloblastoma often arises in the cerebellar vermis and demonstrates gadolinium enhancement. CNS developmental anomalies have been reported in patients with CMMRD, including corpus callosum agenesis, nodular gray matter heterotopia, and developmental venous anomalies [9, 15, 16, 18, 20]. Developmental venous anomalies are typically not adjacent to tumors.

Neuropathologic Findings

Developmental venous anomalies are the most common non-neoplastic CNS pathology observed in patients with CMMRD. Corpus callosum agenesis and nodular gray matter heterotopia have also been reported.

The most prevalent CNS malignancy is high-grade glioma. Gliomas are diffusely infiltrative, causing blurring of the gray-white matter junctions. Mass effect with midline shift, compression of the ventricles and blunting of sulci may be appreciable on gross exam. Microscopically astrocytomas are characterized by infiltrative tumor cells with mild to moderate nuclear atypia and hyperchromatic oval or spindled, irregularly shaped nuclei (Figure 1).

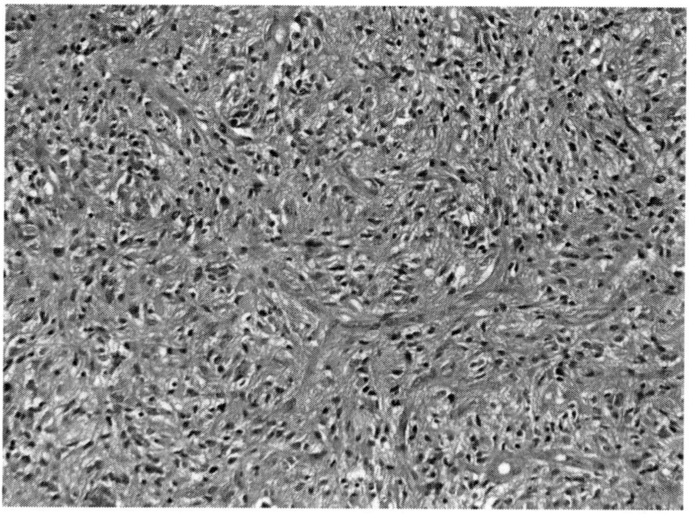

Figure 1. This astrocytoma arising in a patient with constitutional mismatch repair deficiency syndrome is marked by moderate hypercellularity (hematoxylin and eosin, original magnification 200X).

Anaplastic astrocytoma is marked by increased cellularity and more readily identifiable mitotic activity. The presence of microvascular proliferation and/or necrosis defines WHO Grade 4 astrocytoma, or glioblastoma (Figure 2). CMMRD-associated glioblastomas tend to be highly pleomorphic and may display multinucleated giant cells [9]. Astrocytomas are positive for glial fibrillary acidic protein (GFAP) by immunohistochemistry, and most stain positively for p53 protein. Isocitrate dehydrogenase (IDH) is usually wildtype in this disease setting [9].

Oligodendrogliomas often infiltrate the cortex and may have calcifications. Tumor cells with round, well-defined nuclei embedded in a "chicken wire" capillary network are characteristic. Clear perinuclear haloes, referred to as a "fried-egg" pattern, may occur due to fixation artifact in paraffin-embedded tissue. Increased mitoses with or without microvascular proliferation and/or necrosis increase the tumor grade to WHO Grade 3, anaplastic oligodendroglioma. Oligodendrogliomas are usually negative for GFAP and p53 protein staining. Co-deletion of chromosomes 1p/19q and mutations of IDH-1/2 are currently required for the diagnosis of oligodendroglioma. Loss of p16 is common in anaplastic or recurrent oligodendroglioma. Medulloblastoma is the most common embryonal tumor in CMMRD patients. This tumor type is characterized by hypercellularity with necrosis and hemorrhage (Figure 3).

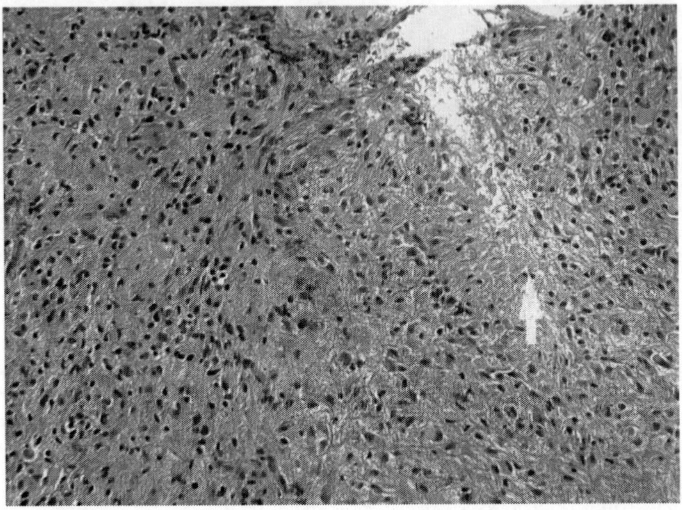

Figure 2. The same tumor as in Figure 1 contained small foci of early necrosis (arrow), consistent with a glioblastoma, WHO grade 4 (hematoxylin and eosin, original magnification 200X).

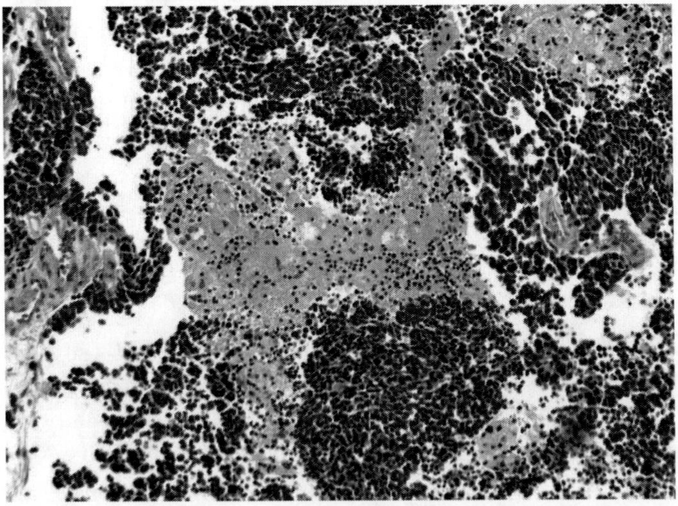

Figure 3. A cerebellar mass in an 8-year-old with marked cellularity and necrosis, consistent with a medulloblastoma, classic type, WHO grade 4 (hematoxylin and eosin, original magnification 200X).

Tumor cells are small, round, and blue due to high nuclear-to-cytoplastic ratio. Mitoses and apoptosis are readily apparent. Approximately one third of cases demonstrate characteristic Homer Wright rosettes. Immunohistochemistry staining is positive for synaptophysin and variably positive for other neural markers.

Immunohistochemistry demonstrates loss of antibody staining for one of the mismatch repair genes in all CMMRD-associated CNS tumors.

Treatment and Prognosis

No specific therapies are available for CMMRD. Prognosis is poor due to the high risk of aggressive cancer during childhood. In one cohort, the median age at death was 13.2 years old, and the most common cause of death was brain tumor [9]. The 3- and 5-year survival rates after the diagnosis of brain tumor were 30% and 22% [9]. Immune checkpoint inhibitor therapy may improve outcomes for patients with mismatch repair deficiency tumors, including CMMRD patients [21, 22]. Imaging and laboratory surveillance is recommended to identify asymptomatic cancers which can be successfully treated if diagnosed promptly [13, 23].

Conclusion

Constitutional mismatch repair deficiency syndrome is a rare autosomal dominant condition resulting from mutations in DNA mismatch repair genes. Loss of mismatch repair function results in microsatellite instability and mutation accumulation. The most common central nervous system manifestation of this disorder is high grade gliomas, especially glioblastoma, WHO grade 4. Cases of oligodendroglioma and medulloblastoma have also been reported in patients with this syndrome.

References

[1] Crail H W. Multiple primary malignancies arising in the rectum, brain, and thyroid. *U S Nav. Med. Bull.* 1949;49:123–8.

[2] Turcot J, Despres J P, St Pierre F. Malignant tumors of the central nervous system associated with familial polyposis of the colon: report of two cases. *Dis. Colon Rectum.* 1959 Oct;2:465–8.

[3] Hamilton S R, Liu B, Parsons R E, et al. The molecular basis of Turcot's syndrome. *N Engl. J. Med.* 1995 Mar 30;332(13):839–47.

[4] Hegde M R, Chong B, Blazo M E, et al. A homozygous mutation in MSH6 causes Turcot syndrome. *Clin. Cancer Res. Off J. Am. Assoc. Cancer Res.* 2005 Jul 1;11 (13):4689–93.

[5] Tan T Y, Orme L M, Lynch E, et al. Biallelic PMS2 mutations and a distinctive childhood cancer syndrome. *J. Pediatr. Hematol. Oncol.* 2008 Mar;30(3):254–7.

[6] Krüger S, Kinzel M, Walldorf C, et al. Homozygous PMS2 germline mutations in two families with early-onset haematological malignancy, brain tumours, HNPCC-associated tumours, and signs of neurofibromatosis type 1. *Eur. J. Hum. Genet.* 2008 Jan;16(1):62–72.

[7] Wimmer K, Kratz C P, Vasen H F A, et al. Diagnostic criteria for constitutional mismatch repair deficiency syndrome: suggestions of the European consortium "care for CMMRD" (C4CMMRD). *J. Med. Genet.* 2014 Jun;51(6):355–65.

[8] Shlien A, Campbell B B, de Borja R, et al. Combined hereditary and somatic mutations of replication error repair genes result in rapid onset of ultra-hypermutated cancers. *Nat Genet.* 2015 Mar;47(3):257–62.

[9] Guerrini-Rousseau L, Varlet P, Colas C, et al. Constitutional mismatch repair deficiency-associated brain tumors: report from the European C4CMMRD consortium. *Neuro-Oncol. Adv.* 2019 Dec;1(1):vdz033.

[10] Chmara M, Wernstedt A, Wasag B, et al. Multiple pilomatricomas with somatic CTNNB1 mutations in children with constitutive mismatch repair deficiency. *Genes Chromosomes Cancer.* 2013 Jul;52(7):656–64.

[11] Wang Q, Lasset C, Desseigne F, et al. Neurofibromatosis and early onset of cancers in hMLH1-deficient children. *Cancer Res.* 1999 Jan 15;59(2):294–7.

[12] Kratz C P, Holter S, Etzler J, et al. Rhabdomyosarcoma in patients with constitutional mismatch-repair-deficiency syndrome. *J. Med. Genet.* 2009 Jun;46(6):418–20.

[13] Bakry D, Aronson M, Durno C, et al. Genetic and clinical determinants of constitutional mismatch repair deficiency syndrome: report from the constitutional mismatch repair deficiency consortium. *Eur. J. Cancer.* 1990. 2014 Mar;50(5):987–96.

[14] Toledano H, Orenstein N, Sofrin E, et al. Paediatric systemic lupus erythematosus as a manifestation of constitutional mismatch repair deficiency. *J. Med. Genet.* 2020 Jul;57(7):505–8.

[15] Shiran S I, Ben-Sira L, Elhasid R, et al. Multiple brain developmental venous anomalies as a marker for constitutional mismatch repair deficiency syndrome. *AJNR Am. J. Neuroradiol.* 2018 Oct;39(10):1943–6.

[16] Cheyuo C, Radwan W, Ahn J, et al. Biallelic PMS2 mutation and heterozygous DICER1 mutation presenting as constitutional mismatch repair deficiency with corpus callosum agenesis: Case report and review of literature. *J. Pediatr. Hematol. Oncol.* 2017 Oct;39(7):e381–7.

[17] Carrato C, Sanz C, Muñoz-Mármol A M, et al. The challenge of diagnosing constitutional mismatch repair deficiency syndrome in brain malignancies from young individuals. *Int. J. Mol. Sci.* 2021 Apr 28;22(9):4629.

[18] Chhabda S, Sudhakar S, Mankad K, et al. Constitutional mismatch repair deficiency (CMMRD) presenting with high-grade glioma, multiple developmental venous anomalies and malformations of cortical development-a multidisciplinary/multicentre approach and neuroimaging clues to clinching the diagnosis. *Childs Nerv. Syst.* 2021 Jul;37(7):2375–9.

[19] Taeubner J, Wimmer K, Muleris M, et al. Diagnostic challenges in a child with early onset desmoplastic medulloblastoma and homozygous variants in MSH2 and MSH6. *Eur. J. Hum. Genet.* 2018 Mar;26(3): 440–4.

[20] Baas A F, Gabbett M, Rimac M, et al. Agenesis of the corpus callosum and gray matter heterotopia in three patients with constitutional mismatch repair deficiency syndrome. *Eur. J. Hum. Genet.* 2013 Jan;21(1):55–61.

[21] Le D T, Uram J N, Wang H, et al. PD-1 Blockade in tumors with mismatch-repair deficiency. *N Engl. J. Med.* 2015 Jun 25;372(26):2509–20.

[22] Bouffet E, Larouche V, Campbell B B, et al. Immune checkpoint Inhibition for hypermutant glioblastoma multiforme resulting from germline biallelic mismatch repair deficiency. *J. Clin. Oncol.* 2016 Jul 1;34(19):2206–11.

[23] Durno C A, Aronson M, Tabori U, et al. Oncologic surveillance for subjects with biallelic mismatch repair gene mutations: 10 year follow-up of a kindred. *Pediatr. Blood Cancer.* 2012 Oct;59(4):652–6.

Chapter 19

Rhabdoid Tumor Predisposition Syndrome: Pathology of a Heritable Syndrome Primarily Affecting the Central Nervous System

Stephanie Njemanze[1], BA, BS
and Richard A. Prayson[2,*], MD, MEd
[1] Cleveland Clinic Lerner College of Medicine, Cleveland, Ohio, USA
[2] Department of Anatomic Pathology, Cleveland Clinic, Cleveland, Ohio, USA

Abstract

Rhabdoid Tumor Predisposition Syndrome (RTPS) is characterized by the development of malignant rhabdoid tumors (MRTs). The most common tumor type found in RTPS is the atypical teratoid and rhabdoid tumor (AT/RT) that occur in the brain, which can co-occur with rhabdoid tumors in other parts of the body, especially the kidney. Patients with RTPS present with an array of neurologic symptoms such as headaches, seizures and cranial nerve palsies. Heterogeneity on imaging studies is characteristic of these large, cystic tumors, which show preference for growth in the cerebellopontine angle region. Constitutional mutations in either the *SMARCB1* or *SMARCA4* gene on chromosome 22q11.2 and 19p13.2 respectively cause RTPS.

Focusing on central nervous system pathology, this chapter will discuss the salient clinicopathologic features of this disorder.

Introduction

Rhabdoid Tumor Predisposition Syndrome (RTPS) is a disorder affecting primarily infants and young children that is characterized by the development

In: Central Nervous System Pathologies in Hereditary Tumor Syndromes
Editor: Richard A. Prayson
ISBN: 979-8-88697-620-5

of malignant rhabdoid tumors (MRTs) [1]. MRTs occur all over the body but most commonly arise in the brain. These central nervous system-based MRTs are referred to as atypical teratoid and rhabdoid tumors (AT/RTs) and are of embryonal origin [1]. The most common location for rhabdoid tumors outside of the brain is the kidney; however, MRTs can also develop in the soft tissues of the head and neck, paravertebral muscles, mediastinum, liver, bladder and ovaries [1-2]. Lynch and colleagues described the first known case of RTPS in 1983 in two sisters who developed paravertebral MRTs and died shortly after [3]. Similar cases of familial tumor disorders have been described since then; however, most cases of RTPS occur de novo. The term RTPS was not coined until 1999, when Sevenet and colleagues described a heritable disorder associated with a constitutional mutation in the *SMARCB1* (hSNF5/INI1) gene that predisposed patients to develop rhabdoid tumors [4].

Genetics

RTPS results from mutations in the *SMARCB1* and/or the *SMARCA4* gene [3]. Located on chromosome 22q11.2, *SMARCB1* is a tumor suppressor gene. These mutations can have an autosomal dominant pattern of inheritance [5]. *SMARCB1* is the first subunit of the SWI/SNF complex, which regulates chromatin remodeling and thus regulates gene expression [5]. Mutations in *SMARCB1* result in a loss of function of this gene that is observed in rhabdoid tumors [6]. *SMARCA4* is also a subunit of the SWI/SNF complex gene. Mutations in *SMARCA4,* which is located on chromosome 19p13.2, have also been identified in rhabdoid tumors expressing *SMARCB1* [7]. Up to 35% of rhabdoid tumors have a germline mutation of *SMARCB1 [8]. SMARCA4* germline mutations in rhabdoid tumors are more rare [9]. Subtypes of RTPS can be described based on the expression of either gene. RTPS1 refers to patients with the *SMARCB1* mutation and RTPS 2 refers to patients with the *SMARCA4* mutation [1].

General Clinical Features

RTPS is clinically aggressive. Children typically present with tumors in the first year of life [2]. The peak incidence of rhabdoid tumors occurs between the ages of birth and 3 years [10]. Between 2000 and 2008, the incidence of rhabdoid tumors in children under the age of 15 years was 0.89 per million for AT/RTs, 0.19 per million for renal tumors, and 0.32 per million for all other rhabdoid tumors [8].

Individuals with RTPS typically present with AT/RTs, which can have a supratentorial or an infratentorial presentation. They commonly arise in the cerebellopontine angle [11, 12]. Other CNS tumors such as choroid plexus carcinomas, infratentorial primitive neuroectodermal tumors (PNETs) and medulloblastomas have been reported in patients with RTPS; however, their inclusion among tumors associated with RTPS is controversial, as they can at times be indistinguishable histologically from AT/RTs [4, 8]. Patients with extra CNS MRTs may present with abdominal distension, soft tissue masses and hematuria [13].

Neurologic Clinical Features

Persons with AT/RTs often present with headache secondary to hydrocephalus due to the tendency of these tumors to obstruct the flow of cerebrospinal fluid. Supratentorial AT/RTs can lead to extremity weakness and seizures caused by cortical compression or direct brain contact [12]. Additional neurologic symptoms include ataxia and cranial nerve palsies such as "extraocular muscle weakness, facial paralysis, and decreased gag reflex" [13].

Imaging Findings

AT/RTs in the brain show heterogeneity on computed tomography (CT) and magnetic resonance imaging (MRI) [14]. Contrast enhancement due to cystic components is seen on T1- and T2-weighted MRI [14, 15]. Multifocal intratumoral calcifications as well as leptomeningeal enhancement are also common [14, 16]. AT/RTs are characteristically large; therefore, imaging can reveal structural changes such as hydrocephalus, mass effect, and invasion of the brain and dura. Skull invasion is also possible due to the aggressive nature of AT/RT [14]. AT/RTs appear similar to medulloblastoma on imaging; however, restricted diffusion can elucidate if a tumor is a medulloblastoma or an AT/RT.

On restricted diffusion, a posterior fossa tumor that is not midline and/or shows involvement of the cerebellopontine angle indicates AT/RT [16].

Furthermore, intratumoral hemorrhage is also associated more with AT/RT than medulloblastoma [16].

Neuropathologic Findings

AT/RTs are normally arranged in dense, highly cellular sheets with variation in the presence of rhabdoid cells. They are often accompanied by areas of necrosis (Figure 1). Characteristic findings include large, polygonal cells with eccentrically placed, vesicular nuclei, prominent nucleoli, and an intracytoplasmic eosinophilic inclusion corresponding to aggregates of intermediate filaments (Figure 2) [17].

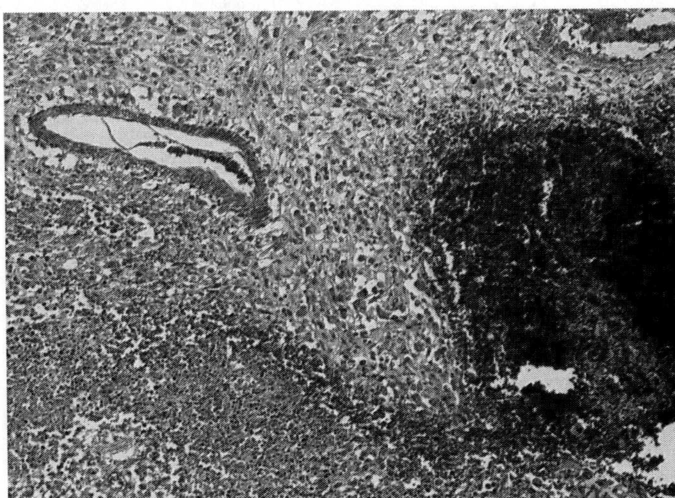

Figure 1. An atypical teratoid/rhabdoid tumor marked by focal hemorrhage (right) and necrosis (bottom) (hematoxylin and eosin, original magnification 100X).

Rhabdoid cells may be intermixed with morphologically diverse cells including large, atypical cells with an irregular border and small spindle shaped cells. Furthermore, rhabdoid cells are also present with poorly differentiated embryonal cells, thus making distinctions between tumors such as PNETs and AT/RTs challenging [17, 18]. Thus, immunostains are useful in providing distinctions between AT/RTs and other tumor types. MRTs such as AT/RTs show distinct "lineage infidelity" [17], expressing markers of different cell origins specifically mesenchymal, neural and epithelial and variably stain with a number of antibodies including vimentin, S-100 protein, cytokeratin, smooth muscle actin, epithelial membrane antigen, neuron-specific enolase, glial fibrillary acidic protein, and Leu7 [18].

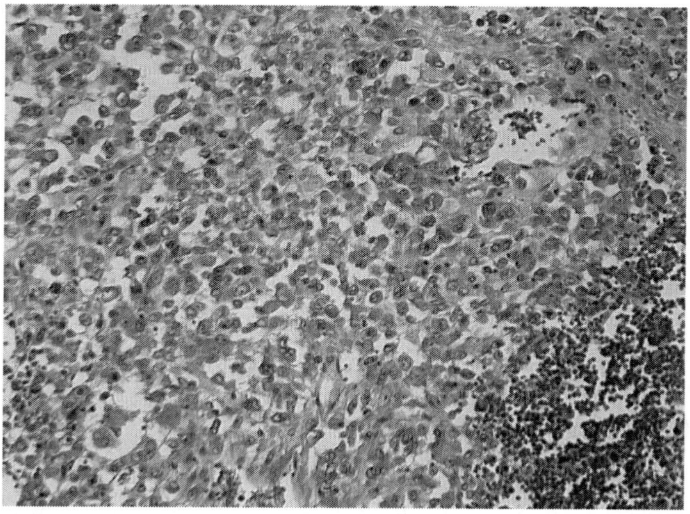

Figure 2. Tumor cells in this atypical teratoid/rhabdoid tumor are marked by eccentric nuclei with nucleoli and prominent eosinophilic cytoplasm (hematoxylin and eosin, original magnification 200X).

AT/RTs stain negatively for desmin and myogenin and germ cell tumor markers. Loss of nuclear staining with antibody to SMARCB1 (INI1) is a highly sensitive marker for AT/RTs.

Treatment and Prognosis

Radiation therapy is an important tool in the treatment of AT/RTs but poses neurocognitive risks for patients under the age of 3 years receiving whole brain therapy [19]. Nevertheless, early focal radiation appears to improve survival. Surgical treatment is provided to nearly all patients presenting with AT/RTs, and high dose chemotherapy can also be employed to extend survival [19, 20]. Unfortunately, the survival of patients with AT/RTs remains poor. AT/RTs are highly, aggressive with a median survival of 17 months [19]. Factors negatively affecting survival include metastatic disease and age <3 years [19].

Thus, early treatment and alternative therapies such as intrathecal chemotherapy could provide breakthroughs in treatment [19, 20].

Conclusion

Rhabdoid tumor predisposition syndrome is due to mutations in the SMARCB1 gene on chromosome 22q or SMARCA4 gene on chromosome 19p. Patients are predisposed to developing atypical teratoid/rhabdoid tumors in the brain.

References

[1] Sredni ST, Tomita T. Rhabdoid tumor predisposition syndrome. *Pediatr Devel Pathol*, 2015; 18(1). https://doi.org/10.2350/՟14-07-1531-MISC.1.

[2] Del Baldo G, Carta R, Alessi I, et al. Rhabdoid tumor predisposition syndrome: from clinical suspicion to general management. *Front Oncol,* 2021; Feb22; 11:586288.

[3] Lynch HT, Shurin SB, Dahms BB, et al. Paravertebral malignant rhabdoid tumor in infancy in vitro studies of a familial tumor. *Cancer,* 1983; 52(2): 290-96.

[4] Sévenet N, Sheridan E, Amram D, et al. Constitutional mutations of the HSNF5/INI1 gene predispose to a variety of cancers. *Am J Hum Genet,* 1999; 65(5):1342-48.

[5] Versteege I, Sévenet, N, Lange, J, et al. Truncating mutations of hSNF5/INI1 in aggressive paediatric cancer. *Nature,* 1998; 394: 203-206.

[6] Biegel JA, Tan L, Zhang F, et al. Alterations of the hSNF5/INI1 gene in central nervous system atypical teratoid/rhabdoid tumors and renal and extrarenal rhabdoid tumors. *Clin Cancer Res,* 2002; 8(11): 3461-7.

[7] Biegel JA, Busse TM, Weissman BE. SWI/SNF chromatin remodeling complexes and cancer. *Am J Med Genet C Semin Med Genet,* 2014; 166(C): 350-356.

[8] Heck JE, Lombardi CA, Cockburn M, et al. Epidemiology of rhabdoid tumors of early childhood. *Pediatr Blood Canc,* 2013; 60(1): 77-81.

[9] Bourdeaut F, Lequin D, Brugières L, et al. Frequent hSNF5/INI1 Germline mutations in patients with rhabdoid tumor. *Hum Cancer Biol*, 2011; 17(1): 31-38.

[10] Biegel JA. Molecular genetics of atypical teratoid/rhabdoid tumors. *Neurosurg Focus,* 2006; 20(1): 1-7.

[11] Rorke LB, Packer RJ, Biegel JA. Central nervous system atypical teratoid/rhabdoid tumors of infancy and childhood: Definition of an entity. *J Neurosurg*, 1996: 85(1): 56-65.

[12] Nesvick CL, Nageswara Rao AA, Raghunathan A, et al. Case-based review: atypical teratoid/rhabdoid tumor. *Neuro-Oncol Pract*, 2019; 6(3): 163-178.

[13] Pinto EM, Hamideh D, Bahrami A, et al. Malignant rhabdoid tumors originating within and outside the central nervous system are clinically and molecularly heterogeneous. *Acta Neuropathol*, 2019; 136(2): 315-326.

[14] Arslanoglu A, Aygun N, Tekhtani D, et al. Imaging findings of CNS atypical teratoid/rhabdoid tumors. *Am JNeuroradiol,* 2004; 25(3): 476-480.

[15] Evans A, Rakesh Ganatra R, Morris SJ. Imaging features of primary malignant rhabdoid tumour of the brain. *Pediatr Radiol,* 2001: 31(9): 631-633.

[16] Koral K, Gargan G, Bowers DC, et al. Imaging characteristics of atypical teratoid–rhabdoid tumor in children compared with medulloblastoma. *Am J Roent,* 2008; 190(3): 809-814.

[17] Hollmann TJ, Hornick JL. INI1-deficient tumors: diagnostic features and molecular genetics. *Am J Surg Pathol,* 2011; 35(10): e47.

[18] Bruggers, CS, Bleyl, SB, Pysher T, et al. Clinicopathologic comparison of familial versus sporadic atypical teratoid/rhabdoid tumors (AT/RT) of the central nervous system. *Pediatr Blood Cancer*, 2011; 56(7): 1026-1031.

[19] Ginn KF, Gajjar A. Atypical teratoid rhabdoid tumor: Current therapy and future directions. *Front Oncol*, 2012; Sept12; 2:114.

[20] Fischer-Valuck BW, Chen I, Srivastava AJ. Assessment of the treatment approach and survival outcomes in a modern cohort of patients with atypical teratoid rhabdoid tumors using the national cancer database. *Cancer,* 2017; 123(4): 682-87.

Chapter 20

DICER1 Syndrome: A Neuro-Clinicopathologic Review

Kiran A. Vaidya[1], BA
and Richard A. Prayson[2,*], MD, MEd

[1] Cleveland Clinic Lerner College of Medicine, Cleveland, Ohio, USA
[2] Department of Anatomic Pathology, Cleveland Clinic, Cleveland, Ohio, USA

Abstract

DICER1 syndrome occurs when the functionality of the endoribonuclease, DICER, is affected either via direct genetic mutations or secondary site mutations, predisposing the individual to developing multiple types of cancers. Of these cancers, the major brain tumor that presents from DICER1 mutations are pineoblastomas. These are highly aggressive, WHO Grade 4 neuroectodermal tumors, which most commonly affect children and adolescents.

The Dicer protein, which regulates miRNA biogenesis, plays an essential role in the development of these tumors. These tumors present with varying mass effect symptoms in the pineal gland region, including vomiting, headache, altered mental status and obstructive hydrocephalus. On imaging, pineoblastomas present as large poorly-defined masses in the pineal gland region with hemorrhagic, necrotic or cystic foci and high rates of seeding to the rest of the neural axis. On histology, these tumors are comprised of poorly differentiated cells with high nuclear to cytoplasmic ratios, frequent mitotic figures, nuclear molding, rosette formation, and sheet-like cells with positive synaptophysin and chromogranin marker staining.

---

* Corresponding Author's Email: praysor@ccf.org.

In: Central Nervous System Pathologies in Hereditary Tumor Syndromes
Editor: Richard A. Prayson
ISBN: 979-8-88697-620-5

Prognosis for the tumor is poor; the tumor is commonly managed with open surgical resection and adjuvant radiotherapy and chemotherapy.

Introduction

DICER1 syndrome is a disorder with a genetic basis that results in susceptibility to multiple cancer types [1]. It is caused by direct mutations within the DICER gene or mutations at secondary sites that affect the functionality of the Dicer protein [1]. Dicer itself is an endoribonuclease that plays a role in miRNA biogenesis and splicing [1]. Because it is ubiquitously expressed, the syndrome results in the development of both benign and malignant tumors in multiple organ systems and tissue types [1].

DICER1 syndrome is also known as pleuropulmonary blastoma familial tumor susceptibility syndrome [1]. The prevalence of the disease is unknown and the full picture of the clinical manifestations that can occur is still unclear. Thus far, DICER1 syndrome is known to be associated with pleuropulmonary blastomas, cystic nephroma, thyroid cancer, ovarian Sertoli–Leydig cell tumors, rhabdomyosarcoma, among other tumors [1]. The most common neurological manifestation of DICER syndrome are the development of pineoblastomas [1].

Genetics

The Dicer-1 and Dicer-2 genes were originally discovered in the Drosophila species in 2001 [2]; the human ortholog is DICER1. DICER1 is located on chromosome 14q32.13 and contains 27 exons and encodes for 1922 amino acids. DICER1 is ubiquitously expressed as a common housekeeping gene for miRNA biogenesis and processing [1]. The Dicer endoribonuclease protein is a component of the RNA-induced silencing complex (RISC) that processes hairpin-folded pre-miRNAs to about 22 nucleotide-sized double stranded RNAs (dsRNAs) [1]. It is hypothesized that Dicer dysfunction may lead to loss-of-function in tumor suppressor genes and gain-of-function in oncogenes [1].

Pathogenic germline mutations that occur within the DICER1 gene involve deletions, duplications, insertions, transitions and transversions [1]. Dicer is not only involved in miRNA processing but also in DNA processing, chromatin structure remodeling and apoptotic pathways among many other mechanisms, but in human disease, Dicer is thought to be primarily related to dysregulation of miRNAs [2]. Arguably, the latest research suggests that DICER1 acts as a haploinsufficient tumor suppressor gene but it has mostly been investigated in those same patients with pathogenic germline mutations involving complete loss of one allele. In these patients, a second somatic mutation is therefore necessary for the clinical phenotype during tumorigenesis and this is often a missense mutation impairing ability of the protein to cleave its targets [1, 2]. The hotspot domain for such a mutation is the RNase IIIb domain during tumorigenesis.

Clinical Features

DICER1 syndrome should be suspected when the thyroid, lungs, ovaries and kidneys are affected [2]. Pleuropulmonary blastoma is the most common neoplastic manifestation [1]. Other manifestations include multinodular goiter, Sertoli-Leydig cell tumor and cystic nephromas [1]. DICER1 was originally identified in 2009 as a germline mutation leading to familial pleuropulmonary blastoma [3]. Subsequently, a study conducted in 2011 elucidated that constitutional DICER1 haploinsufficiency leads to a range of tumors with a predominance of pleuropulmonary blastoma, cystic nephroma and ovarian Sertoli-Leydig tumors and termed the condition, "DICER Syndrome" [4]. This study comprehensively investigated constitutional DNA from 823 unrelated patients with various tumors and in 781 cancer cell lines [4]. Other prevalent tumors included Wilms tumor, seminoma, intraocular medulloepithelioma and thyroid non-toxic goiters/cysts [4]. Familial investigation revealed constitutional DICER1 mutations were found in 19 families with some displaying de novo mutations in a parent [4].

Brain tumors can also develop as a result of DICER1 mutations [5]. DICER1 syndrome has primarily been associated with pineoblastomas and more rarely pituitary blastomas [5]. DICER1 was originally linked to pineoblastomas in 2012, when a case report described a novel germline DICER1 mutation with loss of heterozygosity of the wildtype allele in a young patient with highly aggressive pineoblastoma [6]. The disruption of miRNA processing was later found to be an essential feature to the development of pineoblastomas [7]. Whole exome/genome sequencing revealed that in some cases, pineoblastomas can themselves be characterized by DICER1 or DROSHA mutations, both of which play an important role in the miRNA biogenesis pathway, with DROSHA being upstream of DICER1 [8, 9]. Although extremely rare, Pituitary blastomas were also found to be associated with DICER1 mutations. Out of the 16 cases of this tumor discovered, 14 of the patients that had undergone genetic testing all had DICER1 mutations [10, 11].

Neurological Features

Pineoblastomas are neuroectodermal tumors with a median age at diagnosis of about 13 years [7]. They present with headache, vomiting, ocular symptoms, increased intracranial pressure leading to papilledema and altered mental status[1] [12]. Less common symptoms include ataxia, macrocephaly, seizures, dehydration and irritability [12]. Endocrine labs are normal [12]. Obstructive hydrocephalus is also a common presenting symptom [13]. Pituitary blastomas commonly present with endocrine disorders such as Cushing syndrome or diabetes insipidus [14, 15]. They could also present with ophthalmoplegia [15]. While ACTH is typically elevated, other pituitary hormones may or may not be affected [14, 15]. Altogether, pineoblastomas tend to present with symptoms indicating a mass effect while pituitary blastomas commonly present with endocrine-related symptoms.

Imaging Findings

On imaging, pineoblastomas appear as large masses in the pineal gland region, commonly assessed on computed tomography (CT) or magnetic resonance imaging (MRI) [7]. They may contain hemorrhagic, necrotic or cystic foci, as commonly seen in high-grade tumors [16]. They are infiltrative with ill-defined borders and due to this can sometimes be seen extending into other structures [7, 16].

On T1-weighted MRI, they present as iso- or hypointense but present as iso- or hyperintense on T2-weighted MRI [13 16]. Cystic components, however, will produce increased intensity [16]. With gadolinium, they exhibit inhomogeneous enhancement, which can be useful to differentiate cystic from necrotic components of the tumor [16]. They tend to be at least 3 cm and hyperdense on CT due to the high cellularity [13, 16]. They can appear with calcifications and a cystic appearance but are not to be confused with benign pineal cysts [13].

A clinically significant percentage of patients will present with cerebrospinal fluid seeding, so imaging of the spinal cord is recommended [13, 17].

Pituitary blastomas present on CT and MRI as solid masses in the sellar or suprasellar area and can be differentiated from other tumors by presenting symptoms and endocrine hormone labs [18]. They can also present as a cystic mass [18].

Neuropathologic Findings

Pineoblastomas are characterized as a WHO Grade 4 tumor due to their highly aggressive nature [7]. On histology, they exhibit high cellularity, showing features of anaplasia with hyperchromatic nuclei, cells with a high nuclear-to-cytoplasmic ratio, and frequent mitotic figures (Figure 1) [7, 13]. They can also have areas of necrosis and hemorrhage (Figure 2). Other features include nuclear molding and rosette formation. They typically stain positively for synaptophysin and chromogranin, which are neuronal and neuroendocrine markers, respectively [7, 13]. They are overall comprised of poorly differentiated cells comprising a highly malignant tumor [13].

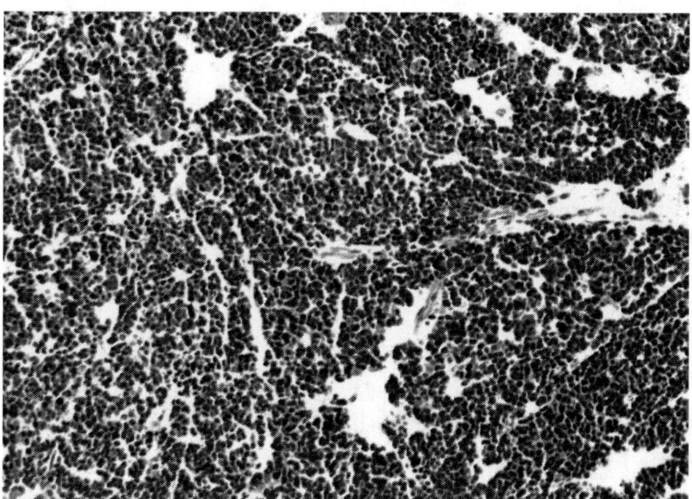

Figure 1. A pineoblastoma, marked by a proliferation of small round "blue cells" with scant cytoplasm (hematoxylin and eosin, original magnification 100X).

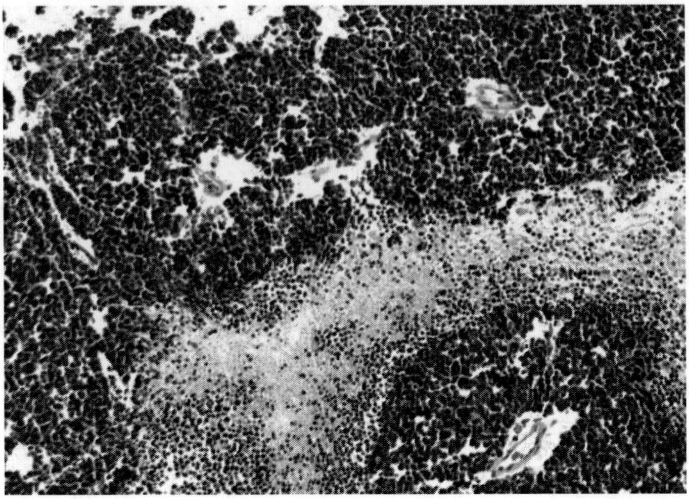

Figure 2. The same tumor as in Figure 1 showing an area of geographic necrosis (hematoxylin and eosin, original magnification 200X).

Pituitary blastomas are comprised of cells arranged in glandular-like structures and resembling secretory-type cells and small blastemal-like cells [7].

There can be areas of necrosis with varying mitotic activity [7]. These tumors stain positively for keratins, galectin-3, annexin-1, S-100 protein, synaptophysin and chromogranin [7].

Treatment and Prognosis

Patients with pineoblastomas have a poor prognosis but complete surgical resection is associated with improved survival [19]. Unfortunately, the 5-year survival rate is 10% with a median overall survival of 20 months [20]. Standard of care is open surgical resection with adjuvant craniospinal irradiation, due to high rates of cerebrospinal fluid seeding, and multi-agent chemotherapy [20, 21]. The most common surgical approach is the supracerebellar infratentorial approach [20]. Adjuvant therapy includes radiotherapy protocols that are 5500 cGy to the tumor region and 3500 cGy to the spinal axis [20].

Common chemotherapy agents employed include vincristine, cisplatin/carboplatin, cyclophosphamide, etoposide and lomustine [20]. Patients presenting with hydrocephalus should receive an endoscopic third ventriculostomy or ventriculoperitoneal shunt [20]. Overall factors that increase survival rates include age at presentation (over 3 years), gross total resection, lack of metastasis, and radiotherapy more than 40 Gy.

Resection and chemotherapy comprise common management for pituitary blastomas with a median survival rate of almost 7 years [22].

Conclusion

DICER1 syndrome results from genetic mutations in DICER1, an endoribonuclease protein encoded for on chromosome 14q. Brain tumors that have been noted to develop in patients with this disorder have included pineoblastomas and pituitary blastomas.

References

[1] Robertson JC, Jorcyk CL, Oxford JT. DICER1 syndrome: DICER1 mutations in rare cancers. *Cancers,* (Basel). 2018; 10(5):143.

[2] Meiklejohn KM, Darbinyan A, Barbieri AL. A review of DICER1: structure, function and contribution to disease. *Diagn Histopathol,* 2022; 28(7):329-336.

[3] Hill DA, Ivanovich J, Priest JR, et al. DICER1 mutations in familial pleuropulmonary blastoma. *Science,* 2009; 325:965.

[4] Slade I, Bacchelli C, Davies H, et al. DICER1 syndrome: Clarifying the diagnosis, clinical features and management implications of a pleiotropic tumour predisposition syndrome. *J Med Genet,* 2011; 48:273-278.

[5] Theotoki EI, Pantazopoulou VI, Georgiou S, et al. Dicing the disease with dicer: The implications of dicer ribonuclease in human pathologies. *Int J Mol Sci,* 2020; 21(19):7223.

[6] Sabbaghian N, Hamel N, Srivastava A, et al. Germline DICER1 mutation and associated loss of heterozygosity in a pineoblastoma. *J Med Genet,* 2012; 49:417-419.

[7] de Kock, L., Priest JR, Foulkes WD, et al. An update on the central nervous system manifestations of DICER1 syndrome. *Acta Neuropathol,* 2020; 139:689-701.

[8] Lee JC, Mazor T, Lao R., et al. Recurrent KBTBD4 small in-frame insertions and absence of DROSHA deletion or DICER1 mutation differentiate pineal parenchymal tumor of intermediate differentiation (PPTID) from pineoblastoma. *Acta Neuropathol,* 2019; 137:851-854.

[9] Snuderl M, Kannan K, Aminova O, et al. Novel candidate oncogenic drivers in pineoblastoma. *Neuro oncology,*-17:iii23.

[10] de Kock L, Sabbaghian N, Plourde F, et al. Pituitary blastoma: A pathognomonic feature of germ-line DICER1 mutations. *Acta Neuropathol,* 2014; 128:111-122.

[11] Gresh R, Piatt J, Walter A. A report of a child with a pituitary blastoma and DICER1 syndrome. 2015 ASPHO Abstracts. *Pediatr Blood Cancer,* 2015; 62:S72-S73.

[12] Cuccia V., Rodríguez F., Palma F, et al. Pinealoblastomas in children. *Childs Nerv Syst,* 2006; 22:577-585.

[13] Lombardi G, Poliani PL, Manara R, et al. Diagnosis and treatment of pineal region tumors in adults: A EURACAN overview. *Cancers,* (Basel). 2022 Jul 27; 14(15): 3646.

[14] Kalinin A, Strebkova N, Tiulpakov A, et al. A novel DICER1 gene mutation in a 10-month-old boy presenting with ACTH-secreting pituitary blastoma and lung cystic dysplasia. Presented at the 19th European Congress of Endocrinology 2017; Lisbon, Portugal. *Endocrine Abstracts,* 49: EP1025.

[15] Sahakitrungruang T, Srichomthong C, Pornkunwilai S, et al. Germline and somatic DICER1 mutations in a pituitary blastoma causing infantile-onset Cushing's disease. *J Clin Endocrinol Metab,* 2014; 99:E1487–E1492.

[16] Solomou AG. Magnetic resonance imaging of pineal tumors and drop metastases: A review approach. *Rare Tumors,* 2017 Oct 23; 9(3):6715.

[17] Fauchon F, Jouvet A, Paquis P, et al Parenchymal pineal tumors: A clinico-pathological study of 76 cases. *Int J Radiat Oncol Biol Phys,* 2000; 46:959-968.

[18] Chhuon Y, Weon YC, Park G, et al. Pituitary blastoma in a 19-year-old woman: A case report and review of literature. *World Neurosurg,* 2020;139:310-313.

[19] Lee JY, Wakabayashi T, Yoshida J. Management and survival of pineoblastoma: An analysis of 34 adults from the brain tumor registry of Japan. *Neurol Med Chir,* 2005; 45(3):132-41.

[20] Tate MC, Rutkowski MJ, Parsa AT. Contemporary management of pineoblastoma. *Neurosurg Clin N Am,* 2011; 22(3):409-12.

[21] Lutterbach J, Fauchon F, Schild SE, et al. Malignant pineal parenchymal tumors in adult patients: Patterns of care and prognostic factors. *Neurosurgery,* 2002; 51 (1):44-56.

[22] Liu APY, Kelsey MM, Sabbaghian N, et al. Clinical outcomes and complications of pituitary blastoma. *J Clin Endocrinol Metab,* 2021 Jan 23; 106(2):351-363.

Chapter 21

Pituitary Gland and Systemic Pathology of Multiple Endocrine Neoplasia Type I (MEN1)

Dhananjay Prakash[1], BS, MS
Precious C. Oyem[2], BA
and Richard A. Prayson[3,*], MD, MEd
[1] Case Western Reserve University, Cleveland, OH, USA
[2] Cleveland Clinic Lerner College of Medicine, Cleveland, OH, USA
[3] Department of Anatomic Pathology, Cleveland Clinic, Cleveland, OH, USA

Abstract

Multiple endocrine neoplasia Type I (MEN1) is a rare autosomal dominant inherited disorder that results from germline mutations of the tumor suppressor gene, MEN1. The MEN1 gene encodes menin, a scaffolding protein implicated in a variety of cell processes, including cell division and transcription. An abnormal MEN1 gene leads to the formation of functioning/non-functioning endocrine tumors involving the pancreas, the parathyroid, anterior pituitary, duodenum, and thymus.

Tumors of the entero-pancreatic axis, anterior pituitary, and parathyroid are more commonly noted in MEN1. Clinically, MEN1 is defined by findings of two or more MEN1-associated neoplasms or by the presence of a single tumor and a first-degree relative diagnosed with MEN1. The histopathological and radiological indications of MEN1-associated tumors are identical to non-MEN1-related counterparts.

* Corresponding Author's Email: praysor@ccf.org.

In: Central Nervous System Pathologies in Hereditary Tumor Syndromes
Editor: Richard A. Prayson
ISBN: 979-8-88697-620-5

Similar to sporadic cases, commonly used stains include Ki-67, Chromogranin A (CgA), and synaptophysin (SYN).

Behind parathyroid-associated MEN1 adenomas, pituitary neuroendocrine tumors (adenomas) make up about 40% of all MEN1 cases, with the majority being functioning pituitary neuroendocrine tumors. They are more commonly found in females compared to males and can cause hyperprolactinemia, acromegaly, and Cushing's disease. Pharmacological approaches have been proven effective in managing the symptoms of certain MEN1 disorders. However, the first line of treatment is surgical intervention due to the drug-resistant and aggressive nature of MEN1 pituitary neuroendocrine tumors. The life expectancy of individuals with MEN1 is substantially less than the general population, averaging 55 years.

This chapter provides an overview of the clinical characteristics of MEN1 with a focus on its pathology, including the impact on the pituitary gland.

Introduction

In 1903, Austrian pathologist Jakob Erdheim documented and published his findings on what is now Multiple Endocrine Neoplasia Type I (MEN1) He wrote about the parathyroid hyperplasia and a pituitary adenoma he found following an autopsy of an acromegalic patient. [1, 2]. In the next quarter century, Cushing and Davidhoff first described the hallmark MEN1 tumor triad consisting of entero-pancreatic, anterior pituitary, and parathyroid adenomas [3]. The almost non-existent imaging and immunohistological techniques of the time made it difficult to further delineate the features of the disorder.

Consequently, most literature on the disorder focused on post-mortem studies. More than 50 years after Erdheim's initial findings, Otto Wermer uncovered the autosomal dominant inheritance pattern of the syndrome, while treating a family in which the father and four of his nine children displayed the characteristic triad [1, 4]. The following year, Zollinger and Ellison discovered a syndrome of peptic ulcers within the jejunum associated with pancreatic islet adenomas. By the late 1960s, technological advancements allowed for clinical guidelines for this disorder and labeled it as Multiple Endocrine Neoplasia Type 1, (MEN1) [5–8].

Genetics

MEN1, a tumor suppressor gene, encodes the protein menin. This 610-amino acid long scaffolding protein is integral to various cellular processes. Menin necessitates critical cellular processes such as transcription, replication, apoptosis, and growth factor signaling. [7, 9] In 1988, Swedish scientists mapped the gene's locus to chromosome 11q13 [10]. MEN1 is transmitted in an autosomal dominant fashion; a parent with the disorder has a 50% chance of transmitting the disease to their children. Approximately 90% of patients inherit the syndrome in this fashion. However, roughly 10% lack family history and are attributed to mutations that arise during embryonic development [1, 11]. Current research implicates menin's role in negative gene expression through suppressed histone acetylation and regulation of miRNA expression [12, 13].

Most MEN1 germline mutations are associated with premature truncation or exon deletion. Frame-shift mutations and nonsense mutations cause premature truncation, while exon deletions are due to splicing defects and extensive deletions [9, 14, 15]. Recent studies have implicated this loss of tumor suppression to an interaction between menin and miR-24-1, a non-coding RNA sequence that disrupts gene expression. Researchers hypothesize that miR-24-1 silences menin expression through a post-transcriptional modification leading to the downstream effect of tumor formation [1, 16].

Non-Neurological Clinical Features

Establishing an MEN1 diagnosis is based on tumor location and family history. Finding two or more neoplasms within the entero-pancreatic axis, anterior pituitary and/or parathyroid glands, or finding a single MEN1-associated neoplasm along with a direct relative with MEN-1 forms the definitive diagnostic criteria [17]. MEN1 includes neoplasms of the duodenopancreatic axis and commonly presents with Zollinger-Ellison syndrome (ZES), through the formation of gastrinomas. Roughly 60-75% of MEN1 patients have either ZES or a marked increase in serum gastrin levels. When compared to their sporadic counterparts, MEN1-related gastrinomas are multifocal and minute [18–21]. Common symptoms of ZES include abdominal pain, diarrhea, and heartburn. The development of severe peptic ulcer disease has been noted in MEN1-associated gastrinoma [22–25].

Insulinomas are another clinical presentation that often raises suspicion of MEN1. They are the second most common MEN1-neoplasm within the enteropancreatic axis and appear in about 10–30% of pancreatic endocrine tumors associated with MEN1 [26]. Autonomic symptoms of insulinoma include tremors, diaphoresis, and palpitation, while neuroglycopenic symptoms consist of confusion, visual disturbances, and sometimes seizures [27]. Insulinomas related to MEN1 tend to appear in patients under 40 years of age, sometimes even before age 20 years, usually with multiple tumors. On the other hand, sporadic instances occur later in life, after the age of 40 years, and mostly present as a single tumor. Furthermore, glucagonoma, VIPoma, and somatostatinoma rarely occur in pancreatic neuroendocrine tumors (pNETs) associated with MEN1 (pNETs) [26–29].

Under normal conditions, menin immunochemistry displays higher nuclear localization than cytoplasmic localization. In pNETs, abnormal menin displays the opposite, with increased aggregation in the cytoplasm. Studies suggest that the dysfunctional protein products from truncating mutations lack a nuclear localization sequence leading to this unique display [30]. A distinct histopathological indication of neuroendocrine tumor is the "salt and pepper" nuclear chromatin pattern under hematoxylin and eosin staining [31]. Other histopathological features of pNETs include a "nest" like formation of cells and "anastomosing ribbon-like" trabecular formations. Well-differentiated and poorly differentiated pNETs are discerned through chromogranin A (CgA) and synaptophysin (SYN) staining. CgA's high specificity and sensitivity for well-differentiated NET allow the distinction. Like most tumors, cell proliferation and prognosis are evaluated using Ki-67 immunostaining [31].

Parathyroid Adenomas in MEN1

Primary hyperparathyroidism (PHPT) due to MEN1-associated parathyroid adenomas is the most common clinical presentation, about 1-18% of PHPT diagnoses link back to MEN1 [32, 33]. The clinical symptoms of parathyroid adenomas associated with MEN1 are similar to those of their sporadic counterparts. Symptoms include hypercalcemia, peptic ulcer disease, hypertension, urolithiasis, and decreased bone mineral density. It is important to note that, hypercalcemia related to PHPT, if uncontrolled, can lead to ZES, peptic ulcer disease, and other gastrointestinal complications. Research has implicated membranous calcium-sensing receptors (CaRs) as a mediator of this calcium-gastrin pathway. The excess CaRs activation and interaction with phospholipase C due to the hypercalcemic state leads to abnormal extracellular calcium influx with the downstream effect of excess gastrin secretion [1, 34–36]. MEN1-related PHPT presents earlier between the ages of 20-25 years compared to sporadic instances, which show up later in life around age 55 years. When comparing tumor characteristics, sporadic parathyroid adenomas localize to a single gland, while MEN1-related parathyroid adenomas are a multi-glandular disease with tumors of varying sizes [1, 17, 37].

Like pNET-MEN1, CgA and SYN stains are used again for parathyroid-associated MEN1. Functioning tumors are stained for hormones in conjunction with keratin and thyroglobulin. In terms of hormonal immunostaining, chief cells stain brightly for parathyroid hormone antibody in parathyroid adenomas, regardless of MEN1 relation. Parathyroid tissue also stains positive for various keratin immunomarkers, with CAM 5.2 being a fairly consistent marker for these tumors. Microscopically, parathyroid adenomas exhibit micro-acinar or palisading formations of chief and oxyphilic cells. Furthermore, tumor cells exhibit hyperchromatic nuclei, mitotic figures, and decreased stromal fat content when compared to normal parathyroid gland cells and tissue [38, 39].

Neuro-Clinical Features

Pituitary neuroendocrine tumors are clinically present in approximately 40% of patients diagnosed with MEN1. However, these findings change depending on the geographical location, with higher incidences reported in Brazil [34]. In about 17% of MEN1 patients, pituitary tumors were the initial clinical manifestation of the disorder; with 38 years being the mean age of onset. MEN1-associated pituitary neuroendocrine tumors are more likely to occur in women than in men. Studies show that about 80% of MEN1-associated pituitary tumors are macroadenomas; among these large tumors, the most commonly appearing subtype are prolactin (PRL)-secreting tumors at 62%, followed by growth hormone (GH) secreting and adrenocorticotropic hormone (ACTH) secreting tumors at 9% and 4%, respectively. Non-secreting tumors were discovered at rates of about 15%. MEN1-associated pituitary neoplasms are radiologically and histopathologically identical to sporadic cases [7, 40, 41].

Symptoms of sporadic and MEN1-associated pituitary neuroendocrine tumors are the same and vary on the type and staging of the tumor [42]. Among functioning tumors, symptoms depend on the specific hormone that becomes dysregulated. In the case of prolactinomas, the downstream suppression of gonadotropins has the effect of decreased libido and infertility. A hallmark of GH-secreting tumors is acromegaly; symptoms include visual abnormalities, diaphoresis, and the formation of prominent facial features. Cushing's disease is linked with ACTH-secreting neoplasms; patients display easy bruising, weight gain, and a round "moon" face. Lastly, patients with TSH-secreting tumors present with weight loss, tremors, and arrhythmia [43]. When comparing MEN1-associated pituitary tumors to the sporadic form, the symptoms remain the same.

Neuropathology

In terms of categorization and histological presentation, MEN1-associated pituitary neuroendocrine tumors are very similar to sporadic cases. MEN1-associated pituitary tumors display a "sheet-like" proliferation of monomorphic appearing cells with a salt and pepper nuclear chromatin pattern [45] (Figures 1 and 2).

Figure 1. A pituitary neuroendocrine tumor (pituitary adenoma) presenting in a patient with MEN 1, marked by a sheet-like proliferation of cells (hematoxylin and eosin, original magnification 100X).

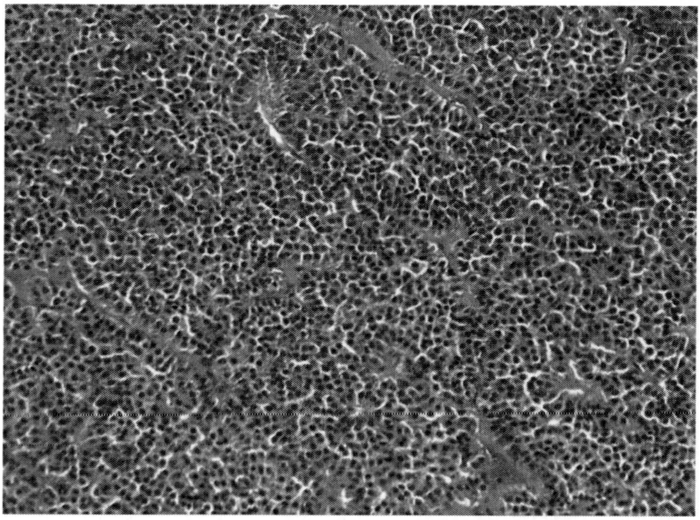

Figure 2. The same tumor as in Figure 1. The tumor cells have a monomorphic appearance with a salt and pepper nuclear chromatin pattern (hematoxylin and eosin, original magnification 200X).

Like sporadic cases, MEN1-associated pituitary tumors may be classified as either sparsely or densely granulated in reference to their cytoplasmic secretory vesicle content. The initial step in evaluating pituitary tumors is to discern neoplasia from hyperplasia. Pituitary neoplasms display prominent degradation of acinar structures when compared to hyperplasia which presents with a relatively preserved acinar or lobular architecture. The test panel for pituitary neuroendocrine tumors is fairly extensive and includes pituitary-specific transcription factor 1 (Pit-1), estrogen receptor alpha (ER-a), T-box transcription factor (Tpit), and steroidogenic factor-1 (SF-1) [44, 45]. Both prolactinomas and GH-secreting, somatotroph adenomas stain positive for Pit-1. While most prolactinomas and gonadotroph adenomas stain positive for ER-a. ACTH-producing pituitary adenomas are positive for Tpit. [44]. Follicle stimulating hormone and luteinizing hormone secreting tumors generally stain with SF-1.

When compared to densely granulated somatotroph adenomas tumors, sparsely granulated somatotroph tumors appear as chromophobic cells with varying cellularity and nuclear aberrations. A histological feature of sparsely granulated tumors is the keratin accumulation, which displays as "pale disks" on hematoxylin and eosin-stained sections. On the other hand, densely granulated somatotroph tumors, lack cellularity and are made up of eosinophilic cells with secretory granule aggregation [46]. Most prolactinomas are of the sparsely granulated subtype; characterized by the presence of "cap-like" formations on prolactin staining and have been linked to calcification and amyloid deposition [46]. Sparsely granulated corticotroph tumors, stain weakly basophilic and often present as clinically asymptomatic. Their dense counterparts stain strongly basophilic and present with symptomatic Cushing's disease. Most dense corticotroph tumors will stain intensely positive for ACTH. Lastly, gonadotroph tumors are often non-functioning, displaying "perivascular rosettes" of neuroendocrine cells with chromophobic staining [46].

Treatment and Prognosis

Treatments for MEN1 are similar to their sporadic non-MEN1 counterparts, both depend on the type of pituitary neuroendocrine tumor and the specific signs and symptoms. The complications of the hypersecretory hormonal state that appear with MEN1 adversely affect patients' quality of life. Therefore, early detection and diagnosis via MEN1 genetic testing allows for prophylactic therapy to reduce the overall morbidity and mortality of MEN1. Currently, there are no curative options, treatment aims to improve patients' quality of life. The overall 20-year mortality rate of MEN1 patients was lower compared to matched populations. Neoplasms associated with the thymus, duodenopancreatic axis, and nonsecreting pancreatic tumors tend to have higher mortality rates. Individuals with this disorder have a significantly lower life expectancy, passing away by their late 50s and early 60s [11, 29, 33, 47].

In the case of MEN1-associated parathyroid tumor treatment, the goals are to reduce hypercalcemia, control hypoparathyroidism, and allow for future surgical procedures, as some patients require multiple surgeries due to persistent PHPT [11]. After a diagnosis of MEN1-associated PHPT, prophylactic surgical intervention is recommended if the patient presents with hypercalcemia, nephrolithiasis, and decreased bone density [26]. The initial procedure is a subtotal parathyroidectomy, removal of 3–3½ parathyroid glands, along with a thymectomy. The thymectomy is performed to reduce the risk of thymic carcinoma. In some instances, a complete parathyroidectomy is performed, followed by a parathyroid autograft in the forearm or neck to reduce hypoparathyroidism that follows gland removal [17, 48]. Pharmacological interventions are recommended for patients who do not meet the criteria for surgical intervention. Cinacalcet, a calcium-sensing receptor agonist which decreases cell proliferation and PTH release, is sometimes used. However, surgical interventions have proven to be far more effective than a pharmacological approach in MEN1 symptom management [11].

While most pituitary neuroendocrine tumors are primarily benign, MEN1 pituitary neuroendocrine tumors are noted to be more aggressive and drug-resistant, patients commonly present with hypopituitarism and visual abnormalities. The clinical presentations of sporadic and MEN1-associated pituitary tumors depend on the tumor size and which hormone(s) release becomes dysregulated. MEN1 pituitary neoplasms are often larger and more aggressive than sporadic cases, requiring early surgical intervention [11, 41, 49]. As previously stated, early detection through genetic tests remains integral to symptom management. For prolactinomas, the initial approach is pharmacological control of PRL hypersecretion via dopamine agonists, trans-sphenoidal surgery, and radiotherapy are indicated for the drug-resistant and symptomatic cases. First-line therapy for GH-secreting and gonadotropin-secreting tumors is trans-sphenoidal surgery. A pharmacological approach using, somatostatin analogs to regulate GH release is reserved for patients unable to undergo surgical intervention. [11, 50].

Gastric tumors within the enteropancreatic axis are hard to treat. Surgery in MEN1-associated gastrinomas is often complicated by the microscopic and diffuse presentation of the tumors. Currently, therapy for MEN1-associated gastrinoma is pharmaceutical, to control acid hypersecretion. The current indications for surgical resection are a tumor diameter of about 2 cm or more or if the tumor has doubled in size in the span of 6 months [11, 26]. In MEN1-associated insulinoma, the number and difficulty localizing pancreatic neoplasms make it harder to treat than sporadic cases. Sporadic variants often present with a single tumor, making surgical intervention the preferred course of action. Treatment for MEN1-associated insulinomas is often corporo-caudal-pancreatectomy or a pancreato-duodenectomy to carefully resect the more diseased pancreatic regions. Depending on the volume of the resected tissue, patients are at an increased risk of dysregulated glucose metabolism and developing diabetes mellitus [11, 51, 52].

Conclusion

Multiple endocrine neoplasia type 1 is an autosomal dominant disorder that is attributable to germline mutations in the tumor suppressor gene MEN1. Pituitary neuroendocrine tumors (pituitary adenomas) may be seen in up to

40% of MEN 1 patents; the majority of these are functional tumors secreting hormones.

References

[1] Marini F, Falchetti A, Luzi E, et al. Multiple Endocrine Neoplasia Type 1 (MEN1) Syndrome. In: Riegert-Johnson DL, Boardman LA, Hefferon T, Roberts M, editors. *Cancer Syndromes [Internet].* Bethesda (MD): National Center for Biotechnology Information (US); 2009 [cited 2022 Aug 11]. Available from: http://www.ncbi.nlm.nih.gov/books/NBK7029/.

[2] Erdheim J. Zur normalen und pathologischen Histologic der Glandula thyreoidea, parathyreoidea and Hypophysis [*On the normal and pathological histologic of the thyroid, parathyroid and pituitary glands*]. *Beitr. Pathol. Anat.* 1903;(33):158–326.

[3] Cushing H, Davidoff L M. *The Pathologic Findings in Four Autopsied Cases of Acromegaly. With a discussion of Their Significance.* The Rockefeller Institute for Medical Research ed. New York.; 1927. (Monograph 22.).

[4] Wermer P. Genetic aspects of adenomatosis of endocrine glands. *Am. J. Med.* 1954 Mar;16(3):363–71.

[5] Zollinger R M, Ellison E H. Primary peptic ulcerations of the jejunum associated with islet cell tumors of the pancreas. *Ann. Surg.* 1955 Oct;142(4):709–23; discussion, 724–8.

[6] Lulu D J, Corcoran T E, Andre M. Familial endocrine adenomatosis with associated Zollinger-Ellison syndrome. Wermer's syndrome. *Am. J. Surg.* 1968 May;115(5): 695–701.

[7] Solomon D A, Perry A. Familial tumor syndromes. In: Perry A, Brat DJ (editors). *Practical Surgical Neuropathology: A Diagnostic Approach - 2nd Editio*n. Elsevier. Philadelphia, PA. 2018. Pp. 505-545.

[8] Nussbaum S R, Potts J T. Immunoassays for parathyroid hormone 1-84 in the diagnosis of hyperparathyroidism. *J. Bone Miner. Res.* 1991 Oct;6 Suppl 2:S43-50; discussion S61.

[9] Wautot V, Vercherat C, Lespinasse J, et al. Germline mutation profile of MEN1 in multiple endocrine neoplasia type 1: search for correlation between phenotype and the functional domains of the MEN1 protein. *Hum. Mutat.* 2002 Jul;20(1):35–47.

[10] Larsson C, Skogseid B, Oberg K, et al. Multiple endocrine neoplasia type 1 gene maps to chromosome 11 and is lost in insulinoma. *Nature.* 1988 Mar 3;332 (6159):85–7.

[11] Marini F, Giusti F, Tonelli F, et al. Management impact: effects on quality of life and prognosis in MEN1. *Endocr. Relat. Cancer.* 2017 Oct 1;24(10):T227–42.

[12] Matkar S, Thiel A, Hua X. Menin: a scaffold protein that controls gene expression and cell signaling. *Trends Biochem. Sci.* 2013 Aug;38(8):394–402.

[13] Agarwal S K, Guru S C, Heppner C, et al. Menin interacts with the AP1 transcription factor JunD and represses JunD-activated transcription. *Cell.* 1999 Jan 8;96(1):143–52.

[14] Lemos M C, Thakker R V. Multiple endocrine neoplasia type 1 (MEN1): analysis of 1336 mutations reported in the first decade following identification of the gene. *Hum. Mutat.* 2008 Jan;29(1):22–32.

[15] Concolino P, Costella A, Capoluongo E. Multiple endocrine neoplasia type 1 (MEN1): An update of 208 new germline variants reported in the last nine years. *Cancer Genet.* 2016 Feb;209(1–2):36–41.

[16] Luzi E, Marini F, Giusti F, Galli G, et al. The negative feedback-loop between the oncomir Mir-24-1 and menin modulates the Men1 tumorigenesis by mimicking the "Knudson's second hit." *PloS One.* 2012;7(6):e39767.

[17] Giusti F, Tonelli F, Brandi M L. Primary hyperparathyroidism in multiple endocrine neoplasia type 1: when to perform surgery? *Clinics.* 2012 Apr;67(Suppl 1):141–4.

[18] Roy P K, Venzon D J, Shojamanesh H, et al. Zollinger-Ellison syndrome. Clinical presentation in 261 patients. *Medicine (Baltimore).* 2000 Nov;79(6):379–411.

[19] Pipeleers-Marichal M, Somers G, Willems G, et al. Gastrinomas in the duodenums of patients with multiple endocrine neoplasia type 1 and the Zollinger-Ellison syndrome. *N. Engl. J. Med.* 1990 Mar 15;322(11):723–7.

[20] Anlauf M, Garbrecht N, Henopp T, et al. Sporadic versus hereditary gastrinomas of the duodenum and pancreas: distinct clinico-pathological and epidemiological features. *World J. Gastroenterol.* 2006 Sep 14;12(34):5440–6.

[21] Donow C, Pipeleers-Marichal M, Schröder S, et al. Surgical pathology of gastrinoma. Site, size, multicentricity, association with multiple endocrine neoplasia type 1, and malignancy. *Cancer.* 1991 Sep 15;68(6):1329–34.

[22] Cho M S, Kasi A. Zollinger Ellison Syndrome. In: *StatPearls [Internet].* Treasure Island (FL): StatPearls Publishing; 2022 [cited 2022 Aug 11]. Available from: http://www.ncbi.nlm.nih.gov/books/NBK537344/.

[23] Arnold R. Diagnosis and differential diagnosis of hypergastrinemia. *Wien. Klin. Wochenschr.* 2007;119(19–20):564–9.

[24] Phan J, Benhammou J N, Pisegna J R. Gastric hypersecretory states: investigation and management. *Curr. Treat Options Gastroenterol.* 2015 Dec;13(4):386–97.

[25] Wermer P. Endocrine adenomatosis and peptic ulcer in a large kindred. Inherited multiple tumors and mosaic pleiotropism in man. *Am. J. Med.* 1963 Aug;35:205–12.

[26] Thakker R V, Newey PJ, Walls GV, et al. Clinical practice guidelines for multiple endocrine neoplasia type 1 (MEN1). *J. Clin. Endocrinol. Metab.* 2012 Sep 1;97(9): 2990–3011.

[27] Cryer PE. Mechanisms of hypoglycemia-associated autonomic failure and its component syndromes in diabetes. *Diabetes.* 2005 Dec 1;54(12):3592–601.

[28] Trump D, Farren B, Wooding C, et al. Clinical studies of multiple endocrine neoplasia type 1 (MEN1). *QJM Mon. J. Assoc. Physicians.* 1996 Sep;89(9):653–69.

[29] Kamilaris CDC, Stratakis CA. Multiple endocrine neoplasia type 1 (MEN1): an update and the significance of early genetic and clinical diagnosis. *Front Endocrinol.* 2019 Jun 11;10:339.

[30] Corbo V, Dalai I, Scardoni M, et al. MEN1 in pancreatic endocrine tumors: analysis of gene and protein status in 169 sporadic neoplasms reveals alterations in the vast majority of cases. *Endocr. Relat. Cancer.* 2010 Sep 1;17(3):771–83.

[31] Kasajima A, Yazdani S, Sasano H. Pathology diagnosis of pancreatic neuro-endocrine tumors. *J. Hepato-Biliary-Pancreat Sci.* 2015;22(8):586–93.

[32] Brandi ML, Gagel RF, Angeli A, et al. Guidelines for diagnosis and therapy of MEN type 1 and type 2. *J. Clin. Endocrinol. Metab.* 2001 Dec;86(12):5658–71.

[33] Goudet P, Dalac A, Le Bras M, et al. MEN1 disease occurring before 21 years old: a 160-patient cohort study from the Groupe d'étude des Tumeurs Endocrines. *J. Clin. Endocrinol. Metab.* 2015 Apr;100(4):1568–77.

[34] Lourenço D M, Toledo R A, Mackowiak II, et al. Multiple endocrine neoplasia type 1 in Brazil: MEN1 founding mutation, clinical features, and bone mineral density profile. *Eur. J. Endocrinol.* 2008 Sep;159(3):259–74.

[35] Burgess J R, David R, Greenaway T M, et al. Osteoporosis in multiple endocrine neoplasia type 1: severity, clinical significance, relationship to primary hyper-parathyroidism, and response to parathyroidectomy. *Arch. Surg.* 1999 Oct;134 (10):1119–23.

[36] Buchan A M, Squires P E, Ring M. Mechanism of action of the calcium-sensing receptor in human antral gastrin cells. *Gastroenterology.* 2001 Apr;120(5):1128–39.

[37] Rizzoli R, Green J, Marx S J. Primary hyperparathyroidism in familial multiple endocrine neoplasia type I. Long-term follow-up of serum calcium levels after parathyroidectomy. *Am. J. Med.* 1985 Mar 1;78(3):467–74.

[38] Juhlin C C, Erickson L A. Genomics and epigenomics in parathyroid neoplasia: from bench to surgical pathology practice. *Endocr. Pathol.* 2021 Mar 1;32(1):17–34.

[39] Erickson L A, Mete O. Immunohistochemistry in diagnostic parathyroid pathology. *Endocr. Pathol.* 2018 Jun 1;29(2):113–29.

[40] Carty S E, Helm A K, Amico J A, et al. The variable penetrance and spectrum of manifestations of multiple endocrine neoplasia type 1. *Surgery.* 1998 Dec 1;124 (6):1106–14.

[41] Vergès B, Boureille F, Goudet P, et al. Pituitary disease in MEN type 1 (MEN1): Data from the France-Belgium MEN1 Multicenter Study. *J. Clin. Endocrinol. Metab.* 2002 Feb 1;87(2):457–65.

[42] Ogra S, Nichols A D, Stylli S, et al. Visual acuity and pattern of visual field loss at presentation in pituitary adenoma. *J. Clin. Neurosci.* 2014 May;21(5):735–40.

[43] Russ S, Anastasopoulou C, Shafiq I. Pituitary Adenoma. In: *StatPearls [Internet].* Treasure Island (FL): StatPearls Publishing; 2022 [cited 2022 Aug 12]. Available from: http://www.ncbi.nlm.nih.gov/books/NBK554451/.

[44] Mete O, Asa S L. Clinicopathological correlations in pituitary adenomas. *Brain. Pathol.* 2012 Jul;22(4):443–53.

[45] Al-Brahim N Y Y, Asa SL. My approach to pathology of the pituitary gland. *J. Clin. Pathol.* 2006 Dec;59(12):1245–53.

[46] Larkin S, Ansorge O. Pathology And Pathogenesis Of Pituitary Adenomas And Other Sellar Lesions. In: Feingold KR, Anawalt B, Boyce A, Chrousos G, de Herder WW, Dhatariya K, et al., editors. Endotext [Internet]. South Dartmouth (MA): MDText.com, Inc.; 2000 [cited 2022 Aug 23]. Available from: http://www.ncbi.nlm.nih.gov/books/NBK425704/.

[47] Dean P G, van Heerden J A, Farley D R, et al. Are patients with multiple endocrine neoplasia type I prone to premature death? *World J. Surg.* 2000 Nov;24(11):1437–41.

[48] Hellman P, Skogseid B, Juhlin C, et al. Findings and long-term results of parathyroid surgery in multiple endocrine neoplasia type 1. *World J. Surg.* 1992 Aug;16(4):718–22; discussion 722-723.

[49] Marx SJ, Nieman LK. Aggressive pituitary tumors in MEN1: do they refute the two-hit model of tumorigenesis? *J. Clin. Endocrinol. Metab.* 2002 Feb 1;87(2):453–6.

[50] Varlamov E V, McCartney S, Fleseriu M. Functioning pituitary adenomas – current treatment options and emerging medical therapies. *Eur. Endocrinol.* 2019 Apr;15(1):30–40.

[51] Brandi M L, Agarwal S K, Perrier N D, et al. Multiple endocrine neoplasia type 1: latest insights. *Endocr. Rev.* 2021 Mar 15;42(2):133–70.

[52] Demeure M J, Klonoff D C, Karam J H, et al. Insulinomas associated with multiple endocrine neoplasia type I: the need for a different surgical approach. *Surgery.* 1991 Dec;110(6):998–1004; discussion 1004-1005.

Chapter 22

Noonan Syndrome: Central Nervous System Manifestations

Precious C. Oyem[1], BA
Dhananjay Prakash[2], BS, MS
and Richard A. Prayson[3], MD
[1] Cleveland Clinic Lerner College of Medicine, Cleveland, Ohio, USA
[2] Case Western Reserve University, Cleveland, Ohio, USA
[3] Department of Anatomic Pathology, Cleveland Clinic, Cleveland, Ohio, USA

Abstract

Noonan syndrome is a multisystem disorder that was first fully described by Dr. Jacqueline Noonan. It is a genetic disorder that displays variable expressivity, and it is generally marked by an autosomal dominant pattern of inheritance, except for the LZTR1 variant which is inherited in an autosomal recessive fashion. The molecular pathway most implicated in Noonan syndrome is the RAS/MAPK pathway which plays a role in cell proliferation, differentiation, survival, and metabolism.

Clinical features described in the condition include short stature, congenital heart defects, hematologic abnormalities, musculoskeletal deformities, and neurological problems. A huge fraction of neuropathologic findings in Noonan are low-grade gliomas/glioneuronal tumors; these include pilocytic astrocytomas, pilomyxoid astrocytomas dysembryoplastic neuroepithelial tumors and rosette forming glioneuronal tumors. High grade gliomas are rare but reported cases have included anaplastic astrocytoma and a case of a spinal cord glioblastoma.

The prognosis of these neurological tumors in Noonan syndrome are fairly similar to those arising outside the syndrome. Treatment often involves a multidisciplinary team approach. This chapter will review the

In: Central Nervous System Pathologies in Hereditary Tumor Syndromes
Editor: Richard A. Prayson
ISBN: 979-8-88697-620-5

clinical features of Noonan syndrome, with an emphasis on the central nervous system-associated pathology.

Introduction

Noonan syndrome has a rich history dating back to the late 19th and early 20th centuries throughout which the condition asked head-scratching questions of the medical and scientific communities. During this period, many publications reported male and female patients with interesting clinical features including webbed necks, short stature, low-set ears, micrognathia, and several other craniofacial abnormalities [1]. This flurry of publications was most likely prompted by Kobylinski's writing in 1883 [2], where he described a 20-year-old male who had marked webbing of the neck, a feature that provoked curiosity in the medical and scientific community back then. In 1902, Funke reported a patient with a constellation of symptoms including webbed neck, micrognathia, short stature, and other deformities [3]. Three decades later in 1930, Ullrich reported an 8-year-old female patient with similar symptoms [4] which was then shortly followed by Turner's report on an older female patient with similar facial findings, but even more remarkably, with sexual infantilism [5].

In his editorial, John M. Opitz who worked under Dr. Jacqueline A. Noonan in the Department of Pediatrics at Iowa, described a 7-year-old boy who was a part of a large study for a congenital heart defect with features consistent with the "male Turner syndrome" [6], a term that caused considerable confusion in the literature. It was not until 1959, when Turner syndrome was found to be a chromosomal abnormality with a 45, X chromosome pattern, bringing the realization that the so-called "male Turner syndrome" was a totally different entity as chromosomal findings showed that Turner syndrome could only occur in females. However, due to poor information dissemination at the time, several reports throughout the 1960s and 1970s still continued the use of the term, "male Turner syndrome." As chromosomal studies become more widely available and several attempts at identifying chromosomal abnormalities in patients with the "male turner syndrome" proved unsuccessful, the label began to fade. In fact, many of the female patients who had previously been diagnosed with Turner syndrome were found to have Noonan syndrome after chromosomal studies found they lacked the characteristic 45, X chromosomal abnormality [1].

In 1962, Dr. Noonan presented her work on the condition at the Midwest Society for Pediatric Research [7] and described 9 patients with the aforementioned clinical features and went on to publish her work in 1968 [8]. Dr. Opitz felt that Dr. Noonan was the first to fully describe this phenomenon and proposed that the eponym "Noonan syndrome" be given to this syndrome [9].

The purpose of this chapter is to review the clinical and pathologic features of Noonan syndrome, focusing on the neuropathologic findings that have been described in this syndrome.

Molecular Genetics

Noonan syndrome is a multisystem disorder that is mostly inherited in an autosomal dominant pattern. This condition displays variable expressivity and has an estimated prevalence of 1 in 1,000 to 2,500 people [10]. Over the past two decades, our understanding of the molecular genetics of this syndrome has grown at an exponential rate which has helped inform today's current knowledge of the pathophysiology and mechanisms underlying the multisystem nature of this disease.

The RAS-MAPK signaling pathway is one that has been heavily studied in Noonan syndrome. It plays a role in cell proliferation, differentiation, survival, and metabolism. RAS acts a molecular switch which acts to stimulate consecutive activation of various kinases in the MAPK pathway, ultimately leading to changes in gene transcription. A ligand binds to cell-surface receptors, leading to phosphorylation of the intracellular subunit. This recruits adaptor proteins (GRB2), which forms complexes with guanosine exchange factors (SOS), leading to a conformational change from the inactive RAS-GDP complex to an active RAS-GTP form [11]. This activated complex then activates the RAF-MEK-ERK cascade through a series of phosphorylation events, culminating in an activated ERK translocating to the nucleus and altering gene transcription [12].

Overall, over 20 genes have been described in association with Noonan Syndrome. Eight of these genes are related to the RAS-MAPK pathway and have been implicated in several related conditions. These genes include PTPN11, SOS1, KRAS, NRAS, RAF1, BRAF, SHOC2, and CBL. Chromosomally, this syndrome has been linked to chromosome 12q24.1 [12]. Of note is the PTPN11 gene that encodes the SHP2 protein which plays an important role in several developmental signal transduction pathways.

Generally, PTPN11 mutations are more likely to be familial than other mutations in the syndrome.

While almost all cases of Noonan syndrome are inherited in an autosomal dominant fashion, there have been several reports of autosomal recessive inheritance [13], particularly caused by the biallelic pathogenic LZTR1 variant [14, 15]. However, very few cases of autosomal dominant inheritance have also been reported for this LZTR1 variant [16].

Non-Neurological Clinical Features

Growth and Development

In up to 80% of patients with Noonan syndrome, there is a presence of postnatal proportionate short stature [17]. This is one of the main features of the syndrome and is often used in diagnosis. This pattern of growth is similar in both male and female patients. Prenatally, patients grow at a similar rate and up to a normal length just like patients without the syndrome. However, growth failure becomes more evident during the first few years of life. Patient's bone maturity is usually delayed by 2 years. PTPN11 and RAF1 mutations were associated with more severely impaired growth than other genotypes [18]. This growth abnormalities can be potentially explained by abnormalities of the growth hormone/insulin-like growth factor (IGF) axis particularly with normal or elevated levels of growth hormone and with low levels of IGF-1. Indeed mutant PTPN11 proteins lead to an impairment in the production of IGF-1, through a hyperactivation of the RAS/MAPK pathway [19].

Another feature of Noonan syndrome described in both sexes is the delayed onset of puberty and an associated decreased pubertal growth spurt [20]. In women, fertility issues have not been reported. However, men sometimes experience gonadal dysfunction with deficient spermatogenesis, partly explaining the observed predominant maternal transmission of the condition [17]. Fertility issues in males may be due to cryptorchidism which is seen in up to 80% of Noonan syndrome males [17].

Cardiovascular System

Over 80% of Noonan syndrome patients have cardiovascular abnormalities [21]. The most common cardiac manifestations in Noonan are the presence of pulmonic valve stenosis (25 to 35%), atrial septal defect (6 to 10%), hypertrophic cardiomyopathy (~20%), and ventricular septal defects [22, 23]. Less common cardiac deformities include aortic valve stenosis, bicuspid aortic valve, patent ductus arteriosus, mitral valve abnormalities, tetralogy of Fallot, and aortic coarctation [24]. About half of patients with Noonan syndrome experience abnormal electrocardiographic patterns in the form of left axis deviation, abnormal R/S ratio over the left precordial leads, and an abnormal Q wave [25].

Hematology and Oncology

In Noonan syndrome patients, 30 to 65% of individuals experience bleeding abnormalities [26]. These bleeding abnormalities occur in the form of excessive bruising, epistaxis, or menorrhagia. This has been explained by coagulation factor deficiency, platelet dysfunction, and sometimes, thrombocytopenia. In fact, a quarter of Noonan patients have a partial factor XI deficiency [26]; however, the level of deficiency has not been found to correlate with symptom severity. Low factor VIII and von Willebrand disease has also been described in Noonan syndrome [24]. Splenomegaly is a common ultrasound finding in up to 52% of patients. This, occasionally combined with hepatomegaly, has been described in the setting of a myeloproliferative disorder, a condition usually seen in infants with monocytosis and thrombocytopenia. A very small minority of these patients go on to develop leukemia [27].

Musculoskeletal System

Noonan syndrome patients often experience various musculoskeletal deformities. Chest deformities, particularly pectus excavatum and pectus carinatum, are perhaps the most common, occurring in 70 to 95% of cases [28]. This is often accompanied by cubitus valgus, genu valgum, and wide-spaced nipples. Spinal defects in the form of scoliosis occur in 10% of patients, as well as other less common deformities such as kyphosis, spina bifida, and other vertebral and spinal abnormalities. Bone mineral density is overall lower in children with the syndrome, but this has not correlated with any significant clinical outcome.

Other Abnormalities

Noonan syndrome also exhibits other various forms of abnormalities. Of note is that patients often have orodental features such as a high-arched palate, micrognathia, and dental malocclusion [11]. Additionally, lymphatic problems are common in the form of lymphedema that usually presents in the early period of life, and in more extreme cases, hydrops fetalis, hypoplastic inguinal and iliac vessels, and rarely, a malformed thoracic duct [24]. Vision and hearing abnormalities are present in a majority of Noonan syndrome patients, with hearing problems less frequent than ocular issues [20].

Neurological Clinical Features

Overall, the neurological features of Noonan syndrome are poorly understood. Most patients with the syndrome have normal levels of intelligence with intelligence quotient scores largely in the normal range. However, it has been found that even among patients with normal intelligence, their quotient score has been shown to be about 10 points less than an unaffected family member or 1 standard deviation below the general population [29]. Sharland et al., described a cohort of 151 patients, and found that 13% had recurrent seizures, 3% had peripheral neuropathy, and that there was delayed motor development with sitting, walking, and speaking 2-word sentences [20]. Cases of subarachnoid hemorrhage have also been reported. Several patients have been found to have spinal problems including myelomeningocele with recurrent tethered cords, spina bifida occulta, and syringomyelia [30]. A highlight of note is that Noonan syndrome is often associated with Neurofibromatosis, often referred to as Neurofibromatosis-Noonan Syndrome (NF-NS). These patients often have features consistent with the type 1 portion of Neurofibromatosis. In these group of patients, there is an association with optic gliomas, medulloblastomas, and malignant as well as benign schwannomas [30].

Psychiatric cases have been reported in patients with Noonan syndrome. Specific behavioral profiles highlighted in this patient population include stubbornness, clumsiness, mood dysregulation, communication difficulties, and faddy eating [31].

Neuropathology

In general, RASopathies have been heavily linked to various central nervous system tumors. Particularly, glial tumors are a common culprit. In Noonan syndrome, most CNS tumors in Noonan are associated with the PTPN11 mutation. In the medical literature, most published cases of brain tumors in patients with Noonan syndrome were low-grade gliomas and glioneuronal tumors [32]. A huge fraction of these low-grade gliomas/glioneuronal tumors were dysembryoplastic neuroepithelial tumors (DNETs). A case series described by Siegfried et. al. showed that the presence of DNETs in Noonan is non-coincidental [33]. While rare and have a prevalence of < 1% in the overall general population, they account for about 40% of brain tumors reported in the syndrome [34]. Microscopy of these DNETs often show a cortical based, multinodular neoplasm marked by a proliferation of rounded oligodendroglial-like cells with intermixed normal appearing neuronal cells. Findings described on immunohistochemistry include positive nuclear staining with Olig2 and pERK in the rounded cells [33].

An "oligoastrocytoma" has also been described in a 22-year-old with Noonan syndrome, in the setting of the autosomal dominant and recessive LZTR1 mutation [35]. In this patient, hematoxylin and eosin staining revealed an astrocytoma component with a gemistocytic pattern, as well as an oligodendrocyte component with the characteristic nuclear roundness and perinuclear halo. On immunochemistry in this patient, there was partial loss of ATRX expression in the astrocytoma component and presence of IDH-1 expression in both the astrocytoma and oligodendrocyte component. The tumor showed a chromosome 19q13 deletion but no evidence of a 1p36 deletion on fluorescent in situ hybridization testing. This same patient experienced recurrence at age 26 years, with the tumor then resembling a glioblastoma. There was diffuse cytoplasmic and nuclear IDH-1 expression, and diffuse loss of ATRX expression.

Interestingly, there has been a report of a spinal cord glioblastoma in a patient with Noonan syndrome [36]. This is particularly noteworthy as almost all the cases of central nervous system tumors in Noonan syndrome reported in the medical literature are located intracranially. Another central nervous system tumor that has been found in patients with Noonan syndrome is pilocytic astrocytoma [37, 38] (Figures 1 and 2).

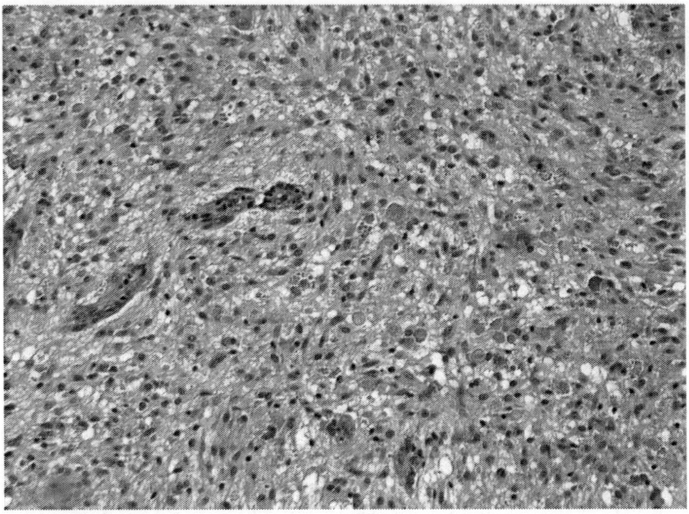

Figure 1. A pilocytic astrocytoma arising in a patient with Noonan syndrome and marked by eosinophilic granular bodies (hematoxylin and eosin, original magnification 200X).

Pilomyxoid astrocytomas, which are a WHO grade 2 neoplasms, are a more recently identified variant of astrocytoma and this has been found involving the optic pathway in a 14-year-old Noonan syndrome patient [39]. Histopathology of the tumor demonstrated a uniform population of tumor cells in a background of microcytic changes and focal perivascular accumulation of tumor cells (Figure 3).

High grade gliomas are a rare occurrence in Noonan syndrome. However, there have been a small handful of cases reported on high grade gliomas in the form of anaplastic astrocytomas [38]. Malignant intracerebral nerve sheath tumors have also been described in Noonan syndrome [40]. Finally, an interesting case of a rosette forming glioneuronal tumor has also been reported in an 18-year-old with Noonan syndrome [41]. These tumors are marked by perivascular pseudorosette-like structures (Figure 4). On immunohistochemistry, this tumor demonstrated strong pERK immunoreactivity which is suggestive of activation of the MAPK/ERK pathway.

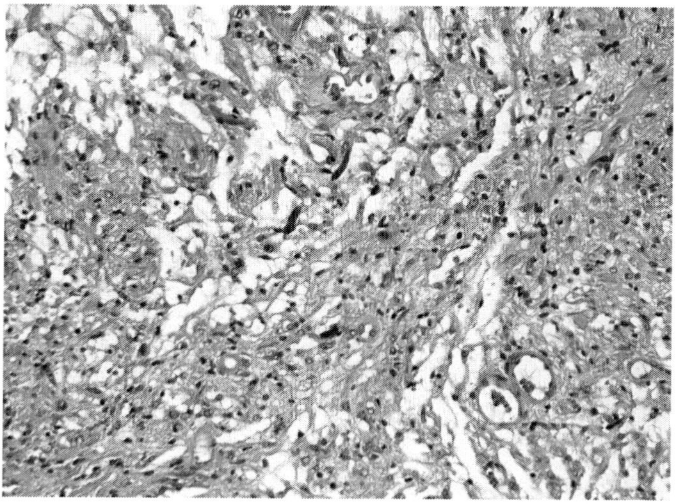

Figure 2. This is the same tumor as in Figure 1. The tumor also showed rare eosinophilic Rosenthal fibers (hematoxylin and eosin, original magnification 200X).

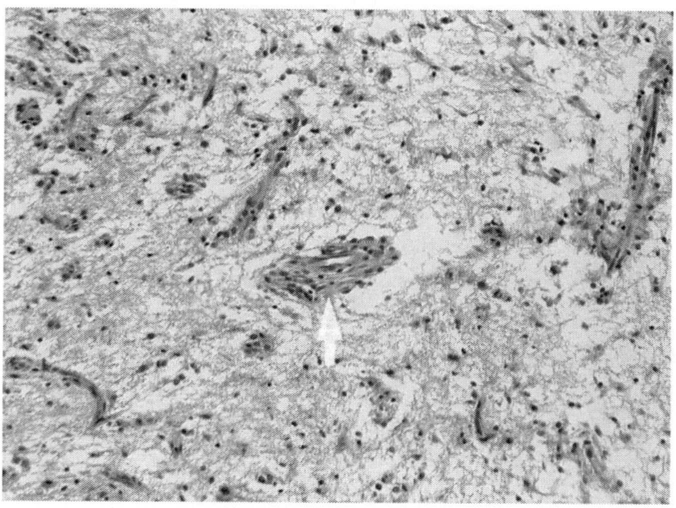

Figure 3. A pilomyxoid astrocytoma marked by a monomorphic proliferation of bipolar fibrillar cells with an angiocentric growth pattern (arrow) (hematoxylin and eosin, original magnification 200X).

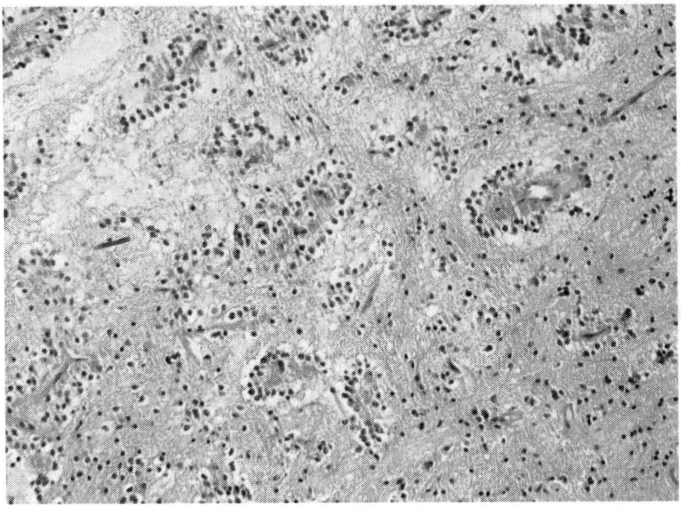

Figure 4. A rosette forming glioneuronal tumor marked by the presence of perivascular pseudorosette-like structures (hematoxylin and eosin, original magnification 200X).

Treatment and Prognosis

The treatment of patients with Noonan syndrome usually involves a multidisciplinary team comprising of various specialists which may include a clinical geneticist, a pediatrician, an endocrinologist, a cardiologist, a neurologist, and sometimes, a neurosurgeon. Because the RAS/MAPK pathway is implicated, some of the strategies for treatment and in development are aimed at decreasing the activity of this pathway. An example of an agent being considered for targeting the RAS/MAPK pathway are 3-hydroxy-3-methylglutaryl CoA reductase inhibitors, also known as 'statins,' which work to decrease RAS activity by reducing its translocation to the plasma membrane [17]. However, these studies have mostly been tested in mouse models of Noonan syndrome. Overall, most of the treatment in this condition is symptomatic including hormone supplementation and regular follow-up [11]. Of note is the use of growth hormone supplementation which is an integral part of management in these patients as almost all patients with the syndrome exhibit short stature. Studies have supported this therapy as it has demonstrated an improvement in growth velocity with a negligible rate of adverse events [42].

Patients with neurological tumors are treated at the discretion of the neurosurgical care team. Central nervous system tumors in the setting of Noonan syndrome are generally treated similarly to their sporadic counterparts. Patients with high grade neoplasms such as malignant intracerebral nerve sheath tumors are often treated surgically with resection [40]. Patients with tumors involving the optic pathways are often treated surgically as well. Biopsy of optic-related tumors is usually not encouraged, unless prompted by suggestive atypical features on imaging that would help guide therapy [43]. However, significant morbidity and complications are not usually encountered with resection or biopsy of these optic pathway tumors with modern surgical techniques. Patients often experience good long-term survival and functional outcomes [44].

Data on long-term outcomes in Noonan syndrome is scarce in the medical literature. However, Shaw et. al. evaluated 112 British patients and found that the mortality rate in a mean follow-up period of 12 years was 9%, with a very wide range of age of death [45].

Conclusion

Noonan syndrome may demonstrate either an autosomal dominant (in the majority of cases) or rarely autosomal recessive (in the case of the LZTR1 variant) pattern of inheritance. Over twenty affected genes have been implicated in the pathogenesis of the syndrome, eight of which are related to the RAS-MAPK pathway. Neuropathologic findings in Noonan syndrome have included low grade glial/glioneuronal tumors including pilocytic astrocytoma, pilomyxoid astrocytoma and rosette forming glioneuronal tumor. Rare cases of high grade gliomas, including WHO grade 3 and 4 astrocytomas, have also been encountered in this clinical setting.

References

[1] Noonan J A. Noonan syndrome. An update and review for the primary pediatrician. *Clin. Pediatr.* 1994 Sep;33(9):548–55.

[2] Kobylinski O. Über eine flughautähnliche Ausbreitung am Halse [*About a wing skin-like spread on the neck*]. *Arch. Anthropol.* 1883;(14:342–348).

[3] Funke O. Pterygium colli [*Pterygium of the neck*]. *Dtsch Zeitschr Chir.* 1902;(63):163–7.

[4] Ullrich O. Über typische Kombinationsbilder multipler Abartungen [*About typical combination pictures of multiple varieties*]. *Z. Kinderheilkd.* 1930;(49):271–6.

[5] Turner H H. A syndrome of infantilism, congenital webbed neck, and cubitus valgus. *Endocrinology.* 1938;(25):566–74.

[6] Flavell G. Webbing of the neck, with Turner's syndrome in the male. *Brit. J. Surg.* 1943 Oct 1;31(122):150–3.

[7] Noonan J, Ehmke D. Associated noncardiac malformations in children with congenital heart disease. *J. Pediatr.* 1963;(31):150–3.

[8] Noonan J A. Hypertelorism With Turner phenotype: a new syndrome with associated congenital heart disease. *Am. J. Dis. Child.* 1968 Oct 1;116(4):373–80.

[9] Opitz J M. The Noonan syndrome. *Am. J. Med. Genet.* 1985 Jul;21(3):515–8.

[10] Mendez H M, Opitz J M. Noonan syndrome: a review. *Am. J. Med. Genet.* 1985 Jul;21(3):493–506.

[11] Carcavilla A, Suárez-Ortega L, Sánchez A R, et al. Noonan syndrome: genetic and clinical update and treatment options. *Anales de Pediatría* (English Edition). 2020 Jul 1;93(1):61.e1-61.e14.

[12] Roberts A E, Allanson J E, Tartaglia M, et al. Noonan syndrome. *Lancet.* 2013 Jan 26;381(9863):333–42.

[13] van Der Burgt I, Brunner H. Genetic heterogeneity in Noonan syndrome: evidence for an autosomal recessive form. *Am. J. Med. Genet.* 2000 Sep 4;94(1):46–51.

[14] Johnston J J, van der Smagt J J, Rosenfeld J A, et al. Autosomal recessive Noonan syndrome associated with biallelic LZTR1variants. *Genet. Med.* 2018 Oct;20(10): 1175–85.

[15] Perin F, Trujillo-Quintero J P, Jimenez-Jaimez J, et al. Two novel cases of autosomal recessive Noonan syndrome associated with LZTR1 variants. *Rev. Esp. Cardiol.* (English Edition). 2019 Nov;72(11):978–80.

[16] Yamamoto G L, Aguena M, Gos M, et al. Rare variants in SOS2 and LZTR1 are associated with Noonan syndrome. *J. Med. Genet.* 2015 Jun;52(6):413–21.

[17] Yart A, Edouard T. Noonan syndrome: an update on growth and development. *Curr. Opin. Endocrinol. Diabetes Obes.* 2018 Feb;25(1):67–73.

[18] Malaquias A C, Brasil A S, Pereira A C, et al. Growth standards of patients with Noonan and Noonan-like syndromes with mutations in the RAS/MAPK pathway. *Am. J. Med. Genet. A.* 2012 Nov;158A(11):2700–6.

[19] Binder G, Neuer K, Ranke M B, Wittekindt N E. PTPN11 mutations are associated with mild growth hormone resistance in individuals with Noonan syndrome. *J. Clin. Endocrinol. Metab.* 2005 Sep;90(9):5377–81.

[20] Sharland M, Burch M, McKenna W M, Paton M A. A clinical study of Noonan syndrome. *Arch. Dis. Child.* 1992 Feb;67(2):178–83.

[21] Burch M, Sharland M, Shinebourne E, et al. Cardiologic abnormalities in Noonan syndrome: phenotypic diagnosis and echocardiographic assessment of 118 patients. *J. Am. Coll. Cardiol.* 1993 Oct;22(4):1189–92.

[22] Ezquieta B, Santomé J L, Carcavilla A, et al. Alterations in RAS-MAPK genes in 200 Spanish patients with Noonan and other neuro-cardio-facio-cutaneous syndromes. Genotype and cardiopathy. *Rev. Esp. Cardiol.* (English Edition). 2012 May;65(5):447–55.

[23] Sznajer Y, Keren B, Baumann C, et al. The spectrum of cardiac anomalies in Noonan syndrome as a result of mutations in the PTPN11 gene. *Pediatrics.* 2007 Jun;119 (6):e1325-1331.
[24] Romano A A, Allanson J E, Dahlgren J, et al. Noonan syndrome: clinical features, diagnosis, and management guidelines. *Pediatrics.* 2010 Oct 1;126(4):746–59.
[25] Raaijmakers R, Noordam C, Noonan J A, et al. Are ECG abnormalities in Noonan syndrome characteristic for the syndrome? *Eur. J. Pediatr.* 2008 Dec;167(12):1363–7.
[26] Witt D R, McGillivray B C, Allanson J E, et al. Bleeding diathesis in Noonan syndrome: a common association. *Am. J. Med. Genet.* 1988 Oct;31(2):305–17.
[27] Kratz C P, Niemeyer C M, Castleberry R P, et al. The mutational spectrum of PTPN11 in juvenile myelomonocytic leukemia and Noonan syndrome/myeloproliferative disease. *Blood.* 2005 Sep 15;106(6):2183–5.
[28] Allanson J E. Noonan syndrome. *J. Med. Genet.* 1987 Jan;24(1):9–13.
[29] van der Burgt I, Thoonen G, Roosenboom N, et al. Patterns of cognitive functioning in school-aged children with Noonan syndrome associated with variability in phenotypic expression. *J. Pediatr.* 1999 Dec;135(6):707–13.
[30] Noonan J. Noonan syndrome. *Clin. Pediatr.* 1994;33(9):548–55.
[31] Wood A, Massarano A, Super M, et al. Behavioural aspects and psychiatric findings in Noonan's syndrome. *Arch. Dis. Child.* 1995 Feb;72(2):153–5.
[32] Lodi M, Boccuto L, Carai A, et al. Low-grade gliomas in patients with Noonan syndrome: case-based review of the literature. *Diagnostics.* 2020 Aug 12;10(8): E582.
[33] Siegfried A, Cances C, Denuelle M, et al. Noonan syndrome, PTPN11 mutations, and brain tumors. A clinical report and review of the literature. *Am. J. Med. Genet A.* 2017 Apr;173(4):1061–5.
[34] Rickert C H, Paulus W. Epidemiology of central nervous system tumors in childhood and adolescence based on the new WHO classification. *Childs Nerv. Syst.* 2001 Sep;17(9):503–11.
[35] Jacquinet A, Bonnard A, Capri Y, et al. Oligo-astrocytoma in LZTR1-related Noonan syndrome. *Eur. J. Med. Genet.* 2020 Jan;63(1):103617.
[36] Khan A, Soliman M A R, Ghannam M M, et al. Spinal cord glioblastoma multiforme in a patient with Noonan syndrome: A clinical report. *Clin. Neurol. Neurosurg.* 2021 Aug;207:106725.
[37] Schuettpelz LG, McDonald S, Whitesell K, et al. Pilocytic astrocytoma in a child with Noonan syndrome. *Pediatr. Blood Cancer.* 2009 Dec;53(6):1147–9.
[38] El-Ayadi M, Ansari M, Kühnöl C D, Bendel A, et al. Occurrence of high-grade glioma in Noonan syndrome: Report of two cases. *Pediatr. Blood Cancer.* 2019 May;66(5):e27625.
[39] Nair S, Fort J A, Yachnis A T, et al. Optic nerve pilomyxoid astrocytoma in a patient with Noonan syndrome. *Pediatr. Blood Cancer.* 2015 Jun;62(6):1084–6.
[40] Allison C M, Shumon S, Joshi A, et al. Malignant intracerebral nerve sheath tumor in a patient with Noonan syndrome: illustrative case. *J. Neurosurg. Case Lessons.* 2021 Jun 28;1(26):CASE21146.

[41] Karafin M, Jallo G I, Ayars M, et al. Rosette forming glioneuronal tumor in association with Noonan syndrome: pathobiological implications. *Clin. Neuropathol.* 2011 Dec;30(6):297–300.
[42] Ogawa M, Moriya N, Ikeda H, et al. Clinical evaluation of recombinant human growth hormone in Noonan syndrome. *Endocr. J.* 2004 Feb;51(1):61–8.
[43] Gnekow A K, Kandels D, Tilburg C van, et al. SIOP-E-BTG and GPOH guidelines for diagnosis and treatment of children and adolescents with low grade glioma. *Klin. Padiatr.* 2019 May;231(3):107–35.
[44] Goodden J, Pizer B, Pettorini B, et al. The role of surgery in optic pathway/ hypothalamic gliomas in children. *J. Neurosurg. Pediatr.* 2014 Jan;13(1):1–12.
[45] Shaw A C, Kalidas K, Crosby A H, et al. The natural history of Noonan syndrome: a long-term follow-up study. *Arch. Dis. Child.* 2007 Feb;92 (2):128–32.

Chapter 23

Neuropathologic Findings in L-2-Hydroxyglutaric Aciduria

Christel M. Kinkopf[1]
and Richard A. Prayson[2,*]**, MD**

[1] Ohio Heritage College of Osteopathic Medicine, Warrensville Heights, OH, USA
[2] Department of Anatomic Pathology, Cleveland Clinic, Cleveland, Ohio, USA

Abstract

L-2-hydroxyglutaric aciduria is a rare autosomal recessive inborn error of metabolism caused by a homozygous or compound heterozygous mutation in the L-2-hydroxyglutarate dehydrogenase (L2HDGH) gene located on chromosome 14q22.1. This disease is associated with elevated L-2-hydroxyglutaric acid levels in the urine, cerebrospinal fluid, and plasma. Patients with this disorder often present early in life with neurologic signs and symptoms including hypotonia, tremors, intellectual disability, macrocephaly, choreodystonia, and seizures. Disease course is slowly progressive, and patients rarely present with acute metabolic disturbances.

Neuroimaging studies demonstrate a distinctive pattern on magnetic resonance imaging T2/FLAIR; abnormalities present as bilateral and symmetric subcortical leukoencephalopathy, atrophy of the cerebellum and signal changes in the putaminal and dentate nuclei. A number of patients have been reported to develop a variety of central nervous tumors in this setting including astrocytomas (low and high grade), anaplastic ependymomas, and medulloblastomas.

This chapter will review the neuropathologic findings described in the setting of this rare metabolic disorder.

---

* Corresponding Author's Email: praysor@ccf.org.

In: Central Nervous System Pathologies in Hereditary Tumor Syndromes
Editor: Richard A. Prayson
ISBN: 979-8-88697-620-5

Introduction

L-2-hydroxyglutaric aciduria is a rare neurometabolic disorder that was first described in 1980 by Duran and colleagues [1]. Duran et al. reported a case of a 5-year-old Moroccan male who presented with psychomotor retardation and dystrophy. It was found that this patient was excreting large amounts of 2-hydroxyglutaric acid in his urine. The authors suspected he suffered from a genetic disorder. Subsequently, similarly elevated urine levels of L-2-hydroxyglutaric acid were documented in seven patients from five families who all demonstrated intellectual disability [2, 3].

The disorder was more formally characterized in 1992 by Barth et al. in a study of eight patients with intellectual disability, from five unrelated families, including three pairs of siblings [4]. Since the initial discovery, only a few hundred cases have been documented in the literature, with even fewer describing neuropathologic findings. This chapter will review the genetics, clinical and neuropathological features of this rare autosomal recessive organic aciduria.

Genetics

A major breakthrough occurred in 2004 when Topçu and colleagues used homozygosity mapping to identify the mutant gene, L2HGDH (C14orf160), responsible for L-2-hydroxyglutaric aciduria [5, 6]. Localized on chromosome 14q22.1, the L2HGDH gene encodes for L-2-hydroxyglutarate dehydrogenase, a FAD-dependent mitochondrial bound metabolite repair enzyme that oxidizes L-2-hydroxyglutarate to α-ketoglutarate [5-8].

Formed via promiscuous (unwanted) malic dehydrogenase reduction of α-ketoglutarate, L-2-hydroxyglutarate (L-2-HG) is considered a damaged metabolite [8, 9]. Over 80 types of novel mutations in the L2HGDH gene have been identified, including missense and frameshift mutations, which occur in an autosomal recessive manner [10]. These mutations lead to defects in the metabolite repair enzyme L2HGDH and buildup of L-2-hydroxyglutarate which has deleterious and oncogenic potential with a predilection for the central nervous system [9, 11, 12].

General Clinical Features and Diagnosis

L-2-hydroxyglutaric aciduria mainly impacts the central nervous system, resulting in chiefly neurological manifestations. Patients that present with early unexplained progressive neurological symptoms of unknown origin should raise concern for an inborn error of metabolism on differential diagnosis. A high degree of clinical suspicion is needed to detect L-2-hydroxyglutaric aciduria; diagnosis is accomplished using genetic analysis, neuroimaging, or examination of bodily fluids. Elevated levels of L-2-hydroxyglutaric acid can be found in urine, cerebrospinal fluid, and to a lesser extent plasma [10, 13]. Although the constellation of neuroimaging findings on computed tomography (CT) and magnetic resonance imaging (MRI) are distinct from other leukoencephalopathies, diagnosis is generally confirmed through either investigation of L2HGD gene mutation or urinary organic acid screening [4, 10, 14]. There exists a small subset of patients whose initial presentation deviates from the norm, with diagnosis of L-2-HGA only occurring after radiological work up for a brain neoplasm. These patients are subsequently diagnosed after a metabolic work-up [15].

2-hydroxyglutaric acid consists of two stereoisomers, L- and D-, each producing a clinically unique disorder that must be differentiated upon testing [4, 16]. Urine in patients with suspected L-2-hydroxyglutaric aciduria is analyzed using gas chromatography-mass spectrometry (GCMS) and chiral differentiation to check for elevated levels of the L-stereoisomer [4, 13]. Urinary levels of L-2-hydroxyglutaric acid are universally elevated in patients with L-2-hydroxyglutaric aciduria, with ranges of 350 to 3,357 μmol/mmol creatinine reported in affected patients [10]. Reported reference ranges in unaffected patients have been reported as 1.3 to 18.9 μmol/mmol creatinine, though sample size was limited [17].

Neurologic Clinical Features

Patients with L-2-hhydroxyglutaric aciduria experience variable degrees of neurologic manifestations including variable pyramidal and extrapyramidal signs, cerebellar dysfunction, seizures, hypotonia, headaches, pseudobulbar signs, behavioral disturbances, loss of milestones, and developmental delay [10, 13, 18, 19]. Progressive macrocephaly is a common physical manifestation that occurs in a significant number of case reports [10, 16]. Early in the disease course, mild psychomotor delay, hypotonia, and seizures were the most common initial presenting symptoms [10]. Seizures are reported as epileptic and febrile in nature [16, 20]. With increasing disease duration, hypotonia was largely replaced with spasticity in a large subset of patients [13]. With sufficient time, nearly all patients develop progressive intellectual disability, increased seizure severity, and cerebellar symptoms such as ataxia and tremor [10, 13, 16]. Progressive neurologic deterioration leads to severe motor impairment, requiring assistance with mobility [20]. Loss of milestones was reported in roughly a quarter of patients, coupled with psychobehavioral disturbances, leading to difficulty in both social and academic environments [13, 14].

Although onset typically occurs within the first year of life, the disease course is generally insidious, slowly progressive, and diagnosis is often delayed, as symptoms may be initially mild and nonspecific [10, 14, 20]. Phenotypic variation may play a role in diagnostic delay. Those with milder phenotypes may go undetected into adulthood; however, numerous L2HGDH mutation types coupled with small sample size has made studying this correlation difficult [10, 18]. In a subset of patients with L2HGA, whose clinical course was found to deviate from the usual progression and experienced a rapid clinical decline, brain neoplasm rather than an acute neurometabolic disturbance was believed to be the cause [10, 13].

Imaging

Neuroimaging of L-2-hydroxyglutaric aciduria produces a distinctive pattern of hyperintense MRI signal abnormalities on T2/FLAIR involving both the gray and white matter. The primary areas involved include subcortical cerebral white matter, dentate nuclei, caudate nuclei, globus pallidus, and the putamen [14, 21, 22]. Imaging changes present in early childhood and may initially appear multifocal in the subcortical white matter. As the disease progresses, subcortical white matter abnormalities spread in a centripetal manner with increasing intensity and confluence on imaging [15, 22]. Both cerebral and cerebellar atrophy may be noted in advanced disease, with the later demonstrating particular involvement of the vermis [4, 14, 15]. Involvement of the gray matter nuclei appear bilateral and symmetric throughout the disease course [15]. Several case reports have indicated that periventricular white matter and brainstem tend to be spared regardless of disease progression; however, there appears to be a discordance in the literature over involvement [14, 18, 21, 22].

Literature review reveals a limited number of case studies that included CT imaging findings. CT imaging of patients from two case studies with L-2-hydroxyglutaric aciduria demonstrated diffuse bilateral hypodensities in subcortical white matter and generalized atrophy of the cerebral hemispheres [18, 21]. White matter located in the deep periventricular area was spared on non-contrast CT imaging [21]. There is little evidence within the literature to correlate severity of abnormalities seen on imaging to clinical presentation and outcomes [23].

Neuropathologic Features

Neuropathological reports of L-2-hydroxyglutaric aciduria are rare and limited in their descriptions within the literature; among the few hundred cases reported, only a few detailed comprehensive postmortem neuropathological changes [9, 18]. Although each report differs slightly in their neuropathological findings, the unifying pathology appreciated in adolescence and adulthood is symmetric demyelination and spongiosis affecting the subcortical regions, and to a lesser extent the cerebellum and basal ganglia [18, 19].

Larnaout et al. was the first to describe such changes in a 30-year-old male with family history of L-2-hydroxyglutaric aciduria and progressively worsening neurological status who became comatose and died after an unexplained fever [9, 19]. Postmortem examination revealed the brain to be slightly underweight with subcortical necrotic foci in all lobes with dilation of the lateral and third ventricles. Extensive damage to the cerebral white matter was noted with diffuse bilateral demyelination, cystic cavitations, and spongiosis occurring primarily in the subcortical regions and cortical convolutions. Cavitations were surrounded by prominent gliosis in the cerebral white matter and were found to be either empty or containing fibrillar material and small blood vessels. Moderate basal ganglia atrophy was present, with pronounced cell loss, spongiosis, and slight astrocytic proliferation present in the globus pallidus. While the striatum was less severely affected, both the striatum and the globus pallidus contained pallor of the myelin fibers. Loss of granular neurons and Purkinje cells were reported in the cerebellum, with notable cell loss and spongiosis in the dentate nucleus. Upon staining with oil red o, toluidine blue, and acid cresyl violet, no abnormal neuronal or glial storage defects were detected [19]. This report remains one of the most thorough neuropathological reports on L-2-hydroxyglutaric aciduria to date.

The neuropathological postmortem analysis from Seijo-Martinez et al. on a 15-year-old male with L-2-hydroxyglutaric aciduria showed diffuse symmetric cerebral white matter demyelination, spongiosis, and cystic cavitations within the subcortical area. A small amount of subcortical neuronal loss was present and staining with glial fibrillary acidic protein (GFAP) revealed prominent gliosis [18]. Although these findings were similar to Larnaout et al., certain notable differences in the cerebellum, basal ganglia, and ventricles are worth mentioning. Neuronal loss was minimal in the cerebellum, with only slight widening of the sulci reported. Changes in the basal ganglia were less profound, with patchy gliosis and spongiosis noted in the basal nuclei near the internal capsule. The dentate nucleus demonstrated minimal neuronal loss, peripheral spongiosis, and vacuolation. Finally, there was an absence of ventricular dilatation upon examination; however, gliosis and spongiosis of the periaqueductal white matter of the fourth ventricle were present [18, 19].

L2HGA has traditionally been described as a slowly progressive neurodegenerative disease that results from accumulated insult of L-2-HGA in the central nervous system over the lifespan and reports of sudden death associated with this disease are rare [10]. Two case reports of sudden death associated with L-2-HGA were found in the literature, an 11-month-old and 28-day-old, which detailed neuropathological changes in postmortem examination [23, 24]. These two reports represent a unique look into the early neuropathologic changes in this disease course.

Gygax et al. reported a case of L-2-HGA associated with sudden death in an 11-month-old female [23]. The previously health patient presented at 10 months with three successive episodes of unresponsiveness followed by what appeared to be post ictal episodes. One week later, the patient developed a fever and diarrhea and died in her sleep 48 hours later without reported signs of distress. Postmortem examination found no signs of trauma, malignancy, infection, or gross malformation. In contrast to the previous neuropathologic findings in the adult and adolescent reports, no evidence of ventricular enlargement, demyelination, or neuronal loss was present. Bilateral vacuolation and spongiosis in the subcortical white matter, putamen, and dentate nuclei was noted. Staining with GFAP revealed significant astrogliosis accompanied by spongiosis in affected areas [23]. It is unclear if this patient died as a result of complications from L-2-HGA or another unknown disease process.

Chen et al. reported the youngest neuropathological report to date of L-2-HGA associated with sudden death in a 28-day old female [24]. The infant, delivered at term, presented with hypotonia and poor respiratory effort that progressed to ventilator dependence. Seizures and lack of several primitive reflexes were noted. Support was withdrawn on day 27 and the patient died on day 28. Postmortem examination found no evidence of subcortical demyelination, vacuolation or spongiosis. Staining with GFAP showed mild diffuse astrogliosis in the cerebrum. Neuronal loss, atrophy, and astrogliosis was noted in the brainstem and cerebellum with particular prominence in the pontine, dentate, and inferior olivary nuclei. Sporadic reactive astrocytes without neuronal drop out were present in Sommer's sector and focal Purkinje cell dropout was found in the cerebellum, concerning for anoxic injury [24].

Differential diagnoses to consider when presented with a patient with the above-mentioned clinical, neuropathological, and imaging findings include but are not limited to other organic acidurias such as D-2-hydroxyglurac acid (D-2-HGA), Canavan disease, and Kearns-Sayre syndrome [18, 21]. D-2-HGA may present similarly to L-2-HGA; chiral differentiation with GCSM is needed for diagnosis [4]. Canavan disease is a spongiform leukodystrophy that shares many similar clinical features with L-2-HGA; however, clinical progression is usually more rapid in Canavan disease [18]. L-2-HGA, Canavan disease, and Kearns-Sayre syndrome all produce abnormalities on imaging in the bilateral subcortical white matter and globus pallidus. In contrast to L-2-HGA, Canavan disease often spares the caudate nucleus and putamen while Kearns-Sayre syndrome often involves the brainstem and thalamus, two structures that are relatively spared in L-2-HGA [21].

CNS Tumor Potential

A growing body of evidence suggests that patients with L-2-hydroxyglutaric aciduria have an increased risk of developing malignant brain tumors, including low and high grade astrocytomas, anaplastic ependymomas, and medulloblastomas [15, 16, 25, 26]. While the exact prevalence is currently unknown, a meta-analysis by Patay et al. suggested a prevalence of between 5 and 40% [15]. The mechanism behind this increase in tumorigenic potential is due to progressive exposure of the central nervous system to increased levels of L-2-hydroxyglutarate over the lifespan [15, 26]. Further evidence for the oncogenic potential of 2-hydroxyglutarate is supported by research on the association between the isocitrate dehydrogenase (IDH-1) enzyme mutation and gliomas [11].

Mutations in IDH-1 and L2HGDH produce unique 2-hydroxyglutarate isomers, D- and L- respectively. Both have been implicated in driving tumorigenesis within the CNS [15]. IDH-1 is an enzyme that catalyzes the formation of α-ketoglutarate from isocitrate. Mutations in this enzyme lead to the inability to convert isocitrate to α-ketoglutarate, resulting in an alternative pathway that reduces α-ketoglutarate to 2-hydroxyglutarate, specifically the D- stereoisomer [11, 26]. Recent advances in sequencing have shown that 80% of grade 2/3 gliomas and secondary glioblastomas contain an IDH-1 mutation [15, 26]. Drastically increased levels of D-2-hydroxyglutarate in the central nervous system has been reported in gliomas that contain an IDH-1 mutation [15]. 2-hydroxyglutarate is associated with increased oxidative stress, alterations in glioma metabolism, differentiation of native T cells, and interference in gene expression, which may collectively promote carcinogenesis [12, 27].

The previous mentioned tumor types that have been described as arising in this clinical setting resemble morphologically similar tumors that arise outside this setting (Figures 1 and 2).

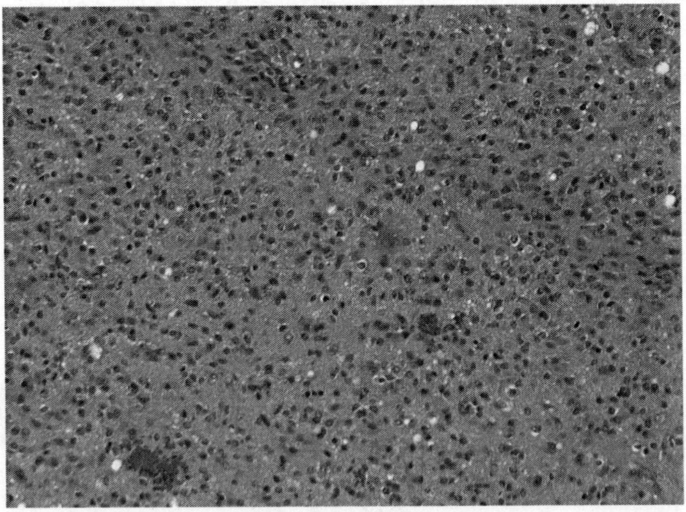

Figure 1. An 8-year-old with an IDH-1 mutated, infiltrating glioma marked by mild to moderate hypercellularity and increased mitotic activity. There was no evidence of vascular proliferation or necrosis. The tumor morphologically was consistent with an astrocytoma, WHO grade 3 (hematoxylin and eosin, original magnification 200X).

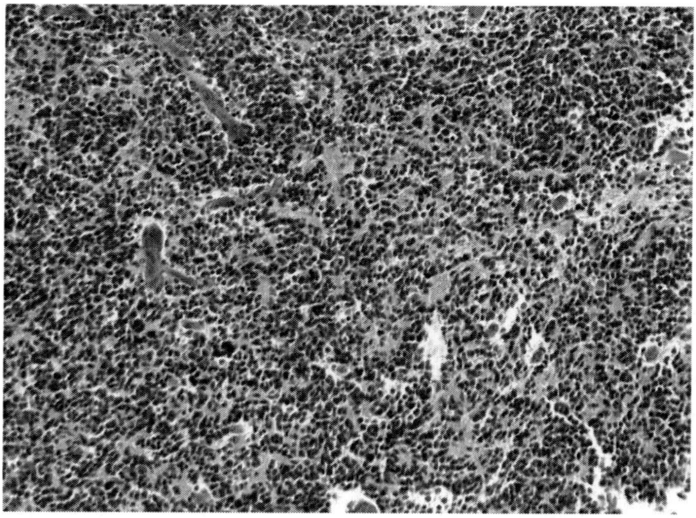

Figure 2. A cerebellar mass in a 3-year-old marked by prominent cellularity and rare Homer Wright pseudorosettes (arrow), consistent with a classic type medulloblastoma, WHO grade 4 (hematoxylin and eosin, original magnification 200X).

Treatment and Prognosis

There currently exists no specific cure for L-2-hydroxyglutaric aciduria. Due to phenotypic variability, clinical presentation may vary among patients and treatment remains largely supportive, tailored to individual symptom management [13, 18, 20]. Although over half of patients develop epilepsy during the disease course, most are generally well controlled with antiepileptic medications; however, this does not slow disease progression [10, 13, 20].

It is theorized that due to L-2-hydroxyglutarate dehydrogenases use of flavin adenine dinucleotide (FAD) as a cofactor, treatment with riboflavin, an essential component of FAD might yield therapeutic effects. There have been a handful of case reports that have investigated the use of riboflavin in patients with L-2-hydroxyglutaric aciduria with varying degrees of success [22, 28, 29]. It is noteworthy to mention that the literature suggests the severity of L2HGDH mutation may impact clinical response, those with milder mutations may have positive clinical responses to riboflavin treatment, whereas severe mutations may be unresponsive [13]. Further research is needed to elucidate these findings.

Prognosis of patients with L-2-hydroxyglutaric aciduria varies, though in general it is poor due to its chronic progressive nature [21, 20]. The suggested increased risk associated with developing malignant brain tumors ranges from 5 to 40% [15]. As the disease course progresses and exposure to L-2-hydrogyglutaric acid increases over the lifespan, patients may benefit from close follow-up and increased imaging surveillance throughout their lifetime in the hopes of early detection of central nervous system malignancies [5, 15].

Conclusion

L-2-hydroxyglutaric aciduria is a rare autosomal recessive inborn error of metabolism that is due to a homozygous or compound heterozygous mutation in the L-2-hydroxyglutarate dehydrogenase gene situated on chromosome 14q. A variety of central nervous system neoplasms have been described to arise in patients with this disorder including astrocytomas, ependymomas and medulloblastomas.

References

[1] Duran, M, Kamerling, JP, Bakker, HD, et al. L-2-hydroxyglutaric aciduria: an inborn error of metabolism? *J Inherit Metab Dis.* 1980; 3(4): 109-112.

[2] Jaeken J, Willekens H, Corbeel L. Leukodystrophy associated with hyperlysinorrhachia and 2-hydroxyglutaric aciduria. *Pediatr Res.* 1988; 24: 266 (Abstract).

[3] Hoffman G, Voss W, Hummeman DH, et al. L-2-hydroxyglutarazidurie: Eine neue enzephalopathie mit leukodystophen veränderungen [L-2-hydroxyglutaric aciduria: a new encephalopathy with leukodystophenic changes]. In: Hannefeld F, Rating D, Christen H-J, eds. *Aktuelle Neuropädiatrie [Current neuropediatrics].* 1989. New York: Springer, 1990: 139-142.

[4] Barth PG, GF Hoffmann, J Jaeken, et al. L-2-hydroxyglutaric acidemia: a novel inherited neurometabolic disease. *Ann Neurol.* 1992; 32: 66-71.

[5] Patay Zoltan, Brent A Orr, Barry L Shulkin, et al. Successive distinct high-grade gliomas in L-2-hydroxyglutaric aciduria. *J Inherit Metab Dis.* 2015; 38(2): 273-277.

[6] Topçu Meral, Florence Jobard, Sophie Halliez, et al. L-2-Hydroxyglutaric aciduria: identification of a mutant gene C14orf160, localized on chromosome 14q22.1. *Hum Mol Genet.* 2004; 13(22): 2803-2811.

[7] Rzem Rim, Maria Veiga-da-Cunha, Gaëtane Noël, et al. A gene encoding a putative FAD-dependent L-2-hydroxyglutarate dehydrogenase is mutated in L-2-hydroxyglutaric aciduria. *Proc Natl Acad Sci U S A.* 2004; 101(48): 16849-16854.

[8] Niehaus TD, Hillmann KB. Enzyme promiscuity, metabolite damage, and metabolite damage control systems of the tricarboxylic acid cycle. *FEBS J*. 2020; 287(7): 1343-1358.

[9] Rzem Rim, Younes Achouri, Etienne Marbaix, et al. A mouse model of L-2-hydroxyglutaric aciduria, a disorder of metabolite repair. *PLoS One*. 2015; 10(3): e0119540.

[10] Steenweg Marjan E, Cornelis Jakobs, Abdellatif Errami, et al. An overview of L-2-hydroxyglutarate dehydrogenase gene (L2HGDH) variants: a genotype-phenotype study. *Hum Mutat*. 2010; 31(4): 380-390.

[11] Du X, Hu H. The roles of 2-hydroxyglutarate. *Front Cell Dev Biol*. 2021; 9: 651317.

[12] Ježek P. 2-hydroxyglutarate in cancer cells. *Antioxid Redox Signal*. 2020; 33(13): 903-926.

[13] Kranendijk Martijn, Eduard A Struys, Gajja S Salomons, et al. Progress in understanding 2-hydroxyglutaric acidurias. *J Inherit Metab Dis*. 2012 Jul; 35(4): 571-87.

[14] Tanyel Zübarioğlu, Cengiz Yalçınkaya, Çiğdem Oruç, et al. Evaluation of clinical, neuroradiologic, and genotypic features of patients with L-2-hydroxyglutaric aciduria. *Turk Pediatri Ars*. 2020; 55(3): 290-298.

[15] Patay Z, JC Mills, U Löbel, et al. Cerebral neoplasms in L-2 hydroxyglutaric aciduria: 3 new cases and meta-analysis of literature data. *AJNR Am J Neuroradiol*. 2012; 33(5): 940-943.

[16] Ozişik Pinar Akdemir, Nejat Akalan, Selçuk Palaoğlu, et al. Medulloblastoma in a child with the metabolic disease L-2-hydroxyglutaric aciduria. *Pediatr Neurosurg*. 2002; 37(1): 22-26.

[17] Struys Eduard A., Erwin EW Jansen, Nanda M Verhoeven, et al. Measurement of urinary D- and L-2-hydroxyglutarate enantiomers by stable-isotope-dilution liquid chromatography-tandem mass spectrometry after derivatization with diacetyl-L-tartaric anhydride. *Clin Chem*. 2004; 50(8): 1391-1395.

[18] Seijo-Martínez Manuel, Carmen Navarro, Maria Castro del Río, et al. L-2-hydroxyglutaric aciduria: clinical, neuroimaging, and neuropathological findings. *Arch Neurol*. 2005; 62(4): 666-670.

[19] Larnaout A, F Hentati, S Belal, et al. Clinical and pathological study of three Tunisian siblings with L-2-hydroxyglutaric aciduria. *Acta Neuropathol*. 1994; 88(4): 367-370.

[20] Nyhan WL, Hoffmann GF. L-2-hydroxyglutaric aciduria. In: Atlas of Inherited Diseases. CRC Press/Taylor & Amp; Francis Group; 2019: 95-99.

[21] Kumar Suresh, Shikha Bhatia, Mukesh Surya, et al. Classic imaging features of L-2-hydroxyglutaric aciduria in young adult presenting as seizures associated with fever. *Ann Indian Acad Neurol*. 2020; 23(3): 352-354.

[22] Steenweg Marjan E, Gajja S Salomons, Zuhal Yapici, et al. L-2-hydroxyglutaric aciduria: pattern of MR imaging abnormalities in 56 patients. *Radiology*. 2009; 251(3): 856-865.

[23] Jequier Gygax Marine, Eliane Roulet-Perez, Kathleen Meagher-Villemure, et al. Sudden unexpected death in an infant with L-2-hydroxyglutaric aciduria. *Eur J Pediatr*. 2009; 168(8): 957-962.

[24] Chen E, WL Nyhan, C Jakobs, et al. L-2-Hydroxyglutaric aciduria: neuropathological correlations and first report of severe neurodegenerative disease and neonatal death. *J Inherit Metab Dis.* 1996; 19(3): 335-343.

[25] Aghili M, Zahedi F, Rafiee E. Hydroxyglutaric aciduria and malignant brain tumor: a case report and literature review. *J Neurooncol.* 2009; 91(2): 233-236.

[26] Dang Lenny, David W White, Stefan Gross, et al. Cancer-associated IDH1 mutations produce 2-hydroxyglutarate. *Nature.* 2009; 462(7274): 739-744.

[27] Perry A, Brat DJ. *Practical Surgical Neuropathology: A Diagnostic Approach: A Volume in the Pattern Recognition Series.* 2nd ed. Philadelphia, PA: Elsevier - Health Sciences Division; 2017.

[28] Samuraki M, K Komai, Y Hasegawa, et al. A successfully treated adult patient with L-2-hydroxyglutaric aciduria. *Neurology.* 2008; 70(13): 1051-1052.

[29] Yilmaz K. Riboflavin treatment in a case with l-2-hydroxyglutaric aciduria. *Eur J Paediatr Neurol.* 2009; 13(1): 57-60.

Index

B

C

D

E

F

I

K

L

M

N

O

P

Q

R

S

T

U

V

W

Z

Editor's Contact Information

Dr. Richard A. Prayson, MD, MEd
Professor of Pathology and Head of Neuropathology
Department of Anatomic Pathology
Cleveland Clinic
Cleveland, Ohio, USA
praysor@ccf.org